Clinical Problem Solving in

Neonatal Emergencies and Intensive Care

Academic Editor
Suraj Gupte

Guest Editor
Neelam Kler

Executive Editor
Shamma-Bakshi Gupte

Foreword
Ajay Gambhir

Clinical Problem Solving in

Neonatal Emergencies and Intensive Care

Suraj Gupte

MD, FIAP, FSAMS (Sweden), FRSTMH (London)

Professor and Head

Postgraduate Department of Pediatrics

Mamata Medical College/Mamata General and Superspeciality Hospitals

Khammam, Telangana, South India

E-mail: *drsurajgupte@gmail.com*

Website: www.drsurajgupte.com

Editor: The Short Textbook of Pediatrics, Recent Advances in Pediatrics (Series), Textbooks of Pediatric Emergencies, Neonatal Emergencies and Pediatric Nutrition, Pediatric Gastroenterology, Hepatology and Nutrition, Pediatric Infectious Diseases, Influenza: Complete Spectrum, Case-based Reviews in Pediatric Emergencies, etc.

Author: Differential Diagnosis in Pediatrics, Instructive Case Studies in Pediatrics, Pediatric Drug Directory, Influenza, Perspectives in Influenza, Speaking of Child Care.

Chief Editor (Gastroenterology Section): International Journal of Gastroenterology, Hepatology, Transplant and Nutrition.

Co-editor: Asian Journal of Maternity and Child Health (Manila, Philippines).

Section and Guest Editor: Pediatrics Today (New Delhi).

Editorial Advisor: Asian Journal of Pediatric Practice (New Delhi).

Editorial Advisory Board Member/Reviewer: Indian Journal of Pediatrics (New Delhi), Indian Pediatrics (New Delhi), Indian J Child Health (Gwalior), Synopsis (Detroit, USA), Maternal and Child Nutrition (Preston, UK), Journal of Infectious Diseases (Turkey), EC Pediatrics (London).

Examiner: Several Universities, including National Board of Examinations (NBE) for DNB, New Delhi; All India Institute of Medical Sciences (AIIMS), New Delhi; Postgraduate Institute of Medical Education and Research (PGIMER), Chandigarh; Sher-i-Kashmir Institute of Medical Sciences (SKIMS), Srinagar; Indira Gandhi Open University (IGNOU), New Delhi.

Pediatric Faculty Selection Expert: All India Institute of Medical Sciences (AIIMS), Punjab Public Service Commission, Jammu and Kashmir Public Service Commission, Union Public Service Commission.

PEEPEE

PUBLISHERS AND DISTRIBUTORS (P) LTD.

Clinical Problem Solving in Neonatal Emergencies and Intensive Care

Published by
Pawaninder P. Vij and Anupam Vij

Peepee Publishers and Distributors (P) Ltd.
Head Office: 160, Shakti Vihar, Pitam Pura
Delhi-110 034 (India)

Correspondence Address:

7/31, First Floor, Ansari Road, Daryaganj
New Delhi-110002 (India)
Ph: 65195868, 23246245, 9811156083
e-mail: peepee160@yahoo.co.in
e-mail: peepee160@gmail.com
www.peepeepub.com

First Edition: **2019**

ISBN: 978-81-8445-214-3

Dedicated to
everybody contributing to an intact neonatal survival

Foreword

In recent years, neonatology in India has come of age thanks to the initiatives taken at various levels, including the Indian Academy of Pediatrics (IAP), National Neonatology Forum (NNF) of India, Ministry of Health and Family Welfare and such international organizations as WHO and UNICEF.

Effectively dealing with neonatal emergencies and providing specialized and intensive care is mandatory to meet the goal of 'intact neonatal survival'. This should involve clinical problem-solving skills on the part of the attending doctors.

The appearance of the **Clinical Problem Solving in Neonatal Emergencies and Intensive Care,** by Dr Suraj Gupte, therefore, needs a warm welcome from the academic circles. Dr Gupte, a well-known pediatric educationist, author and innovator, is credited for giving us *Neonatal Emergencies, RAP Special Vol. 4 and 5: Neonatology', RAP Special Vol. 21: Neonatal and Pediatric Intensive Care, RAP Special Vol. 25: Neonatology, etc.* With Dr Neelam Kler, a noted neonatologist as the Guest Editor and over 40 experts in neonatology as contributors, the book stands out as a unique and innovative treatise.

It has a wide spectrum of coverage including common neonatal emergencies and complex problems like arrhythmias, endocrinal emergencies and inborn errors of metabolism. All chapters are dealt with in a comprehensive, lucid and easy-to-follow manner.

Each case scenario is followed by critical analysis of the case in a nutshell and interactive topic discussions which are very pertinent, providing clarity of the subject. At the end of each chapter, take home messages are listed to drive home the key learning points. Each and every chapter bears a testimony to simplistic yet rational, clear, to-the-point and precise thought process of the authors and editors.

In my considered opinion, Dr Suraj Gupte's **Clinical Problem Solving in Neonatal Emergencies and Intensive Care** should prove an important tool for professionals involved in emergency and intensive care of the newborn. The unique book indeed deserves a warm welcome from the professionals, especially the pediatric and neonatology residents and budding neonatologists. Even established neonatologist will find considerable material of interest in the book.

Ajay Gambhir
MD, FNNF, FIAP, FIAMS
President
National Neonatology Forum (NNF) of India

Preface

Years ago, I had a unique opportunity of addressing an august gathering of neonatologists and pediatricians from all over the world at an international conference held in Hong Kong.

As I was in the thick of building up a case for enhancing emphasis on clinical scenarios, stood up Prof Brown, a doyen in the field, saying,

> "*Not just that. You have to bank considerably on the actual clinical cases you saw,*
> *you are seeing, or you will be seeing, to streamline and refine your management...*
> *The errors committed and the strong positives attained become a stepping*
> *stone in your clinical delivery of optimal care.*"

The new book, **Clinical Problem Solving in Neonatal Emergencies and Intensive Care,** draws its inspiration from this philosophy. Each of the 33 chapters authored by 40 experts in neonatology gets off the ground with a one or more case scenario, focusing on presentation and management of the problem. It is followed by a critical appraisal of the case and developments in its management in brief. The errors, if any, and important therapeutic points are particularly brought to light. Finally, there appears an extensive interactive discussion on the topic as such. In this discussion, such important points that remain elusive in the textbooks receive special attention.

Clinical-orientation and practical applicability receive central stage in each and every chapter. In order to enhance the impact of the narration, a large number of illustrations (including Algorithms, Tables, Boxes) stand incorporated. In addition to the core matter, an 'Abstract with Key Words' at the outset and 'Conclusions' and 'Take Home Messages' at the fag-end are given. Also incorporated is 'Further Reading' providing some key references for more probing readers.

Here's hoping that the **Clinical Problem Solving in Neonatal Emergencies and Intensive Care** emerges as a welcome and significant educational treatise for the target readers, especially the postgraduates, residents and upcoming neonatologists.

Suraj Gupte
MD, FIAP, FSAMS (Sweden), FRSTH (London)
Academic Editor

Acknowledgements

Grateful acknowledgement is due to:

- Prof. RE Brown, Former WHO Adviser, for providing inspiration for this project.
- Dr. Rita Fernandes (Hong Kong), Michael Davidson (Buffalo) and Bonita William (London), for initial discussions on the layout of the book and for reviewing the drafts and making useful suggestions.
- Dr. Neelam Kler (New Delh), renowned neonatologist, for accepting our invite to be the Guest Editor.
- The contributing authors, for providing excellent state-of-the-art chapters on various topical issues in neonatal emergencies and intensive care and reposing confidence in our editorship.
- The peer-reviewers for critically reviewing the contributions and providing us the benefit of their expertise.
- Dr. Gagan Hans, Assistant Professor (Psychiatry), All India Institute of Medical Sciences, New Delhi, for voluntarily helping us in various ways in taking the project to its logical conclusion.
- Dr. Novy Gupte, Project Director, Cliniminds for valuable help in so many ways.
- Manu Gupte and Shivani-Mahendru for their help at various stages.
- World Health Organizaton (WHO), Center for Disease Control and Prevention (CDC), American Academy of Pediatrics (AAP), Indian Academy of Pediatrics (IAP), National Neonatology Forum (NNF) of India, etc. for access to their recommendations.
- A number of journals, periodicals and websites for including their references under "Further Reading".
- Dr. Ajay Gambhir, President National Neonatology Forum (NNF), for heart-warming compliments for the project and for generously recommending the book.

Finally, hats off to the publishers, Mr. Pawaninder Pal Vij and Anupam Vij and their studious staff at the Peepee Publishers and Distributors (P) Ltd. for the skillful and praiseworthy production qualities of the book.

Suraj Gupte
Academc Editor
Shamma-Bakshi Gupte
Executive Editor

Introductory Note by the Guest Editor

"Sometimes the smallest things take up the most room in your heart." **–Anonymous**

Newborns are very fragile and vulnerable. Neonatal emergencies are a fundamental part of neonatal medicine and underpinning the science of handling neonatal emergencies timely will result in intact neonatal survivals. Despite the strides made in evidence-based neonatology, the real challenge remains in managing patient at the bedside, and, often, at odd hours.

This book, **Clinical Problem Solving in Neonatal Emergencies and Intensive Care,** by Dr Suraj Gupte, a noted pediatric educationist, researcher and author of national and international standing, envisages a vision to help residents and clinicians in day-to-day management of neonatal emergencies. The goal although ambitious and challenging has been turned into reality by a team of experts in neonatal–perinatal medicine.

This is not a comprehensive textbook of neonatology but stands out for being able to incorporate common neonatal emergencies and case scenarios in a crisp question answer based format. The discussions are relatively brief, but interactive and the points made are very pertinent providing clarity of the subject. Although the emphasis has been on management, yet the recent literature has been adequately reviewed and incorporated at appropriate places. At the end of each chapter, take-home messages are given to understand the implications of their use in the NICU. The chapters are testimony to simplistic yet clear and precise thought process of authors and editor.

This book has a wide spectrum of coverage including common neonatal emergencies like neonatal seizures, electrolyte imbalance, neonatal surgical problems and cardiac disorders. Even complex problems like arrhythmia, endocrinal emergencies and inborn errors of metabolism have been dealt with in a comprehensive and lucid manner.

I sincerely hope that this problem solving book in neonatal emergancies and intensive care turns out to be an important tool for residents and budding neonatologists to manage sick neonates in NICU.

Neelam Kler
MD
Chairperson
Department of Neonatology
Institute of Child Health
Sir Ganga Ram Hospital
New Delhi, India

Contributors

1. **Neeraj Aggarwal**
Consultant in Pediatric Cardiology
Sir Ganga Ram Hospital
New Delhi, India
Ch 21: Acyanotic Heart Disease with Congestive Heart Failure
Ch 22: Critical Cyanotic Congenital Heart Disease

2. **Mridul Aggarwal**
Consultant Pediatric Cardiologist
Sir Ganga Ram Hospital
New Delhi, India
Ch 21: Acyanotic Heart Disease with Congestive Heart Failure
Ch 22: Critical Cyanotic Congenital Heart Disease

3. **Asif Ahmed**
Lecturer
Department of Neonatology
Sher-i-Kashmir Institute of Medical Sciences
Srinagar, Jammu and Kashmir, India
Ch 26: Hemorrhagic Disease of the Newborn

4. **Susanta Kumar Badatya**
Fellow DNB Neonatology
Sir Ganga Ram Hospital
New Delhi, India
Ch 14: Inborn Errors of Metabolism
Ch 16: Neonatal Hypoglycemia
Ch 27: Rhesus Isoimmunization

5. **Sriparna Basu**
Associate Professor in Neonatology and Perinatology
Department of Pediatrics
Institute of Medical Sciences
Banaras Hindu University (BHU)
Varanasi, UP, India
Ch 5: Neonatal Apnea
Ch 11: Necrotizing Enterocolitis
Ch 13: Neonatal Sepsis

6. **Nitasha Bagga**
Consultant Neonatologist
Rainbow Children's Hospital
Hyderabad, Telangana, India
Ch 8: Persistent Pulmonary Hypertension of the Newborn

7. **Bijay Laxmi Behera**
Fellow, DM Neonatology
Maulana Azad Medical College
New Delhi, India
Ch 1: Perinatal Asphyxia

8. **Elizabeth Bell**
Associate Professor
Neonatal-Perinatal Medicine Fellow Program
State University of New York
Buffalo, New York, USA
Ch 24: Acute Renal Failure in the Newborn

9. **Rahul Bhamkar**
Associate Consultant
Department of Pediatrics and Neonatology
Sir HN Reliance Foundation Hospital
Mumbai, Maharashtra, India
Ch 3: Cyanosis in the Newborn

10. **Bashir A Charoo**
Professor
Department of Neonatology
Sher-i-Kashmir Institute of Medical Sciences
Srinagar, Jammu and Kashmir, India
Ch 26: Late Hemorrhagic Disease of the Newborn

11. **Rajib Chatterjee**
Professor and Unit Head
Incharge Neonatology
Department of Pediatrics
Pravara Institute of Medical Sciences
Loni, Maharashtra, India
Ch 25: Bleeding Neonate

12. Dinesh Chirla
Consultant Neonatologist
Rainbow Children's Hospital
Hyderabad, Telangana, India
Ch 8: Persistent Pulmonary Hypertension of the Newborn
Ch 10: Pulmonary Hemorrhage in the Neonates

13. Abhishek Chopra
Fellow, DNB (Neonatology)
Sir Ganga Ram Hospital
New Delhi, India
Ch 15: Infant of Diabetic Mother
Ch 28: Polycythemia in the Newborn

14. Anupam Chawla
Assistant Professor in Pediatric Neurology
Institute of Child Health and Adolescence
London, England
Ch 3: Neonatal Seizures

15. Rita Chawla
Fellow in Neonatology
Institute of Child Health and Adolescence
London, England
Ch 3: Neonatal Seizures

16. Monica Dutta
Senior Clinical Research Fellow
Neonatal-Perinatal Medicine Fellow Program
State University of New York
Buffalo, New York, USA
Ch 24: Acute Renal Failure

17. Michael Davidson
Assistant Professor
Neonatal-Perinatal Medicine Fellow Program
State University of New York
Buffalo, New York, USA
Ch 23: Acute Renal Failure in the Newborn

18. Rita Fernandes
Neonatologist
Hospital for Sick Children
Hong Kong
Ch 9: Meconium Aspiration Syndrome

19. Pankaj Garg
Senior Consultant in Neonatology
Sir Ganga Ram Hospital
New Delhi
Ch 27: Rhesus Isoimmunization

20. Suraj Gupte
Professor and Head
Department of Pediatrics
Mamata General and Superspeciality Hospitals
Khammam, Telangana, India
Ch 2: Neonatal Meningitis
Ch 9: Meconium Aspiration Syndrome

21. Raja Joshi
Chairman and Senior Consultant
Pediatric Cardiac Sciences
Sir Ganga Ram Hospital
New Delhi, India
Ch 21: Acyanotic Heart Disease with Congestive Heart Failure
Ch 22: Critical Cyanotic Congenital Heart Disease

22. Reena Joshi
Consultant, Pediatric Cardiac Anesthetist
Department of Pediatric Cardiac Sciences
Sir Ganga Ram Hospital
New Delhi, India
Ch 22: Critical Cyanotic Congenital Heart Disease

23. Jay Kishore
DNB (Neonatology) Fellow
Sir Ganga Ram Hospital
New Delhi, India
Ch 4: Intraventricular Hemorrhage
Ch 18: Hyperthyroidism
Ch 19: Congenital Adrenal Hyperplasia

24. Neelam Kler
Chairperson
Department of Neonatology
Institute of Child Health
Sir Ganga Ram Hospital
New Delhi, India
Ch 28: Polycythemia in the Newborn

25. Anjali Kulkarni
Ex-Head
Department of Pediatrics
Sir HN Reliance Foundation Hospital
Mumbai, Maharashtra, India
Ch 6: Cyanosis in the Newborn

26. Ashok Kumar
Professor in Neonatology and Perinatology
Department of Pediatrics
Institute of Medical Sciences
Banaras Hindu University (BHU)
Varanasi
Ch 5: Neonatal Apnea
Ch 13: Neonatal Sepsis
Ch 11:Necrotizing Enterocolitis

27. Ajit Kumar
Consultant Neonatologist
Sir Ganga Ram Hospital
New Delhi, India
Ch 17: Electrolyte Imbalance in the Newborn

28. Manoj Modi
Consultant Neonatology
Sir Ganga Ram Hospital
New Delhi
Ch 4: Intraventricular Hemorrhage
Ch 16: Neonatal Hypoglycemia

29. Nancy Nelson
Associate Professor Neonatology
University School of Medicine
Philadelphia, USA
Ch 2: Neonatal Meningitis

30. James Nelson
Senior Consultant Neonatologist
Hospital for Sick Children
Hong Kong
Ch 9: Meconium Aspiration Syndrome

31. P Preetham
Consultant Neonatologist
Rainbow Hospital
Hyderabad, Telangana, India
Ch 10: Pulmonary Hemorrhage in Neonates

32. Alpana Prasad
Consultant Neonatal Surgery
Sir Ganga Ram Hospital
New Delhi, India
Ch 29: Congenital Diaphragmatic Hernia
Ch 30: Abdominal Wall Defects
Ch 31: Intestinal Obstruction
Ch 32: Hirshsprung Disease
Ch 33: Esophageal Atresia and Tracheoesophageal Fistula 9

33. Satish Saluja
Senior Consultant Neonatologist
Sir Ganga Ram Hospital
New Delhi
Ch 18; Neonatal Hyperthyroidism
Ch 19: Congenital Adrenal Hyperplasia

34. RK Sharma
Assistant Professor, Neonatology
University School of Medicine
Philadelphia, USA
Ch 2: Neonatal Meningitis

35. Anita Singh
Consultant Neonatologist
Sanjay Gandhi Postgraduate Institute of Medical Sciences
Lucknow, UP, India
Ch 12: Neonatal Hyperbilirubinemia
Ch 20: Neonatal Shock

36. Poonam Singh
DNB (Neonatology) Fellow
Sir Ganga Ram Hospital
New Delhi
Ch 23: Neonatal Arrhythmia

37. Utpal Kant Singh
Professor and Head (Ex)
Nalanda Medical College
Patna, Bihar, India
Ch 9: Meconium Aspiration Syndrome

38. Arun Soni
Consultant Neonatologist
Sir Ganga Ram Hospital
New Delhi, India
Ch 15: Infant of Diabetic Mother

39. Anup Thakur
Consultant in Neonatology
Sir Ganga Ram Hospital
New Delhi
Ch 1: Perinatal Asphyxia
Ch 12: Neonatal Hyperbilirubinemia
Ch 14: Inborn Errors of Metabolism
Ch 17: Electrolyte Imbalance in the Newborn
Ch 20: Neonatal Shock
Ch 23: Neonatal Arrhythmia

40. Bonita William
Associate Professor in Pediatric Neurology
Institute of Child Health and Adolescence
London, England
Ch 3: Neonatal Seizures

Contents

PART 4: Infections

PART 5: Metabolic Disorders

PART 6: Endocrinology

PART 7: Cardiovascular Disorders

PART 8: Renal Disorders

PART 9: Hematology

Chapter

1 Perinatal Asphyxia

Bijay Laxmi Behera, Anup Thakur

ABSTRACT

Perinatal asphyxia results from decreased oxygen supply that occurs due to various perinatal events. Though most babies recover, some develop permanent neurological sequelae. Based on a case scenario, the pathophysiology, timing, severity, the clinical feature, investigation, management and outcome of perinatal asphyxia are discussed in this chapter.

Key Words: Cerebral blood flow (CBF), Hypoxic-ischemic encephalopathy (HIE), Perinatal asphyxia (PA), Therapeutic hypothermia.

INTRODUCTION

The term, *perinatal asphyxia*, refers to a condition during first and second stage of labor in which impaired gas exchange leads to fetal hypoxemia and hypercarbia. It remains one of the three most common causes of neonatal deaths along with prematurity and bacterial infections. The incidence is about 1 to 1.5% of live births in developed countries and is inversely related to birth weight and gestation. It occurs in 9.0% of infants younger than 36 weeks gestation and in 0.5% in infants older than 36 weeks of gestation. Out of 2.7 million stillbirths globally, approximately 1.2 million occur during intrapartum period, largely owing to asphyxia. National Neonatal Perinatal Database (NNPD-2002–2003) reported perinatal asphyxia to be the most common cause of still-births, accounting for 45.1% of all such cases.

CASE SCENARIO

A woman with full-term pregnancy was admitted with labor pains in a hospital for safe confinement. She had regular checkups with her obstetrician. The antenatal period so far had been uneventful. She was progressing well but she developed vaginal bleeding 5 hours after admission. USG abdomen was suggestive of abruption placentae. Cardiotocography (CTG) was suggestive of late decelerations indicating fetal compromise. Emergency Cesarean section was performed. Baby didn't cry after

Contd.

Contd.

birth, was limp, with poor respiratory efforts, required intubation and positive pressure ventilation (PPV). Apgar score was 1 at 1 min, 3 at 5 min, 6 at 10 min and 7 at 15 mins. Cord pH was 6.9 with mixed metabolic acidosis. Baby was transported to NICU for post-resuscitative care. Ventilation was continued and intense monitoring of vital parameters was done. Baby developed shock at 1 hour of age-dobutamine was started @ 10 mcg/kg/min. At 2 hours of age, baby had multi-focal clonic seizures. A loading dose, 20 mg/kg, of phenobarbitone was given. Seizures were controlled. Baby's oxygenation and perfusion was managed. Metabolic parameters-blood sugar and serum calcium were maintained. Ionotrope was tapered and stopped after 48 hours. Baby was weaned gradually and was extubated on day 3 of life. Tube feeds were started and gradually built up. MRI Brain done on day 7 showed evidence of hypoxic-ischemic injury. Early stimulation therapy was started. Serial neurological examination showed some improvement. Since the baby had poor sucking and swallowing co-ordination, breast feeds could be started on day 14 only. Baby was discharged on day 16 of life. Neurological examination at discharge showed some truncal hypotonia and poor eye contact. Parents were counseled about risk of neurological sequelae and advised regular follow-up.

CRITICAL CASE ANALYSIS

In the present case, the fetus suffered acute placental insufficiency leading to severe perinatal asphyxia. The CTG was abnormal, Apgar score was low and cord gas showed mixed metabolic acidosis. This baby required resuscitation at birth and immediate supportive management in the NICU. The mainstay of management comprised supportive management-adequate ventilation, maintenance of perfusion, control of seizures, metabolic control and management of associated organ dysfunction. MRI and neurological examination at discharge was abnormal. Parents were rightly counseled about risk of sequelae and need for long-term follow-up.

INTERACTIVE TOPIC DISCUSSION

What are the definitions of perinatal asphyxia?

There is no universally-accepted definition of perinatal Asphyxia (PA). The definitions given by World Health Organization, Neonatal Perinatal Database and American Academy of Pediatrics for prediction of its long-term outcome are given in Table 1.1.

Table 1.1: Definitions of perinatal asphyxia

World Health Organization	**Failure to initiate and sustain breathing**
American Academy of Pediatrics and American College of Obstetrics and Gynecology	Presence of all of the following criteria: • Profound metabolic or mixed acidemia (pH < 7.00) in umbilical cord blood • Persistence of low Apgar scores less than 3 for more than 5 minutes • Signs of neonatal neurologic dysfunction (e.g., seizures, encephalopathy, tone abnormalities) • Evidence of multiple organ involvement (such as that of kidneys, lungs, liver, heart and intestine).

What should be the clinical and laboratory monitoring of an asphyxiated infant?

Stringent clinical monitoring is required during post-resuscitative care of an asphyxiated baby (Table 1.2). Clinical deterioration in the form of shock or multi-organ dysfunction can occur hence, these babies require close monitoring for prompt management of these complications.

The laboratory investigations (Table 1.3) should be guided by the clinical course. For example, a baby who required PPV at birth but remained in room air with no features of hypoxic-ischemic encephalopathy or any organ dysfunction may require little laboratory investigations. On the other hand, an infant who suffered severe HIE and has multi-organ dysfunction may require extensive serial laboratory monitoring.

Table 1.2: Clinical monitoring

Parameter	Frequency
Heart rate, Respiratory rate, Saturation and temperature	Continuously
Blood pressure, Capillary refill time, Peripheral pulses	Hourly
Neurological examination	6 hourly
Weight, Urine output	12 hourly
Anterior fontanel, Occipitofrontal circumference	Daily
Other systemic examination	As clinically indicated

Table 1.3: Lab monitoring

Parameter	Frequency
Blood sugars	At admission and then 6 hourly
Blood gas	At admission and then as required
Hematocrit	2 hourly, 12 hourly and then as required
Serum Na, K, BUN, Creatinine	Daily, clinically required
Urine osmolality/specific gravity	6 hourly or as indicated
ECG	Continuous
Serum calcium	As clinically required
Chext X-ray, ECHO	As clinically required

What is hypoxic-ischemic encephalopathy (HIE)?

Hypoxic-ischemic encephalopathy implies an abnormal neurobehavioral state consisting of decreased level of consciousness and usually other signs of brain stem and/or motor dysfunction with objective data to support a hypoxic-ischemic mechanism as underlying cause for the encephalopathy.

Discuss the various clinical staging and scoring systems of HIE?

Two staging systems (Tables 1.4 and 1.5) are classically used for categorizing, monitoring and prognosticating infants who suffer from HIE. Sarnat and Sarnat is more extensive while Levene staging system has lesser parameters but is well-validated. Thomson scoring system (Table 1.6) for progress of HIE is derived from Sarnat and Sarnat staging and is useful in a way that it objectively gives a score to infants neurological status, can be used to monitor progress and helps in prognostication. An infant with a score of >14 beyond first week of life is likely to suffer long-term neurological sequelae.

Table 1.4: Classification of HIE as per Levene (term and preterm babies)

Feature	Mild	Moderate	Severe
Consciousness	Irritable	Lethargy	Comatose
Tone	Hypotonia	Marked hypotonia	Severe hypotonia
Seizures	No	Yes	Prolonged
Sucking/respiration	Poor suck	Unable to suck	Unable to sustain spontaneous respiration

Table 1.5: Sarnat and Sarnat staging (>36 weeks)

Sign	Stage 1	Stage 2	Stage 3
Tone	Normal	Mild hypotonia	Flaccid
LOC	Hyperalert; irritable	Lethargic or obtunded	Stuporous, comatose
Posture	Mild distal flexion	Strong distal flexion	Decerebrate
Stretch reflexes	Overactive	Overactive, disinhibited	Decreased or absent
Segmental myoclonus	Present or absent	Present	Absent
Moro	Strong; low threshold	Weak; incomplete, high threshold	Absent
Oculovestibular reflex	Normal	Overactive	Weak or absent
Suck	Weak	Weak or absent	Absent
Tonic neck	Slight	Strong	Absent
Autonomic function	Generalized sympathetic	Generalized parasympathetic	Both systems depressed
Pupils	Mydriasis	Miosis	Midposition, often unequal; poor light reflex
Respirations	Spontaneous	Spontaneous, occasional apnea	Periodic, apnea
Heart rate	Tachycardia	Bradycardia	Variable
Bronchial and salivary secretions	Sparse	Profuse	Variable
GIT motility	Normal or decreased	Increased; diarrhea	Variable
Seizures	None	Common; focal or multi-focal (6–24 hours of age)	Uncommon (excluding decerebration)
EEG findings	Normal (awake)	*Early:* Generalized low voltage slowing (continuous delta and theta) *Later:* Periodic pattern (awake) *Seizures:* Focal or multi-focal, 1–1.5 Hz spike and wave	*Early:* Periodic pattern with Isopotential phases *Later:* Totally isopotential
Duration	<24 hours	2–14 days	Hours to weeks
Outcome	About 100% normal	80% normal, abnormal if lasting >5–7 days	About 50% die, remainder with severe sequelae

Table 1.6: Thomson score

Sign	0	1	2	3
Tone	Normal	Hypertonia	Hypotonia	Flaccid
Consciousness	Normal	Hyperalert	Lethargic	Comatose
Fits	None	< 3 per day	> 2 per day	
Posture	Normal	Fisting, cycling	Strong distal flexion	Decerebrate
Moro	Normal	Partial	Absent	
Grasp	Normal	Poor	Absent	
Suck	Normal	Poor	Absent ± bites	
Respiration	Normal	Hyperventilation	Brief apnea	IPPV (apnea)
Fontanel	Normal	Full, not tense	Tense	

What is the pathophysiology of HIE?

Pathophysiology of HIE is depicted in Figure 1.1.

The principal pathogenic mechanism underlying the neuropathology of intrapartum hypoxia–ischemia is impaired cerebral blood flow (CBF) which most likely occurs as a consequence of interruption in placental blood flow and gas exchange either acute or intermittent. Disrupted cerebral blood flow leads in sequence to the phase of primary energy failure, the immediate reperfusion period, the latent phase and finally, the secondary phase of energy failure.

At the cellular level, the disruption of CBF leads to a primary energy failure and the activation of cell death processes. During primary phase energy failure, decreased levels of high-energy phosphate compounds, such as phosphocreatine (PCr), the principal storage form of high-energy phosphate, and adenosine triphosphate (ATP), promote mitochondrial dysfunction. Under healthy conditions, the cell's ATP is mitochondrially generated via oxidative phosphorylation, which is tightly coupled to glucose metabolism. After energy failure, ATP production relies primarily on anerobic glycolysis. A critical function of ATP is to maintain sodium (Na), potassium (K), and calcium (Ca) ionic gradients across membranes. After ATP loss, K leaks out of the affected cell, inducing depolarization and a massive release of glutamate, an excitatory amino acid. Energy failure induced by severe, acute asphyxia rapidly results in neuronal death via necrosis, characterized by plasma membrane swelling and rupture, which releases intracellular toxins into the local milieu. In contrast, energy loss after less severe or prolonged hypoxic-ischemic insult leads to apoptosis, a slower form of neuronal death often described as cell suicide.

Primary Energy Failure

- Decrease in CBF, O_2 substrates, high-energy phosphate compounds
- Excitotoxic-oxidative cascade
- Loss of ionic homeostasis across membranes, entry of intracellular calcium, mitochondrial disruption, brain acidosis, apoptosis followed by necrosis.

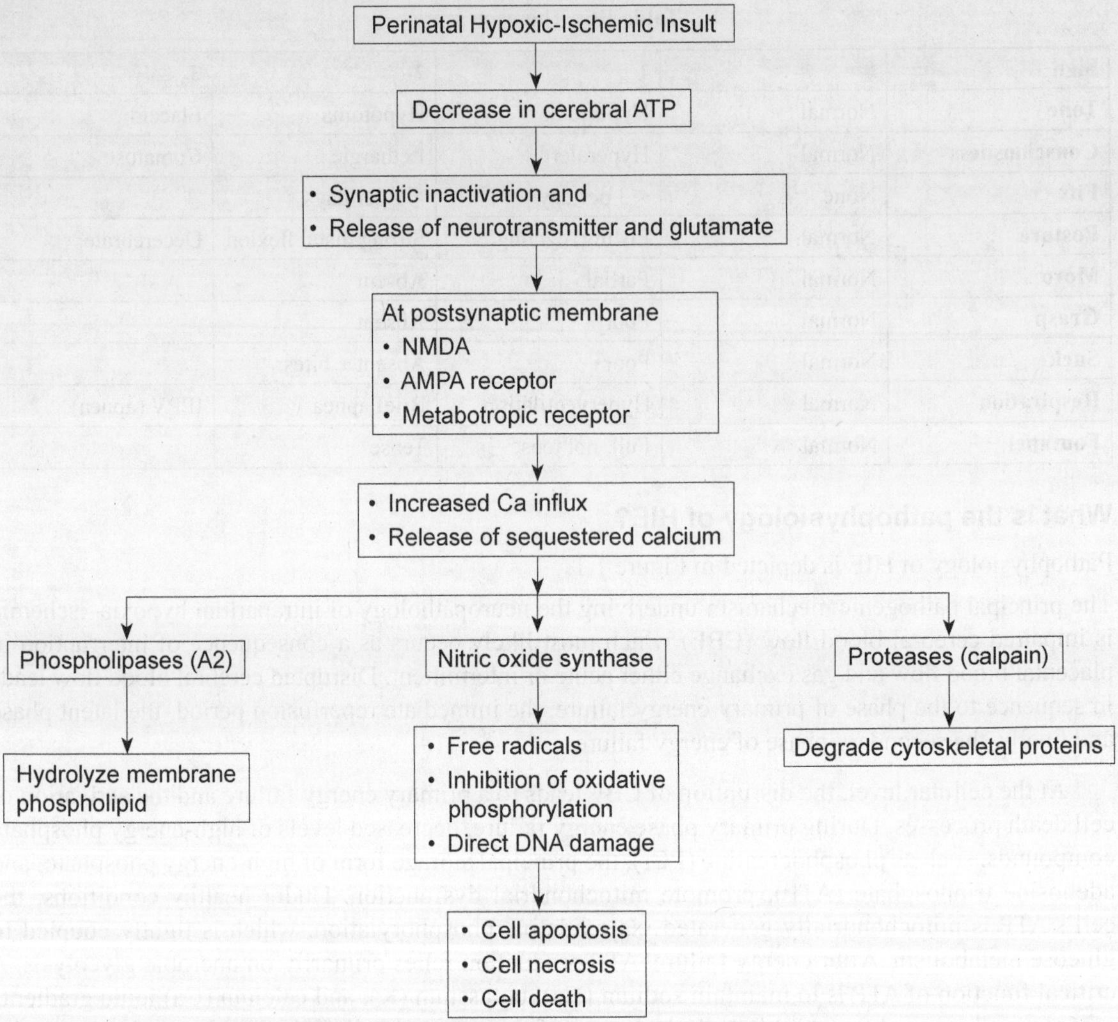

Fig. 1.1: Pathophysiology of perinatal asphyxia

Secondary Energy Failure

- Continuation of excitotoxic-oxidative cascade.
- Activation of microglia—inflammatory response.
- Activation of caspase proteins.
- Reduction in levels of growth factors, protein synthesis.
- Apoptosis–necrosis continuum.

The return of CBF demarcates the *immediate reperfusion period*. This period is characterized by normal blood pressure and intracellular pH, a transient improvement in cytotoxic edema and an absence of seizures. The immediate reperfusion period rapidly transitions into the *latent phase* during which within the cell, mitochondrial metabolism is nearly restored. Neuro-protective strategies are most effective if implemented during the first 6 hours after reperfusion. After this temporal window, however, the affected infant experiences a second phase of energy failure. Once again, levels of ATP as well as PCr decrease, whereas cytotoxic edema increases. The cellular response to *secondary phase energy failure* is similar to that of the primary phase energy failure in that excitatory amino acids are released from cells, leading to necrotic and apoptotic cell death. Much of the cell death is delayed, occurring slowly (hours to days) during the infant's recovery period.

What are the consequences of asphyxia on various organ systems?

Table 1.7 lists the said consequences. In minority of cases (<15%), the brain may be the only organ exhibiting dysfunction following asphyxia. In more severe cases, multi-organ dysfunction occurs as a result of systemic hypoxia-ischemia.

Table 1.7: Effects of perinatal asphyxia

Central Nervous System	Hypoxic-ischemic encephalopathy, intracranial hemorrhage, seizures, long-term neurological sequelae
Cardiac	Myocardial dysfunction, valvular dysfunction, rhythm abnormalities, congestive cardiac failure
Renal	Hematuria, acute tubular necrosis, renal vein thrombosis
Pulmonary	Delayed adaptation, respiratory failure, meconium aspiration, surfactant depletion, primary pulmonary hypertension
Gastrointestinal tract	Necrotizing enterocolitis, hepatic dysfunction
Hematological	Thrombocytopenia, coagulation abnormalities
Metabolic	Acidosis, hypoglycemia, hypocalcemia, hyponatremia

Discuss the evolution of HIE in time-frame.

Table 1.8 lists the evolution of HIE in time-frame.

Table 1.8: Evolution of HIE in time-frame

Birth to 12 hours	Depressed level of alertness, periodic breathing or respiratory failure, intact pupillary and occulomotor responses, hypotonia, seizures
12–24 hours	Variable change in level of alertness, more seizures, apnoeic spells, jitteriness, weakness in proximal limbs, upper > lower (full term), hemiparesis (full term), lower limbs (premature)
24–72 hours	Stupor or coma, respiratory arrest, brainstem pupillary and occulomotor disturbances, catastrophic deteoriation with severe intraventricular hemorrhage and periventricular hemorrhagic infarction (premature)
After 72 hours	Persistent yet diminishing stupor, disturbed sucking, swallowing, gag and tongue movements, hypotonia > hypertonia, weakness in proximal limbs, upper > lower (full term), hemiparesis (full term), lower limbs or hemiparesis (premature)

How should one manage a neonate with perinatal asphyxia?

The management of asphyxiated babies is mainly supportive and involves maintaining optimum oxygenation, ventilation, perfusion, metabolic milieu and control of seizures (Fig. 1.2).

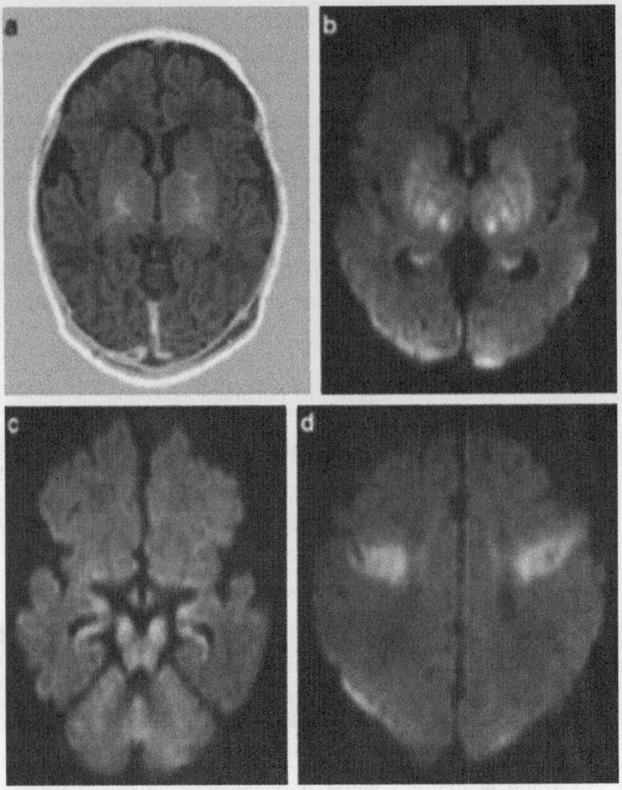

Fig. 1.2: (a) MRI pattern suggestive of acute near total asphyxia, (b-d) DWI shows restricted diffusion in the ventrolateral thalami, lentiform nuclei, cerebral peduncles and in the perirolandic cortex

Delivery Room Management

All neonates at birth should be resuscitated in delivery room as per national resuscitation program guidelines. Every delivery should be attended by at least one person trained in all steps of resuscitation including endotracheal intubation. One should seek additional help in situations when a baby is born depressed. Presence of metabolic acidosis (pH < 7.00 and base deficit greater than 16 mmol/L) in cord blood indicates relatively long standing asphyxia (many minutes to hours), while presence of respiratory acidosis in absence of metabolic acidosis indicates presence of acute asphyxia (minutes) as in cord prolapse, acute abruption of placenta etc. One should try to obtain cord gas and in cases when this was not done, arterial blood gas should be obtained after admission to NICU, preferably within an hour. All infants who require positive pressure ventilation should be preferably shifted to NICU for post-resuscitative care.

Management in NICU

1. **Temperature:** Normal body temperature of the baby should be maintained and hyperthermia should be avoided.

2. **Oxygenation and Ventilation:** Assess for adequate spontaneous breathing and need for oxygenation and ventilation support as needed. Assisted ventilation is required if baby is apneaic, there is inadequate spontaneous respiration or there is continuing hypoxia or hypercarbia. Hypoxia or hyperoxia and hypocarbia or hypercarbia should be avoided. Hypocarbia would reduce the cerebral perfusion and hypercarbia can increase intracranial pressure and predispose the baby to intracranial bleed.
3. **Maintain Normal Tissue Perfusion:** Normal tissue perfusion should be maintained. If the tissue perfusion is inadequate, ionotropic support of dobutamine or dopamine to maintain adequate cardiac output is required. Echocardiography in infants with shock may help to guide appropriate management strategy and to assess cardiac contractility. Fluid restriction is needed there is hyponatremia secondary to syndrome of inappropriate secretion of ADH (SIADH) or if there is renal failure.
4. **Maintain Normal Hematocrit and Metabolic Milieu:** Maintain blood glucose and hematocrit. Maintain pH above 7.30 and maintain serum calcium concentration in the normal range.
5. **Treatment of Seizures:** Metabolic alteration such as hypoglycemia, hypocalcemia, and hyponatremia that can cause or exacerbate seizures should be corrected. Seizures caused by HIE can be extremely difficult to control.
   - Phenobarbitone is the initial drug of choice and is given as a loading dose of 20 mg/kg IV. If seizures continue, additional loading doses of 5–10 mg/kg IV may be needed to control seizures. Maintenance dose of phenobarbitone is 3–5 mg/kg/day. It should be started 12–24 hours after the loading dose. Therapeutic levels are to 15–40 mg/dL. Because of prolonged serum half-life, which may be increased in the presence of renal and hepatic dysfunction, serum levels should be monitored and maintenance dosing adjusted accordingly.
   - Phenytoin may be added when seizures are not controlled by phenobarbitone. The loading dose is 15–20 mg/kg IV followed by maintenance dose of 4–8 mg/kg divided q8 hourly. Fosphenytoin may be used instead of phenytoin in equivalent doses as risk of hypotension and extravasation is less.
   - Bendodiazepines are considered third line drug. Lorazepam 0.05–1 mg/kg/dose IV can be given. Midazolum infusion may be another alternative. Recently, there are a few series reporting benefit of Levertiracetam in neonatal seizures.
6. **Nutrition:** Feeding should be withheld until baby is hemodynamically stable, off vasopressors and has a normal abdominal examination (no distension, passing stool and normal bowel sounds).
7. **Others:** Renal dysfunction should be monitored by measuring urine output, serum electrolytes and urine specific gravity. In the presence of oliguria/anuria fluids should be restricted. Hematological abnormalities should be monitored and corrected.

What should be algorithmic approach for management of HIE?

Figure 1.3 is the flowchart for the algorithmic approach for management of HIE.

What are the newer modes of therapy?

Therapeutic Hypothermia (TH)

Application of therapeutic hypothermia (33–34°C) in infants of at least 36 weeks gestation with moderate to severe encephalopathy in intensive care unit settings, initiated within 4–6 hours and continued for 72 hours of age has shown to reduce mortality and neuro-morbidity by 18 months of age. TH can be instituted by selectively cooling the head or the whole body. It is a safe modality in settings where intensive care facilities to manage sickest neonates are available. A cochrane review (8 RCTs; 638 term infants with moderate/severe encephalopathy and evidence of intrapartum asphyxia) showed that TH reduced combined outcome of mortality or major neuro-developmental disability by 24% to 18 months of age.

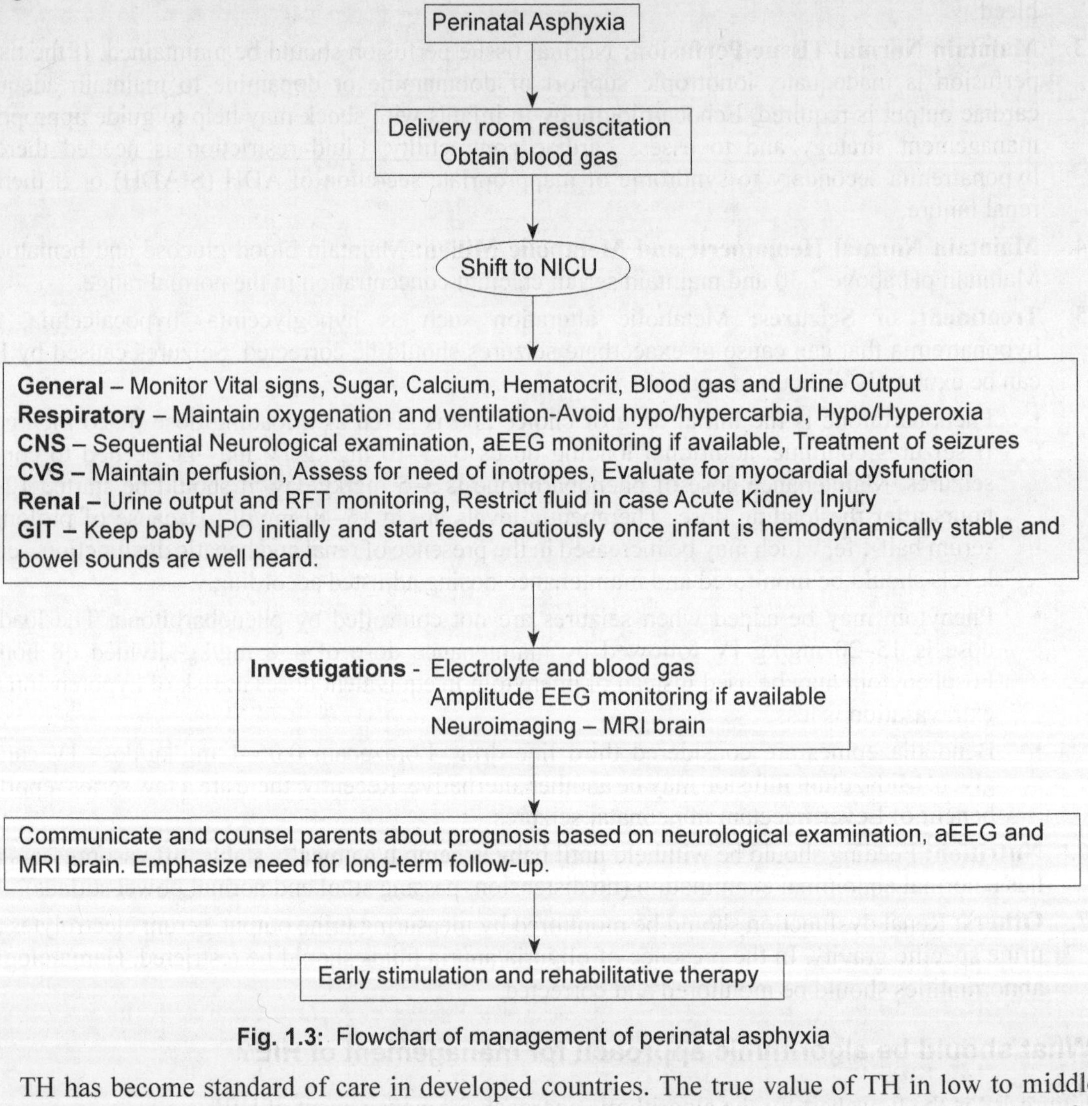

Fig. 1.3: Flowchart of management of perinatal asphyxia

TH has become standard of care in developed countries. The true value of TH in low to middle income countries is yet to be tested. In India, rehabilitative program is weak and national registry for TH is lacking. There are problems related to high sepsis rates, lack of adequate manpower, diversity of care and lack of integrated national follow-up program. Besides many asphyxiated infants are born in far-flung areas and due to lack of a dedicated neonatal transport system, the therapeutic window of 6 hrs may be missed. These issues need to be resolved and data should be generated in randomized control trial before it becomes a standard of care in our country.

Certain drugs are under investigation for neuro-protection which can be used in thc carly period of hypoxic ischemic injury. They act by causing blockade of free radical generation (allopurinol, oxypurinol), scavenging of oxidants (superoxide dismutase, glutathione, N-acetyl cysteine and alpha tocopherol), and calcium channel blockade (flunarizine, nimodipine).

What is the role of Imaging in HIE?

USG Cranium can diagnose cerebral edema, any bleed, ventricular dilatation or any cystic lesion first few days of life but MRI is the method of choice to obtain more detailed and accurate information about the HI insult. It is important to rule out intracranial bleed before opting for therapeutic hypothermia.

CT scan can detect the same abnormalities as USG but it is only recommended where ultrasound and MRI are not available. In acute stage of HIE in term babies generalized low attenuation of brain parenchyma may be seen.

MRI: The best timing to detect brain lesions is usually after 7–10 days after the insult.

Diffusion-weighted imaging (DWI) has improved ability to detect time of onset of brain lesions. A reduced apparent diffusion coefficient (restricted diffusion) during the first few days after the insult, with pseudonormalisation by the end of the first week is seen.

Main patterns of injury:

1. Basal ganglia–thalamus pattern (BGT) – Involves ventrolateral thalami, perirolandic cortex, hippocampus and brainstem. It occurs in 'acute near total asphyxia'.
2. Watershed predominant pattern of injury (WS) is the other pattern of injury which is also referred to as a pattern seen following 'prolonged partial asphyxia'.

What is the role of EEG in HIE?

Electroencephalography (*EEG*) helps in the diagnosis and management of seizures and prognosticating the babies for long-term outcomes. The prognosis is likely to be poor if the EEG shows:

1. Long periods of inactivity (more than 10 seconds).
2. Brief period of bursts (less than 6 seconds) with small amplitude bursts.
3. Interhemispheric asymmetry and asynchrony.
4. Isoelectric and low voltage (less than 5 microvolts).

The cerebral function monitor or amplitude-integrated electroencephalography (*aEEG*) is a simplified, continuous EEG that uses a limited number of electrodes and provides an overall impression of cerebral activity. Both background pattern and the presence of sleepwake Cycles (SWCs) are useful aEEG measures in predicting neurodevelopmental outcomes of asphyxiated infants. Burst suppression on flat tracing or continuous low-voltage patterns on aEEG without recovery at 24 hours are predictive of a poor outcome. The onset of SWCs correlates well with severity of HIE, with milder forms of injury demonstrating earlier SWCs. The presence of seizures is associated with a delay in SWC onset. Following abnormalities would indicate poor prognosis:

- Wide fluctuations in the amplitude with the baseline voltages dropping to near zero.
- Peak amplitudes under 5 mV.
- Seizure spikes.

While a normal aEEG may not necessarily mean that the brain is normal, a severe or moderately severe aEEG abnormality may indicate brain injury and poor outcome. The time of onset of sleep wake cycling (SWC) has a prognostic value. If SWC returns before 36 hours then the outcome is good.

Discuss the prognosis of HIE.

Up to 80% of infants who survive severe HIE develop serious complications, 10–20% develop moderately serious disabilities, and up to 10% are normal. Among the infants who survive moderately severe HIE, 30–50% may suffer from serious long-term complications, and 10–20% with minor neurological morbidities.

- Stage 1–98–100% have normal neurological outcome.
- Stage 2–20% die or have abnormal developmental outcomes.
- Stage 3–Death and disability such as cerebral palsy, intellectual disability, visual impairment and epilepsy are common.

Poor prognostic factors for neuro-developmental disability are:

- Severe encephalopathy.
- Presence of seizures-risk of cerebral palsy is 50–70 folds.
- Abnormal low voltage or isoelectric EEG/persistent burst suppression pattern.
- Abnormal MRI especially with significant cortical or sub-cortical brain injury.

CONCLUSIONS

Perinatal asphyxia still constitutes a major etiology for morbidity and mortality during neonatal period and infancy. Along with enforcement of steps to prevent asphyxia, postnatal management (including delivery room resuscitation and NICU care) play important role in determining intact survival. Although neuroprotective strategies like therapeutic hypothermia has became standard of care in developed countries, its applicability in developing and underdeveloped world is yet to be established. Prognostication and prediction of sequelae by neuromonitoring and neuroimaging is important. Follow-up and rehabilitation is essential to minimize the effects long-term sequelae.

TAKE HOME MESSAGES

- Perinatal asphyxia remains one of the three most common causes of neonatal deaths along with prematurity and bacterial infections.
- Supportive care is important in management of perinatal asphyxia.
- Neuro-monitoring is important for prognostication and predicting sequelae.
- Therapeutic Hypothermia is a promising therapy to decrease the risk of cerebral palsy and has become the standard of care in developing country.
- Long-term follow-up and rehabilitative therapy are essential to minimize risk of sequelae in these infants.

FURTHER READING

1. Black RE, Cousens S, Johnson HL, Lawn JE, Rudan I, Bassani DG, *et al.* (For Child Health Epidemiology Reference Group of WHO and UNICEF). Global, regional, and national causes of child mortality in 2008: A systematic analysis. *Lancet* 2010;375(9730):1969–1987.
2. Delivoria-Papadopoulos M, Marro PJ. Biochemical basis of hypoxic-Ischemic encephalopathy. *NeoReviews* 2010;11;e184–e193.
3. de Vries LS, Groenendaal F. Patterns of neonatal hypoxic-ischaemic brain injury. *Neuroradiology* 2010; 52:555–566.
4. Hill A,Volpe J. Hypoxic Ischcmic cerebral injury in the newborn. In: Swaiman KF, Ashwal S, (eds). *Pediatric Neurology: Principles and Practice*. St Louis: Mosby 1999:191–204.
5. Lawn JE, Blencowe H, Pattinson R, Cousens S, Kumar R, Ibiebele I, *et al.* Lancet's Stillbirths Series steering committee. Stillbirths: Where? When? Why? How to make the data count? *Lancet* 2011;377(9775):1448–1463.
6. National Neonatology Forum, India. *Report of the National Neonatal Perinatal Database* 2003. *Available at:* http://www.nnfiorg/images/NNPD_2002-03.pdf on 1/6/2015. Accessed on: 25 June 2016.

Chapter

2 Neonatal Meningitis

Suraj Gupte, RK Sharma, Nancy Nelson

ABSTRACT

Neonatal meningitis, usually in preterm and low birthweight neonates, is predominantly caused by gram-negative pathogens, especially E. coli, in India. Brain injury in the form of diffuse neuronal insult and periventricular leukomalacia results from reduced cerebral blood flow and ischemia. Encephalopathy, subdural effusion and empyema are present in all cases. Neurologic signs/complications are more common in late-onset bacterial meningitis than in early-onset meningitis. High index of clinical suspicion needs to be supported by evidence from CSF, blood and urine culture, ultrasonography and imaging studies for establishing diagnosis. Appropriate antibiotic therapy in correct dose and for correct period of time together with supportive therapy is mandatory for positive outcome. Neuropathologic sequelae include hydrocephalus, multicystic encephalomalacia and cerebral atrophy (both cortical and white matter). Hence, follow-up must include neurodevelopmental assessment.

Key Words: Antibiotic therapy, Empyema, Encephalopathy, Hydrocephalus, Lumbar puncture, Neonatal meningitis, Neurodevelopmental assessment, Neuropathologic sequelae, Subdural effusion.

INTRODUCTION

Neonatal meningitis continues to contribute substantially to neurological disability globally, in source-limited countries in particular. A multitude of factors contribute to its continuing occurrence.

Bacterial and viral (HSV, VZV) infections dominate the scene in causation of neonatal meningitis. Nonetheless, infrequently fungal meningitis also occurs in neonates. Among the emerging pathogens that may cause neonatal meningitis are enteroviruses with considerably virulent strains.

Meningitis in neonates, being an emergency, needs early diagnosis and aggressive treatment. Else, risks of morbidity and mortality are considerable.

CASE SCENARIO

A 3-week-old neonate was admitted with refusal of feeds, fever, and seizures. He was born by normal delivery at 37 weeks and 5 days of gestation to a healthy mother. His birth weight was

Contd.

Contd.

2.9 kg. Subsequently, he had been doing fine but developed umbilical sepsis for which he was on oral amoxicillin in a sub-therapeutic dose. ***Physical examination:*** *Sick-looking neonate with subtle/focal seizures and bulging anterior fontanel; weight 2.8 kg; heart rate 140/min, respiratory rate 66/min; fluctuation in blood pressure; umbilicus septic; multiple pustules over neck and back of trunk; bilateral widespread coarse crepitations.* ***Investigations:*** *TLC 10700/cmm; CSF Glucose 12 mg/dL, protein 450 mg/dL, cells 3800 WBC/cmm with ploys 90%. CXR: Bilateral bronchopneumonia.* ***Diagnosis:*** *Late-onset neonatal sepsis with meningitis and bronchopneumonia.* ***Treatment:*** *He was started on ampicillin and amikacin on top of anticonvulsive therapy and supportive measures. However, on the intervention of the senior consultant, within hours, amoxicillin was replaced with cefotaxime plus amikacin.* ***Outcome:*** *He was discharged as cured after 6 weeks stay in the hospital.*

CRITICAL CASE ANALYSIS

The presenting manifestations and physical examination were consistent with late-onset neonatal sepsis with bronchopneumonia. The presence of seizures strongly suggested the diagnosis of meningitis. The clinical impression was supported by the characteristic CSF biochemistry and cellularity showing 90% polymorphonuclear cells.

Presence of pustules pointed that the most probable cause of meningitis was bacterial. There are two major kinds of bacteria that my cause neonatal meningitis: *Listeria monocytogenes* and *Streptococcus agalactiae* in newborn.

Since this neonate was born by a vaginal delivery and it was a late-onset disease, *Streptococcus agalactiae* (which exists in vagina canal) was the most likely cause of meningitis in him. In Cesarean births, *Listeria monocytogenes* is the predominant cause of neonatal meningitis. The senior consultant was, therefore, fully justified in changing the antibiotic from ampicillin to cefotaxime.

INTERACTIVE TOPIC DISCUSSION

What are the factors contributing to continuing occurrence of mortality in neonatal meningitis?

The factors include:

- Increasing numbers of infants surviving premature delivery.
- Limited access to medical resources in developing countries.
- Usually, absence of specific neurologic clinical findings making diagnosis of meningitis more difficult in neonates.
- A wide variety of pathogens encountered in neonates because of immaturity of their immune systems and intimate exposure to possible infection from their mothers.
- Changing pattern of the etiologic pathogens.
- Emergence of resistant strains.

What is etiopathogenesis of neonatal meningitis?

Since, there is an intimate relationship of neonatal meningitis with sepsis, the causative bacterial flora are more or less same. Similarly, there is variation in the frequency of various pathogens from nursery to nursery.

As a rule, gram-negative bacteria (especially E. coli from maternal genitourinary infection) dominate the scene in Indian subcontinent though Group B Streptococcus (GBS) is the dominant pathogen encountered in neonatal meningitis in western countries.

Other causative organisms include *Klebsiella, Pseudomonas aeruginosa, Citrobacter koseri, Staphylococcus aureus, Staphylococcus epidermis, Group D Streptococcus* (both enterococcal and nonenterococcal), etc.

Listeria monocytogenes, though the third most common cause of neonatal meningitis in the west, is an infrequent cause of neonatal meningitis in developing countries. It stands out among the various pathogens for exhibiting transplacental infection.

In addition to bacteria, neonatal meningitis may occur secondary to viral and fungal infections.

Are there any factors that indeed have an impact on pattern of neonatal meningitis?

The pattern of neonatal meningitis is dependent on certain factors which may be in relation with

- Pregnancy and delivery
- Infant
- Neonatal environment
- Pathogen(s)

Table 2.1 lists these factors in some details.

Table 2.1: Factors influencing pattern of neonatal meningitis

Pregnancy and delivery
• Complications during labor and delivery
• Maternal peripartum genitourinary infection
• Prolonged rupture of membranes
• Chorioamnionitis.
Infant
• Deficiency of non-specific immunity: Impaired leukocyte, chemotaxis, phagocytosis and bactericidal activity
• Deficiency of specific humoral immunity: IgM, IgG antibodies.
Neonatal environment
• Inhalation therapy equipment
• Aerosols
• Indwelling catheters (vascular, umbilical, intraventricular)
• Exposure to infected individuals in nursery.
Microorganisms
• Serotype III in case of GBS, K1 strains in case of *E. coli* and serotype IVb in case of *Listeria monocytogenes* are predominant specific types causing neonatal meningitis.

How does CNS invasion by the etiologic pathogens behave subsequently?

Following sepsis, CNS invasion occurs leading to:

- Blood-brain barrier (BBB) permeability
- Endothelial injury
- Release of PAF, thromboxanes and free radicals.

Thereafter, there is occurrence of vasogenic edema, vasculitis and hydrocephalus due to ventriculitis-arachnoiditis, diminished cerebral blood flow and ischemia. Diffuse neuronal injury, periventricular leukomalacia and thrombotic cerebral infarction finally result.

What is its neurophysiology?

Neonates are at greater risk of sepsis and meningitis than other age groups. This is because of deficiencies in humoral and cellular immunity and in phagocytic function in neonatal period.

Inefficiency in the neonates' alternative complement pathway compromises their defense against encapsulated bacteria. T-cell defense and mediation of B-cell activity also are compromised. Deficient migration and phagocytosis by neutrophils contribute to neonatal vulnerability to pathogens of even low virulence.

Preterm infants < 32 weeks' gestation are more vulnerable to invasion by the microorganisms.

What is the neuropathology?

In terms of neuropathology, acute changes include arachnoiditis, ventricultis, vasculitis, cerebral edema, infarction and associated encephalopathy.

The notable chronic changes are hydrocephalus, multi-cystic encephalomalacia and cerebral cortical and white matter atrophy.

What is its epidemiology?

The incidence of neonatal meningitis worldwide cannot be accurately determined because of testing limitations. According to conservative estimates, neonatal meningitis occurs in roughly 0.3 per 1000 live births. It is almost always associated with neonatal sepsis. The latter is estimated to be 5 times as common as neonatal meningitis. In other words, 1 in 5 neonates suffering from sepsis develop meningitis.

Though there has been considerable fall in mortality from neonatal meningitis, occurrence of neurologic deficit continues to be of high magnitude.

What are clinical manifestations?

Conventionally, neonatal meningitis, like its parent illness (sepsis/septicemia) may be:

1. Early onset: < 72 hours
2. Late onset: > 72 hours.

Early Onset NM (<72 Hours)

This, usually occurring in first 24–48 hours is mostly secondary to obstetrical infection and premature birth. This is a vertical infection straight from mother close to delivery time. It is important to bear in mind the role of maternal infection suggested by prolonged rupture of membranes, fever and chorioamnionitis. Not all maternal infection need be symptomatic.

Manifestations are usually non-specific (those of sepsis) and include unstable temperature (hyperthermia alternating with hypothermia), apnea, hypotension, feeding difficulties, icterus, hepatomegaly, and respiratory distress. The last-named is especially outstanding in GBS meningitis but may occur in E. coli meningitis as well.

Less frequently, petechiae, sclerema and overt focal infection may occur.

Late Onset NM (>72 Hours)

Here, neurologic signs of meningitis (change in sensorium, irritability, seizures, bulging anterior fontanel, extensor rigidity, focal cerebral signs, cranial nerve involvement, and neck rigidity) are dominant though pyrexia, irritability and feeding difficulties may also be present. Occurring usually after the 1st week, mode of transmission of infection is usually horizontal and from contaminated equipment.

Usual neurologic signs pointing to meningitis are lethargy (stupor), and irritability. Meningeal signs occur in only one-third cases.

It is noteworthy that the course of late-onset disease is less dramatic than that of early-onset disease (Table 2.2).

Table 2.2: Early onset versus late onset neonatal meningitis

	Early onset	**Late onset**
Time factor	< 72 hours	> 72 hours
Nature of manifestations	Non-specific, usually referable to systemic illness (sepsis) rather than meningitis	Neurologic signs are predominant
Common manifestations	Temperature instability Feeding difficulty, irritability alternating with lethargy, episodes of apnea, episodes of bradycardia, hypotension, jaundice, respiratory symptoms (in GBS, and less frequently in *E.coli* and *L. monocytogenes*).	Neurologic symptoms include irritability, stupor Neurologic signs include seizures, bulging fontanel, extensor posturing, opisthotonos, cranial nerve palsies, gaze deviation, hemiparesis (from cerebral involvement), neck (nuchal) rigidity.

All said and done, regardless of the specific pathogen involved, neonatal meningitis is most often caused by vertical transmission during labor and delivery. It occurs most frequently in the days following birth and is more common in premature infants than term infants.

Is it true that skin lesions are invariably present in HSV and VZV meningitis? What are clinical clues to its diagnosis?

A high index of suspicion is central to the diagnosis of neonatal meningitis. Though in each and every case of neonatal sepsis, clinical suspicion of meningitis should remain high in mind, a spectrum of neurologic signs such as change in sensorium, irritability and refusal to feed strongly points to this early enough. Other meningeal/neurologic signs may be noticed fairly late during the course of meningitis.

What is the role of lumbar puncture?

Lumbar puncture must be done in each and every newborn suspected of having meningitis.

Three classic finding in CSF for confirming diagnosis of meningitis are:

- Reduced CSF glucose.
- Elevated CSF protein.
- Pleocytosis.

Magnitude of pleocytosis is more in gram-negative meningitis and late gram-positive meningitis. This combination also is suggestive of viral meningitis, especially by HSV.

Likewise, only if all three parameters are normal does the lumbar puncture provide evidence against infection.

Does it mean that no single CSF parameter can reliably rule out the presence of meningitis in a neonate?

That is right. No single CSF value can be relied upon to exclude neonatal meningitis. Hence, it is important to consider the findings as a group.

Table 2.3 gives CSF findings suggestive of neonatal bacterial meningitis.

Table 2.3: CSF findings suggestive of neonatal bacterial meningitis

WBC > 30/mm^3 (usually > 100/mm^3) with predominance of polymorphs
Protein > 100–200 mg/dL (in preterms, it should be yet higher)
Glucose < 20–30 mg/dL (< 50% of blood glucose)

In neonates with viral meningitis, pleocytosis is not as dramatic. Viral meningitis, say HSV meningitis, particularly, may demonstrate a large number of RBCs in the CSF.

What about the CSF culture?

In order to confirm the diagnosis of meningitis, it is mandatory to do the CSF culture, preferably along with blood culture.

Does a negative CSF culture rule out meningitis?

A positive blood culture is certainly helpful. However, a negative one doesn't exclude the presence of meningitis.

What are the factors contributing to culture negative CSF?

Table 2.4 lists the factors contributing to culture negative CSF.

Table 2.4: Causes of culture negative CSF in suspected meningitis in newborns

Prior treatment with antibiotics
Brain abscess
Such bacteria as *M. hominis*, *U. urealyticum*, *Bacteroides fragilis*
Viruses

Any nonculture method of diagnosis?

Examination of a stained smear of CSF for bacteria.

How About Imaging Studies

Chest X-ray, Cranial ultrasonography, CT scan and MRI are also helpful during treatment and follow-up (Table 2.5).

Table 2.5: Role of neuroimaging in neonatal meningitis

Modality	Role
Chest radiography	Chest radiograph provides important information about the lung parenchyma and cardiac silhouette.
Ultrasonography	Useful for monitoring ventricular size for hydrocephalus during the acute phase of meningitis.
CT Scan	Useful in decision-making for potential neurosurgical interventions, such as ventriculostomy for hydrocephalus or surgical drainage of empyema or abscess.
MRI	Delineates all CNS changes very clearly + early and clear detection of ischemic changes and brain edema, cortical or white matter infarcts; MR spectroscopy can add important information on the metabolic function of the neonatal brain.

What is the role of PCR?

PCR is useful in identifying GBS antigen in urine or in CSF, and HSV and enteroviral infection in CSF.

Any other tests?

- Latex particle agglutination (LGA) test of urine.
- Fluid culture from skin lesions.
- Cultures from swabs of conjunctiva, nasopharynx and rectum for HSV, VZV, etc.

How about EEG?

EEG is indicated in neonates who are unresponsive or have seizures presenting as episodes of apnea, bradycardia, or rhythmic focal movements. EEG monitoring provides useful information to guide treatment with anticonvulsant drugs.

What is the specific antibiotic therapy?

Most often, a combination of antibiotics is needed.

Initially, the recommendation is to use ampicillin + an aminoglycoside). Alternatively, cefatoxamine (as such or in combination with an aminoglycoside) may be employed.

Once the CSF culture and sensitivity report is available, a change in antibiotic therapy may be made if warranted.

Tables 2.6 and 2.7 give pathogen-specific antibiotics and the dosage of the commonly employed antibiotics, respectively.

Table 2.6: Pathogen-specific antibiotics for neonatal meningitis

Pathogen	Recommended antibiotic(s)
Bacteria	
E. coli and other gram-negative	Ampicillin + aminoglycoside*
	Ampicillin + aminoglycoside
	Cefotaxime ± aminoglycoside/ampicillin
L. monocytogenes	Ampicillin + aminoglycoside
Group B *Streptococcus*	Ampicillin/penicillin G + aminoglycoside
Group D *Streptococcus* (nonenterococcal)	Ampicillin
Group D *Streptococcus* (enterococcal)	Ampicillin + aminoglycoside
Staphylococcus aureus/epidermidis	Cloxacillin, methicillin, oxacillin or vancomycin
P. aeruginosa	Ceftazidime + aminoglycoside
Citrobacter koseri	Cefotaxime + aminoglycoside
	Cotrimoxazole
	Imipenem
	Cilastatin
Group B *Streptococcus*	Ampicillin/penicillin G + aminoglycoside
Viruses	Acyclovir
Fungus	Amphotericin B

* Gentamicin, netilmicin, amikacin

Table 2.7: Dosage of the commonly employed antibiotics in neonatal meningitis

Antibiotic	Dose	Comments
Ampicillin	<7 days: 200–300 mg/kg/day (IV) divided q8h >7 days: 300 mg/kg/day (IV) divided q4-6h	Doses as high as 4–5 mg/kg (IV) every 8 h have been recommended to achieve therapeutic levels in CSF
Gentamicin* Amikacin	2.5 mg/kg (IV) every 8h. < 7 days 15 mg/kg/day (weight < 2 kg) and 10 mg/day (weight > 2 kg) divide q12h	
Cefotaxime	150–200 mg/kg/d IV/IM divided q4-6h	

* Intraventricular gentamicin therapy in gram-negative bacillary meningitis may be considered. In case of viral and fungal meningitis, the drugs of choice are acyclovir and amphotericin B, respectively.

What about Intralumbar/Intrathecal/Intraventricular Antibiotic Therapy?

Though once recommended, this therapy does not seem to be of any added benefit. Hence, it need not be given as a routine in neonatal bacterial meningitis.

How much should be the duration of antibiotic therapy?

Recommended duration of antibiotic therapy is given in Table 2.8.

Table 2.8: Duration of antibiotic treatment in neonatal meningitis

Gram-negative pathogens	At least 2 weeks after sterilization of CSF OR A total of 3 weeks (whichever is greater)
Gram-positive pathogens	3 weeks

What should be the guideline for empirical antibiotic therapy?

Empirical antimicrobial therapy must be such as covers all likely pathogens, i.e., both gram-positive and gram-negative organisms.

LP for Re-evaluation: Yes or No?

According to one school of thought, after 48 hours of initiating appropriate therapy, repeat lumbar puncture is advisable. If the response is poor (pathogens seen on grams staining), a change in antibiotic therapy should be considered. In such a case, it is advisable to carry out a diagnostic tap of the lateral ventricle and imaging studies should be performed to determine development of complications such as ventriculitis.

What are the recommendations for antiviral agents?

For treatment of HSV and VZV meningitis, acyclovir (Zovirax) is considered the best.

It is administered in a dose of 60 mg/kg/day (IV) in 3 divided doses for 21 days, each dose best given as an infusion over a span of 1 hour. In very premature neonates, it is advisable to reduce the dose.

What are the recommendations for antifungal agents?

Amhotericin B is the drug of choice for fungal meningitis.

It is administered in a dose of 1 mg/kg/day (IV) up to a total dose of 20 mg/kg.

Anticonvulsants

In order to terminate clinical and electrical seizure activity and to prevent recurrence of seizures, an anticonvulsant is usually required (Table 2.9). Phenobarbital and phenytoin remain the current drugs of choice.

Table 2.9: Anticonvulsant therapy in neonatal meningitis

Drug	Dosage
Phenobarbital	10–20 mg/kg/dose (IV) 5 mg/kg/day (IV,O) as maintenance dose
Phenytoin	10–20 mg/dose (IV) 5 mg/kg/day (IV, O) as maintenance dose
Lorazepam	0.05 mg/kg/dose (IV)

Any role of steroids?

None, except in Hib infection which is rare in neonates.

What are salient features of supportive therapy?

Supportive care is focused on:

- Supporting blood pressure to maintain adequate cerebral perfusion.
- Preventing secondary brain injury.
- Meticulous fluid management to minimize cerebral edema and to respond to inappropriate antidiuretic hormone (ADH) secretion.

The syndrome of inappropriate ADH secretion may cause hyponatremia and hypo-osmolality, which may increase lethargy and seizures while further increasing intracranial pressure.

Any role of surgical intervention?

Ventriculostomy with external drainage may be required with the development of acute hydrocephalus secondary to obstruction of CSF flow.

Ventriculostomy with intermittent administration of intraventricular antibiotic may be required for the management of ventriculitis.

Any pitfalls in treatment.

The pitfalls in treatment are listed in Table 2.10.

Table 2.10: Pitfalls in treatment of neonatal meningitis

• Delay in diagnosis and initiation of treatment.
• Failure to perform a lumbar puncture and detect infection in a neonate with mild fever and minimal, non-specific clinical findings is problematic. Hence, all neonates in whom meningitis is suspected as the cause of symptoms should undergo CSF examination.
• Delay in treatment because of equivocal laboratory screening tests or because findings are altered by prior partial treatment.
• Inappropriate initial treatment in respect of drug(s), dosage and duration.
• Failure to make appropriate change in antibiotic therapy when warranted by clinical profile and/or culture and sensitivity report.

List the Neurologic Complications

Regardless of etiology, meningitis in neonates can progress rapidly to serious complications (Table 2.11). These include cerebral edema; hydrocephalus; hemorrhage; ventriculitis, especially with bacterial infection; and cerebral infarction. Cerebral edema, hydrocephalus, and hemorrhage, each may cause increased intracranial pressure, with potential for secondary ischemic injury to the brain because of decreased brain perfusion.

Table 2.11: Complications of neonatal meningitis

Increased ICP/Cerebral Edema
It results from vasogenic changes, cytotoxic cell injury, and, at times, inappropriate antidiuretic hormone (ADH) secretion.
Acute Hydrocephalus
It develops as a result of debris obstructing CSF flow through the ventricular system or dysfunction of arachnoid villi.
Hemorrhage
It occurs in regions of infarction or necrosis and should be suspected in a neonate with new focal neurological findings or clinical deterioration.
Ventriculitis
It results in sequestration of infection to areas poorly accessible to systemic antimicrobial drugs. Inflammation of the ependymal lining of ventricles often obstructs CSF flow. Thus, all of these complications are interactive, making effective management difficult.
Cerebral Infarction
Cerebral infarction, both focal (arterial) and diffuse (venous), may complicate recovery.
Necrotizing Lesions
These lesions, secondary to HSV meningitis, can be deleterious to the developing brain.

What is outcome and prognosis?

Despite availability of effective treatment, mortality from neonatal meningitis at present revolves round 10%. More importantly, neurologic morbidity leading to disability is common.

Table 2.12 gives the factors contributing to poor outcome.

Table 2.12: Factors contributing to poor outcome in neonatal meningitis

Etiologic type	Factors
GBS meningitis	Comatose or semicomatose state
	Poor perfusion
	TLC > 5000/mm^3
	Absolute neutrophil count < 1000/mm^3
Gram-negative bacillary	CSF protein > 500 mg/dL
Meningitis	CSF leukocyte count >1000/mm^3
	Persistence of positive culture
	Persistence/presence of 1L-1B and tumor necrosis factor
E-coli meningitis	K_1 capsular polysaccharide antigen
	Endotoxin concentration in CSF

Notwithstanding a remarkable fall in mortality to the present level of 10%, 2–30% survivors suffer from neurologic sequelae such as:

- Chronic/recurrent seizures.
- Cognitive impairment/learning difficulties/behavioral problems which may not be detected until the child enters school.

- Mental retardation.
- Hearing loss is more common in bacterial meningitis (30%) than in viral meningitis (12–16%).
- Language disorders.
- Hydrocephalus.
- Various paresis.
- Motor impairment.

It is important to carry follow-up of these infants for neuro-developmental assessment and appropriate advice.

Is follow-up necessary?

Yes, all neonates treated for meningitis need a follow-up in the outpatient or neonatal special clinic. It is important to conduct careful screening for neurological deficits as a part of routine pediatric care over the period of many years with special attention to problems of perception, learning, and behavior.

The risk for hearing loss being high, brainstem auditory evoked response assessment (BAERA) should be done at 4–6 weeks after discharge.

CONCLUSIONS

Clinical suspicion of neonatal meningitis, a fatal condition, needs to be supported by evidence from CSF, blood and urine culture, ultrasonography and imaging studies. The central pillar of treatment is appropriate antibiotic therapy (depending on the microbial pattern of the nursery), correct dose and for correct period of time. Supportive therapy includes maintenance of nutrition and fluid-electrolyte balance, control of seizures, reduction of cerebral edema and other neurologic complications. Follow-up need to include neurodevelopmental assessment.

TAKE HOME MESSAGES

- Neonatal meningitis, usually having a bacterial origin, occurs more frequently in preterm and low birthweight neonates.
- In India, Gram-negative pathogens, especially E. coli, dominates the etiologic scenario.
- Factors concerning the neonate (immunity), environment (indwelling catheters, aerosols, inhalation therapy equipment, and infected caretakers in nursery) and factors related to pathogens have beariung on its occurrence.
- Brain injury (diffuse neuronal insult and periventricular leukomalacia) is the outcome of reduced cerebral blood flow and ischemia.
- Encephalopathy, subdural effusion and empyema are consistently present in all cases.
- Neuropathologic sequelae include hydrocephalus, multicystic encephalomalacia and cerebral atrophy (both cortical and white matter).
- Neurologic signs/complications are more common in late-onset bacterial meningitis than in early-onset meningitis.

Contd.

Contd.

- Clinical suspicion needs to be supported by evidence from CSF, blood and urine culture, ultrasonography and imaging studies for establishing diagnosis.
- Appropriate antibiotic therapy in correct dose and for correct period of time together with supportive therapy is mandatory for positive outcome.
- Neurodevelopmental assessment is the cornerstone of follow-up.

FURTHER READING

1. Gupte S, Sharma RK, Smith WE, Nelson N. Neonatal meningitis. In: Gupte S, Gupte SB (eds): *Recent Advances in Pediatrics* (Special Vol 21: Neonatal and Pediatric Intensive Care). New Delhi: Jaypee 2011:190–203.
2. Malbon K, Mohan R, Nicholl R. Should a neonate with possible late-onset infection always have a lumbar puncture? *Arch Dis Child* 2006;91:75–76.
3. Malik GK. Neonatal bacterial meningitis. In: Gupte S (ed): *Recent Advances in Pediatrics* (Special Vol 18: Pediatric Neurology). New Delhi: Jaypee 2008:199–212.
4. Nair MK, Jain N. *The High Risk Newborn*. New Delhi: Jaypee 2008.
5. Suresh G, McKenney W. Neonatal sepsis. In: Bhandari V (ed): *Manual of Neonatology*. New Delhi: Jaypee 2008:346–356.

Chapter

3 Neonatal Seizures

Bonita William, Anupam Chawla, Rita Chawla

ABSTRACT

Neonatal seizures are usually subtle and often symptomatic of a serious neurological disorder. The most frequent etiology is hypoxic-ischemic encephalopathy which is often associated with poor neurodevelopmental outcome. Early identification, determination of the triology and management is mandatory for favorable outcome. Conventional anticonvulsants are effective in around 60% of cases, warranting the need for newer agents. Prolonged seizures can result in permanent lowering the seizure threshold. A proportion of survivors are likely to develop long-term sequelae such as future cerebral palsy, mental retardation, cognitive and learning impairment.

Key Words: Acute brain injury, Cerebral palsy, Cognitive impairment, Learning impairment, Mental retardation, Phenobarbital, Phenytoin, Pyridoxine, Seizures, Subtle seizures.

INTRODUCTION

Seizure is the most frequent clinical manifestation of central nervous system dysfunction in the newborn with an incidence varying from 1–5%. Subtle seizures are the most common type of neonatal seizures, other types being tonic, clonic and myoclonic seizures. Myoclonic seizures have the worst neurodevelopmental outcome. Most common cause of neonatal seizures is hypoxic-ischemic encephalopathy.

Appropriate workup and management of neonatal seizures is complex.

CASE SCENARIO

A 3-day-old neonate, with history of perinatal asphyxia, born early term (38 weeks) to a primigravida mother by vaginal delivery, developed subtle seizures in the form of horizontal sustained deviation of the eyes. His weight was 2.9 kg. Icterus was present up to umbilicus.

Investigations: *Hemoglobin 17 g/dL,*

Serum bilirubin 8.5 mg/dL (conjugated 1 mg/dL, unconjugated 7.5 mg/dL)

Serum calcium 7.2 mg/dL, glucose 20 mg/dL

Lumbar puncture: Normal biochemistry as well as cellularity.

Contd.

Contd.

Therapy: *Since response to IV glucose and calcium as also 10 mg/kg of IV Phenobarbital failed to control the seizures, he was given IV phenytoin, 20 mg/kg. Response to this therapy was gratifying.*

Outcome: *There was no recurrence of seizures and he remained well with gradual regression of icterus. He was discharged on phenobarbital for 2 weeks.*

CRITICAL CASE ANALYSIS

The subtle seizures in this neonate with history of perinatal asphyxia appear to be the outcome of stage 2 HIE. No response to IV glucose and calcium despite their documented somewhat low levels certainly justified therapy with phenobarbital. However, poor response to a sheer 10 mg/kg of phenobarbital (given to this subject) was not an acceptable ground for shifting to therapy with phenytoin. As per standard norms, after a loading dose of 20 mg/kg, further smaller doses of phenobarbital can be given. The total dose of phenobarbital should not exceed 40 mg/kg. Only then, change over to phenytoin is recommended.

This was a good decision to continue phenobarbital for 2 weeks only since the baby remained neurologically stable.

INTERACTIVE TOPIC DISCUSSION

What is clinical classification of neonatal seizures?

Following is the clinical classification of neonatal seizures:

1. Subtle seizures (most common)
2. Clonic seizures
3. Tonic seizures
4. Myoclonic seizures (responsible for poor neurodevelopmental outcome).

The predominant type of seizures in neonates is subtle which is often very difficult to identify.

Why are generalized seizures rare in neonates?

Newborns only rarely have generalized tonic clonic seizure. Even partial seizures with secondary generalization are rare.

This is because of the immaturity of the neocortical networks at birth. Programmed synaptogenesis, apoptosis and myelination which occur later are a "must" for development of generalized seizures.

Why neonatal seizures are often not picked up by EEG?

Mediation of many seizures by brainstem or subcortical structure is responsible for their not being picked up by surface EEG monitoring.

What are subtle seizures?

Subtle seizures are the most common type of seizures in neonates, constituting about 50% of all seizures. Subtle seizures such as ocular movements, lip smacking, bicycling movements and apnea are more frequently seen in preterm infants than term infants. Ocular movements are the most common type seen in both preterm and term neonates. In full-term infants, there is often horizontal sustained deviation of the eyes. In preterm infants, the most common manifestation is sustained eye opening with unresponsiveness and eye fixation. These seizures usually do not have any electroencephalographic correlate.

Whether the subtle seizures represent subcortical seizure activity or brainstem release phenomenon is controversial. The present accepted hypothesis is that subtle seizures is predominantly subcortical in origin and may spread to involve cortical neurons.

What about neonatal apnea? Is it always a manifestation of seizures?

Apnea as a seizure manifestation requires special consideration. Apnea in a premature neonate is rarely an epileptic event. This is most often due to prematurity per se, sepsis, hypoxia or respiratory problems. Apnea due to seizure activity is associated with a normal heart rate or tachycardia. Apnea due to other causes is associated with bradycardia. However, prolonged seizures may be associated with bradycardia as a result of hypoxemia.

In term infants, apnea as a seizure manifestation occur more often associated with other manifestations such as eye deviation, mouth movements or eye opening.

What are neonatal clonic seizures?

These, rhythmic movements of muscle groups, can either be focal or multifocal with a fast and slow component. Occurrence is with a frequency of 1 to 3 jerks per second.

Clonic seizures are more frequently seen in term infants than preterm infants and are almost invariably associated with surface EEG rhythmic electrographic seizure activity.

What is the usual abnormality in clonic seizures?

The usual abnormality seen is that of trains of theta and alpha range frequencies.

Nevertheless, in multifocal clonic activity, the electrographic seizures will be of a certain frequency to start within one region followed by a different rhythmic frequency in a different part of the brain. This again reflects the immaturity of the neonatal cortical circuit immaturity.

Do neonates show typical Jacksonian march?

Newborns do not demonstrate a classical Jacksonian march or a partial seizure with secondary generalization.

But, why?

This is because cortical neurons are not sufficiently connected to achieve such an electrical evolution.

What are neonatal tonic seizures?

These are sustained flexion or extension of axial or appendicular muscle groups. These may be may be focal or generalized. EEG correlate is more frequent when tonic seizures contain focal features like unilateral involvement or eye deviation.

Manifestations include stereotyped, abrupt or slower tonic posturing of limb, and/or trunk or eyes, often accompanied by apnea, flushing, or mild cyanosis.

What are neonatal myoclonic seizures?

Lightning fast jerks of upper and lower limbs are distinguished from clonic seizures by the greater rapidity of the jerks, absence of the slow component and a predilection for flexor muscle groups. Myoclonic seizures are seen in both preterm and term neonates.

Do myoclonic seizures have EEG correlates?

- Myoclonic seizures may or may not have EEG correlates.
- Myoclonus seizures in relation to sleep or hypoxic-ischemic injury usually have no EEG correlate.

Any neonatal syndromes related to myoclonic seizures?

Neonatal syndromes related to myoclonus include Otahara syndrome and early myoclonic epileptic encephalopathy. These two syndromes are associated with burst suppression pattern in EEG and are associated with poor prognosis.

What is role of EEG in neonatal seizures?

The presence of marked abnormality in EEG background activity implies substantial EEG abnormality that can predict possibility of future electrographic seizures. Yet better is a video EEG which may be required in situations where a seizure is strongly suspected but uncertainty prevails clinically.

What is the special benefit of video EEG?

Video EEG provides simultaneous video image of the patient with time-synchronized coincident EEG.

What are the normal activities mistaken as seizures during awake or somewhat drowsy state?

- Roving and, sometimes, disconjugate eye movements.
- Sucking, puckering mouth movements without tonic eye deviation.

What are the normal activities mistaken as seizures during sleep?

- Fragmentary myoclonic jerks (may be multiple) is often normal during sleep.
- Benign neonatal sleep myoclonus, mainly seen in preterm babies during first week of life, occurs during NREM sleep. These are usually abolished when the baby is aroused. The movements tend to increase with restraint and benzodiazepines. As a rule, EEG is normal.

What about jitteriness? Should it be considered a seizure?

No, jitteriness, though often confused with seizures, is seen in HIE, hypoglycemia, hypocalcemia, and drug withdrawal.

Then what are the special features of jitteriness?

- Tremors, 4–6/second, are the characteristic finding.
- The movement lacks the fast and slow component that is characteristic of clonic seizures.
- No associated abnormality of gaze or eye movement.
- No associated autonomic changes.
- Stimulus-sensitivity, i.e., it can be provoked by stimulation of the infant or by stretching of the limb.
- Cessation of the movements with passive limb flexion.
- EEG normal.

Why is neonate's immature brain more vulnerable to seizures?

The neonate's immature brain has a unique neurobiology with an abundance of excitatory circuits and sparse inhibitory circuits. This renders him vulnerable to seizures. Additionally, there are an increased number of excitatory receptors, sensitivity to neurotransmitters and decreased inhibitory neurotransmitter binding.

Is it true that HIE is the most common cause of neonatal seizures?

Yes, undoubtedly, hypoxic-ischemic encephalopathy is the most common etiology of neonatal seizures. Around 50–60% of neonatal seizures are secondary to it.

What is characteristic about seizures in HIE?

Seizures associated with HIE usually manifests in the first 12 hours of life; only a small proportion have an onset within 24–48 hours.

HIE seizure can manifest as subtle seizures, multifocal clonic seizures and focal clonic seizures. Of these, subtle seizures are the most common presentation.

Status epilepticus is a relatively common manifestation. These seizures are often very difficult to treat.

What are other systemic manifestations in severe HIE cases?

Acute renal failure deranged liver functions and cardiomyopathy.

How does hypoxic-ischemic encephalopathy cause seizures?

Hypoxia and ischemia, the most common cause of neonatal seizures, result in a sharp decrease in energy production, causing a failure of the sodium-potassium pump. In addition, hypocalcemia and hypomagnesemia that may be associated can alter membrane potential, producing sodium influx and depolarization.

Other Common Causes of Neonatal Seizures

Stroke, intraventricular hemorrhage or intraparenchymal hemorrhage, meningitis, sepsis or metabolic disorders.

Neonatal seizures could be due to intracranial or extracranial causes. Various intracranial causes could be related to HIE, meningitis, congenital intracranial infections, intraventricular hemorrhage or subarachnoid hemorrhage.

Extracranial cause could be conditions like sepsis or metabolic conditions. Intracranial infections probably constitute 5–10% of all cases of neonatal seizures.

Any Peripartum Events that Predispose to Neonatal Seizures

Nulliparity, hydramnios, post-term pregnancy, oxytocin augmentation of labor, prolonged second stage of labor, emergency cesarean section, and assisted vaginal delivery are associated with neonatal seizures in term infants.

What is role of congenital infections in causation of neonatal seizures?

Toxoplasmosis, cytomegalovirus, herpes simplex and less frequently rubella are well-known causes of neonatal seizures. Toxoplasmosis and cytomegalovirus infection is transplacentally acquired while herpes simplex is acquired while passage through the infected birth canal.

In cytomegalovirus infection, the most common and most serious congenital infection in neonates, seizures usually occur in the first 3 days of life. Congenital cytomegalovirus infection is often associated with intrauterine growth restriction, microcephaly, meningoencephalitis, hepatosplenomegaly, hyperbilirubinemia and thrombocytopenia. Periventricular calcification is very common.

Clinical features of congenital toxoplasmosis include intrauterine growth restriction, meningoencephalitis, seizures, chorioretinitis, hepatosplenomegaly, hyperbilirubinemia and anemia.

Neonatal herpes simplex infection usually presents with meningoencephalitis, seizures, irritability and coma. Herpes simplex-1 encephalitis usually present in the second week of life.

In addition to meningoencephalitis, what are other manifestations of neonatal herpes simplex infection?

Multifocal brain parenchymal necrosis usually hemorrhagic which later on leads to diffuse encephalomalacia causing developmental delay, seizures and neurological sequela.

How about bacterial infections?

These include group B. streptococcus, E. coli and Listeria. Seizures due to these agents tend to occur later. They usually occur towards the end of 1st week or even as late as 3 months of life. The most manifestations include fever, irritability, seizures and features of meningoencephalitis.

Can maternal fever cause neonatal seizures?

Intrapartum maternal fever has 3 to 4-fold greater risk for unexplained neonatal seizures. Maternal fever more than 38°C has been associated with future cerebral palsy as well.

Any other effects of maternal fever?

Birth depression, neonatal encephalopathy, and increased neonatal mortality and morbidity.

What about intracranial hemorrhage?

Intracranial hemorrhage responsible for 10–12% cases of seizures in neonates. Most typical seizures in intracranial hemorrhage are generalized tonic seizures.

In subarachnoid hemorrhages, seizures occurs on the 2nd day of life in an otherwise healthy-looking baby ("well baby with seizures"). Resolution occurs quickly with no major sequelae.

In subdural hemorrhage, occurring secondary to trauma (cerebral contusion), seizures are usually focal. Such seizures develop in the first 48 hours of the traumatic event.

What is role of metabolic conditions?

Seizures secondary to hypoglycemia, hypocalcemia and hypomagnesemia are more common in infant of diabetic mother and in small-for-gestational age babies. Occasionally, hyponatremia and hypernatremia too can cause neonatal seizures.

How frequently do inborn errors of metabolism cause neonatal seizures?

IEMs causing neonatal seizures include aminoacidopathies, urea cycle disorders, biotinidase deficiency, mitochondrial disorders, and defects in beta oxidation, glucose transporter deficiency and peroxisomal disorders.

Amino acid and organic acid metabolism disturbances are frequent causes of neonatal seizures.

Pyridoxine dependency produces severe seizures that are resistant to anticonvulsant medication.

What about severe catastrophic epilepsy syndromes?

Ohtahara's syndrome and early myoclonic encephalopathy begin in the neonatal period, often in the first 10 days of life. The profile is in the form of severe encephalopathies associated with severe neurological illness, developmental delays and intractable seizures.

What is Ohtahara's syndrome?

Ohtahara's syndrome is characterized by brief repetitive episodes of tonic spasms akin to infantile spasms which may be isolated or present in clusters. Poor cognition is usually associated.

Interictal EEG shows a persistent burst suppression pattern. During the ictal phase, electro-decremental response is seen.

What is its cause?

The underlying etiology is often cortical brain malformations.

What about its treatment?

Despite therapy with drenocorticotropic hormone (ACTH), prednisolone, sodium valproate, topiramate or felbamate, response is poor. Around 30% cases die during infancy per se.

What is early myoclonic encephalopathy?

It is characterised by fragmentary myoclonic jerks or violent myoclonic spasms with severe neurological impairment.

Interictal EEG shows burst suppression pattern. Ictal EEG shows bursts of generalized polyspike, spike and slow wave discharges followed by electrodecremental pattern.

What is its etiology?

IEMs such as propionic academia, nonketotic hyperglycinemia and D-glyceric academia are responsible for most cases.

What is its therapy and prognosis?

Most of these babies any die in early infancy.

What are fifth day fits?

Fifth day fits, supposedly to be related to zinc deficiency, account for about 5% of seizures in full-term infants.

Typical onset is in the first week of life in otherwise healthy neonates. Seizures are usually clonic and tend to alternate between left and right side. Duration of seizures is usually less than 24 hours.

Often, these are related to apnea and cyanosis.

Anticonvulsants have only doubtful role in controlling these episodes.

What should be the investigative approach in neonatal seizures?

The following investigations are in order in most cases:

- Serum glucose, electrolytes, Ca and Mg.
- Sepsis screen.
- CSF.
- Toxicology screen.
- Maternal and fetal titers for TORCH infection.
- Neuroimaging (neurosonogram/CT/MRI of the brain).
- EEG.

What special tests are needed in IEMs?

- Blood lactate, pyruvate and ammonia.
- VBG.
- Biotinidase level.
- Quantitative aminoacids and very long chain fatty acids.
- Urine quantitative organic acids.
- CSF-pyruvate, lactate, glucose (with simultaneous blood glucose) and quantitative amino acids.

What should be the approach in a given case?

The two major goals are:

1. Identifying the cause.

2. Treating cause and seizures, e.g., treat hypoglycemia in case of hypoglycemic seizures.

If workable, continuous EEG monitoring is advised in order to avoid missing subclinical seizures.

It is ideal to treat all seizures in view of the potential harm caused.

Administration of phenobarbital or other antiepileptic agents can cause cessation of clinical seizures. However, the electrical activity may continue referred to as uncoupling.

Does it mean greater relevance of EEG?

Yes, present concept is to aim at elimination of electroencephalographic seizures. Clinical seizures are very difficult to identify. EEG not only helps to identify and quantify the seizure, it also helps to demonstrate the efficacy of the treatment offered.

Then, what should the therapeutric approach in a given neonate with seizure?

The initial step to obtain sugar estimation by dextrostix. If there is hypoglycemia, 10% dextrose should be administered followed by continuous infusion. If seizure persists, phenobarbitone is administered in a dose of 20 mg/kg slowly over 20 minutes. Repeat doses can be administered in aliquots of 5 or 10 mg/kg to a maximum of 40 mg/kg ideally until clinical and electrographic seizures cease.

What is the special benefit of fosphenytoin?

It has special advantage that it can be administered with glucose solution, can be administered rapidly and is virtually devoid of the side effect 'purple glove syndrome' which is frequent in case of IV phenytoin.

What is purple glove syndrome?

Purple glove syndrome refers to the soft tissue injury and necrosis that can occur with administration of highly alkaline phenytoin.

What are the ADRs of phenytoin and fosphenytoin?

ADRs include hypotension, cardiac *arrhythmias*, CNS adverse events (*nystagmus*, dizziness, sedation/somnolence, *ataxia* and *stupor*), and local dermatological reactions.

Purple glove syndrome probably occurs with fosphenytoin but possibly at lower frequency than with intravenous phenytoin.

Fosphenytoin can cause *hyperphosphatemia* in end-stage *renal failure* patients.

What about other anticonvulsants?

Benzodiazepines, lorazepam, diazepam and midazolam can be used but they carry risk of apnea, respiratory deporession and bradycardia.

Lidocaine may be effective in aborting some of the neonatal seizures. A starting infusion of about 4–6 mg/kg/hour has been found to be useful in the management of neonatal seizures, with or without a preceding bolus. The drug may be tapered and stopped following adequate response. Doses in premature infants are low compared to term infants. It should not be administered with phenytoin.

Felbamate, levetiracetam and lamotrigene may also be useful in the management of neonatal seizures. Felbamate is associated with acute liver failure and aplastic anemia. Rapid titration of lamotrigene in neonates may result in life threatening allergic rash.

What should be the maintenance therapy once the acute seizures are controlled?

- **Phenobarbitone:** 3–4 mg/kg/24 hours PO/IV/IM.
- **Phenytoin:** 3–4 mg/kg/24 hours IV.

Additionally,

- **Calcium gluconate:** 500 mg/kg/24 hours, PO.
- **Magnesium sulphate (50%):** 0.2 ml/kg/24 hours, IM.

Any role of EEG during follow-up.

Yes. If the infant is neurologically abnormal at discharge and neurologic examination remains abnormal, EEG should be repeated. Meanwhile, AED therapy needs to be continued. If EEG is normal but neurologic status is abnormal, AED therapy should be tapered. If EEG still shows epileptiform abnormalities, AED must be continued. Repeat EEG is required after 3 months.

Precisely, what should be the guidelines for discontinuing anti-convulsant therapy?

The requisite guidelines are listed in Table 3.1.

Table 3.1: Guidelines for discontinuing anticonvulsant therapy in neonatal seizures

Status	Action
Clinical examination normal	Discontinue phenobarbital just 2 weeks after last seizure.
Clinical examination abnormal	Continue phenobarbital for an additional month.
At 1 month, if clinical examination still abnormal	Obtain an EEG.
If EEG is normal	Wean phenobarbital.
If EEG shows abnormality	Continue AED for an additional 3 months and repeat EEG.
Every 3 months, reassess until one year of age	

Finally, what is the outcome?

High morbidity (50%) and mortality (30%) are well-known in neonatal seizures.

Outcomes is worst in

- HIE.
- Meningitis.
- Cerebral dysplasia.

What is the future risk of epilepsy in survivors?

Around 10–30% survivors are likely to have epilepsy.

Any other sequelae?

- Cerebral palsy.
- Mental retardation.

What are the good predictors of outcome?

- Interictal EEG.
- Neurological exam.
- Neuroimaging.

Is it true that neonatal seizures related to hypoxic ischemic encephalopathy with a seizure frequency of greater than 5 hours have invariably developmental delay?

Yes, it is true.

There is clear relationship between the outcome and the underlying etiology of neonatal seizures.

What are the factors/conditions in which risk of epilepsy is high?

1. Status epilepticus.
2. Abnormal neurosonography.
3. Severe abnormalities in background EEG.

Are the neonates with metabolic aberrations likely to have significant morbidity?

Yes, neonates with metabolic defects stand higher risk of having severe morbidity, especially if the underlying metabolic abnormality is not recognized.

What about neonates with pyridoxine-dependent seizures?

Infants with pyridoxine dependent seizures, if effectively managed with pyridoxine administration, usually have normal neurodevelopmental outcome.

What are the most important causes of fulminant intractable seizures?

Fulminant intractable seizures are usually to Sturge weber syndrome, hemimegelencephaly or encephalomalacia due to perinatal infarctions. They often benefit from epilepsy surgery done early in life.

CONCLUSIONS

Neonatal seizures, usually subtle and symptomatic of serious neurological disorder such as hypoxic-ischemic encephalopathy, are often associated with poor neurodevelopmental outcome. Their early identification and determination of the etiology is important. In high-risk neonates, though overt clinical manifestations are missing, electrographic seizures may be present. Institution of management to control them is mandatory. Future cerebral palsy, mental retardation, cognitive and learning impairment are serious long-term problem in survivors.

TAKE HOME MESSAGES

- Neonatal seizures are usually subtle and symptomatic serious neurological disorder.
- Hypoxic-ischemic encephalopathy, often associated with poor neurodevelopmental outcome, is the most common cause of neonatal seizures.
- Early identification, determination of the triology and management is mandatory.
- Electrographic seizures without overt clinical manifestation remains a distinct possibility in high-risk neonates, thereby highlighting the value of video EEG suspicious cases.
- Since conventional anticonvulsants are ineffective in more than 35% of cases, newer antiepileptics need serious consideration.
- In prolonged seizures, there is a considerable risk of in permanent lowering the seizure threshold.
- Future cerebral palsy, mental retardation, cognitive and learning impairment are serious long-term problem in survivors.

FURTHER READING

1. Bassan H, Bental Y, Shany E, Berger I, Froom P, Levi L, Shiff Y. Neonatal seizures: Dilemmas in workup and management. *Pediatr Neurol* 2008;38:415–421.
2. Bartha A, Shen J, Katz KH, *et al*. Neonatal seizures: Multicenter variability in current treatment practices. *Pediatr Neurol* 2007;37:85–90.
3. Ben-Ari Y, Holmes GL. Neonatal seizures. *Lancet Neurol* 2006;5:1055–1063.
4. Gopakumar H, Puthenveettil V. Neonatal seizures. In: Gupte S, Gupte SB (eds): *Recent Advances in Pediatrics* (*Special Vol 21: Neonatal and Pediatric Emergencies and Intensive Care*). New Delhi: Jaypee 2011:290–312.
5. Guillet R, Kwon J. Seizure recurrence and developmental disabilities after neonatal seizures: Outcomes are unrelated to use of Phenobarbital prophylaxis. *J Child Neurol* 2007;22:389–395.

Chapter

4 Intraventricular Hemorrhage

Jay Kishore, Manoj Modi

ABSTRACT

Intraventricular hemorrhage (IVH) is mainly seen in preterm babies. Currently, 20–25% preterm babies develop IVH. Intravascular, vascular and extravascular factors contribute in the pathogenesis of intraventricular hemorrhage. Clinically, it can manifest in three ways: most commonly silent presentation followed by saltatory and very rarely catastrophic presentation. Cranial USG is the most ideal way to diagnose IVH. Complications following IVH result into germinal matrix destruction, periventricular hemorrhagic infarction and post-hemorrhagic hydrocephalus. Most effective antenatal preventive strategy is use of antenatal steroid. Postnatal interventions comprise meticulous newborn resuscitation, correction of fluctuating cerebral blood flow velocity, correction or prevention of other major hemodynamic disturbances and correction of abnormalities of coagulation. Management includes maintenance of cerebral perfusion, prevention of cerebral hemodynamic disturbances, supportive care, serial ultrasound scans and management of post-hemorrhagic hydrocephalus.

Key Words: Hemodynamic disturbances, Intraventricular hemorrhage, Periventricular hemorrhagic infarction, Post-hemorrhagic hydrocephalus, Preterm babies, Silent saltatory catastrophic.

INTRODUCTION

Most common intracranial hemorrhage in preterm baby is intraventricular hemorrhage. The incidence is directly related to the prematurity. About 50% had onset of hemorrhage on the first postnatal day, an additional 25% on the second day, and an additional 15% on the third day. Increased incidence of IVH in preterm babies has been ascribed to many factors.

A pressure-passive state due to the lack of autoregulation of cerebral blood flow in the cerebral arterioles in the premature brain is an important predisposing factor.

Highly vascularised subependymal germinal matrix, the lack of a supporting basement membrane in the blood vessels of the germinal matrix and an increased amount of fibrinolytic activity in the germinal matrix region are contributory factors in the pathogenesis of IVH.

Elevation of venous pressure or an increase in fluctuations in cerebral blood flow velocity from a variety of factors is also important culprits in the causation of intraventricular hemorrhage.

CASE SCENARIO

Baby A was a 750 gm, 25-week premature male infant born to a 29-year-old gravida 1, para 0 (G1P0) mother whose pregnancy was complicated by the onset of premature labor. The mother received single dose betamethasone approximately 5 hours prior to a vaginal delivery. The infant was delivered with no respiratory effort and a heart rate of 70/min, required intubation at birth because of poor respiratory efforts. The infant was admitted to the intensive care unit and was given one dose of a surfactant preparation for respiratory distress syndrome (RDS). At 6 hours of life, baby developed a pneumothorax that required chest tube drainage on day of life (DOL) 1. On DOL 2 there was worsening of respiratory distress with evidence of pulmonary hemorrhage, associated hypoxic respiratory failure and significant metabolic acidosis. A head ultrasound scan showed a grade III intraventricular hemorrhage on the right with dilation of the ventricle.

CRITICAL CASE ANALYSIS

The above case scenario highlights many risk factors for IVH. First of all, baby was of just 25 weeks of gestational age which is a very important risk factor for IVH development. Mother received single dose antenatal steroid 5 hours prior to delivery. Antenatal steroid complete course is one of the effective preventive treatments for IVH. Resuscitation and respiratory distress are other contributory factors in the evolution of IVH. Development of pneumothorax and hypoxia due to pulmonary hemorrhage are other predisposing factors for IVH as these factors cause fluctuation in cerebral blood flow.

INTERACTIVE TOPIC DISCUSSION

What are the risk factors for development of IVH?

The risk factors are: intravascular, vascular and extravascular.

- *Intravascular risk factors*: Fluctuating cerebral flow, increase in cerebral blood flow due to systemic hypertension, use of colloid, normal saline bolus, sodium bicarbonate, hypercarbia, anemia, hypoglycemia, decrease in cerebral blood flow due to systemic hypotension, increase in cerebral venous pressure, Platelet and coagulation abnormality.
- *Vascular factors*: Tenuous capillary integrity, vulnerable matrix capillaries to hypoxic-ischemic injury.
- *Extravascular factors*: Deficient vascular support, increased fibrinolytic activity.

What are the clinical manifestations of intraventricular hemorrhage?

Clinically, it can manifest in three ways:

- *Silent presentation*: Most common presentation is silent in which clinical features are subtle, most important clue is unexplained fall in hematocrit.
- *Saltatory presentation*: Slow evolution, altered sensorium, change in quantity and quality of movement, hypotonia, subtle change in eye position and movement.
- *Catastrophic presentation:* Dramatic presentation–deep stupor or coma, respiratory abnormalities as apnea or hypoventilation, generalized tonic seizures, decerebrate posturing, pupils fixed to light and flaccid quadriparesis.

Which modality is ideal for IVH detection?

Cranial ultrasound is the diagnostic modality of choice. It is easily available and can be done at the bedside.

How do we classify IVH grades?

There are two classifications: Papile classification is based on CT scan and Volpe classification is based on Ultrasound.

Papile classification of IVH

Grade 1: Subependymal hemorrhage with minimal or no IVH.

Grade 2: Definite IVH without distention of the ventricles.

Grade 3: Enlargement of the ventricles secondary to distention with blood.

Grade 4: Extension of the hemorrhage into the parenchyma along with IVH and enlargement.

Volpe classification of IVH

Grade 1: Germinal matrix hemorrhage with no or minimal intraventricular hemorrhage (<10% of ventricular area on parasagittal view).

Grade 2: Intraventricular hemorrhage (10–50% of ventricular area on parasagittal view).

Grade 3: Intraventricular hemorrhage (>50% of ventricular area on parasagittal view; usually distends lateral ventricle).

Separate notation: Periventricular echodensity (location and extent).

What are the antenatal measures to prevent IVH?

Effective interventions are:

- Prevention of premature delivery: Progesterone or 17(OH) progesterone has a role in preventing preterm labor.
- In utero transportation.
- Antenatal administration of glucocorticoids: Most effective antenatal intervention-decreases risk of IVH by 50%.
- Optimal management of labor and delivery.
- No role of antenatal phenobarbitone, vitamin K and magnesium sulphate.

What are the postnatal interventions to prevent IVH?

- Proper resuscitative measures: Avoidance of volume expanders and sodium bicarbonate.
- Correction of fluctuation of cerebral blood flow velocity.
- Correction of hemodynamic disturbances: Minimal handling, avoidance of tracheal suctioning, avoidance of hypoxia and hypercarbia, avoidance of pneumothorax, slow infusion of colloid and normal saline.

- Role of indomethacin: Prophylactic treatment in infants <1000 gm for patent ductus arteriosus did show a decrease in major IVH.
- No consistent result with phenobarbitone, vitamin E and etamsylate.

What should be the strategy of acute management of IVH?

- Maintenance of Cerebral Perfusion–Meticulous control of blood pressure.
- Correction of hemodynamic disturbance by avoidance of high blood pressure, acidosis, hypoxia, hypercarbia, rapid volume expansion, pneumothorax, sodium bicarbonate and seizure.
- Supportive care, correction of anemia, thrombocytopenia and coagulation profile.
- Control of seizures.
- Head circumference monitoring.
- Serial USG scan.
- Management of post-hemorrhagic hydrocephalus.

What are the complications of intraventricular hemorrhage?

Common complications of IVH are germinal matrix destruction, periventricular hemorrhagic infarction and post-hemorrhagic hydrocephalus.

What is the fate of slowly progressive post-hemorrhagic hydrocephalus?

- Spontaneous arrest: 40%.
- Persistent slowly progressive ventricular dilatation: 20% develop arrest, 30% rapid progressive ventricular dilatation.
- Rapid progressive ventricular dilatation: 10%.

What should be the management strategy of post-hemorrhagic hydrocephalus?

For management strategy, post-hemorrhagic hydrocephalus is classified into four groups:

- **Type I:** Slowly progressive ventricular dilatation: moderate dilation, normal rate of head growth, duration <2 weeks.
- **Type II:** Persistent slowly progressive ventricular dilatation: duration is >2 weeks and rate of head growth may begin to increase.
- **Type III:** Rapidly progressive ventricular dilatation: moderate to severe dilation, excessive rate of head growth.
- **Type IV:** Arrested progression: spontaneous arrest of ventricular dilatation or arrest following lumbar puncture.

In group I: Close surveillance required.

In group II: Close surveillance for 2 more weeks if IVH grade I/II, serial lumbar puncture (Controversial).

In group III:

A. Serial lumbar punctures-controversial

B. Ventricular drainage

C. Ventriculoperitoneal shunt: After CSF clears and CSF protein level <1.5 g/L.

In group IV: Close surveillance for 1 year.

What should be the algorithmic approach for the prevention and treatment of IVH?

Figure 4.1 provides such an approach.

CONCLUSIONS

VH is a problem of preterm babies. Antenatal strategy to prevent IVH includes prevention of preterm birth, in utero transport, use of antenatal steroid, optimum management of labor and delivery. Preventive strategies during postnatal period include proper resuscitative measures, avoidance of volume expanders and sodium bicarbonate, correction of fluctuation of cerebral blood flow velocity, correction of hemodynamic disturbances, minimal handling, avoidance of tracheal suctioning, avoidance of hypoxia and hypercarbia, avoidance of pneumothorax, slow infusion of colloid and normal saline, indomethacin administration, etc. Management includes maintenance of cerebral perfusion, correction of hemodynamic stability, supportive measure, serial USG scan and appropriate handling of post-hemorrhagic hydrocephalus.

TAKE HOME MESSAGES

- Antenatal steroid is the most effective antenatal strategy to prevent IVH.
- Judicious use of volume expander and hyperosmolar solution, correction of hypoxia, acidosis, and hypercarbia, adequate management of seizure are effective postnatal strategy to prevent IVH.
- Regular OFC measurement and serial cranial USG are important for detection of post-hemorrhagic hydrocephalus management of labor and delivery. Postnatal preventive strategy includes: proper resuscitation, avoidance of fluctuation in cerebral blood flow velocity by judicious use of muscle paralytic agent, correction of hemodynamic stability and correction of coagulation abnormality. Management of IVH includes maintenance of cerebral perfusion, correction of hemodynamic stability, supportive measure, serial USG scan and management of post-hemorrhagic hydrocephalus.

FURTHER READING

1. Bonifacio SL, Gonzalez F, Ferriero DM. Central Nervous System Injury and Neuroprotection. In: Gleason, Christine A (eds): *Avery's Diseases of the Newborn,* 9th edn. Philadelphia: Elsevier 2012:869–891.
2. De Vries LS. Intracranial hemorrhage and vascular lesions in the neonate. In: Martin, Richard J (eds): *Fanaroff and Martin's Neonatal-Perinatal Medicine,* 10th edn. Philadelphia: Elsevier 2015:886–903.
3. Volpe JJ. Intracranial Hemorrhage: Germinal Matrix–Intraventricular Hemorrhage of the Premature Infant. In: Volpe JJ (ed): *Neurology of Newborn,* 5th edn. Philadephia: Elsevier 2008:483–516.
4. Whitelaw A. Posthemorrhagic hydrocephalus: Management strategies. In: Pan, Jeffry M (ed): *Neurology: Neonatal Questions and Controversies,* 2nd edn. Philadelphia: Elsevier 2012:47–62.

Intravascular hemorrhage

Antenatal preventive strategy:

- Prevention of preterm birth: use of progesterone
- In utero transport
- Antenatal steroid: betamethasone preferred
- Optimum management of labor and delivery

↓

Postnatal preventive strategy:

- Proper resuscitation: Avoid normal saline bolus and sodium bicarbonate
- Avoid fluctuating cerebral blood flow: Use muscle paralytic agent judiciously
- Correction of hemodynamic instability

↓

Management of IVH:

Maintain cerebral perfusion

- Correction of hemodynamic stability by prompt management of acidosis, hypoxia, hypercarbia, seizure, avoid volume expander and hyperosmolar solution
- Supportive management
- Serial USG
- Management of post-hemorrhagic hydrocephalus

Management of post-hemorrhagic hydrocephalus

- Weekly cranial USG in grade I–II IVH

Twice weekly cranial USG in grade III IVH

- Action line: Ventricular width 4 mm higher than the 97th centile width for age
- Other parameters: Anterior horn width (95th centile – 3 mm) + 1 mm, thalamo-occipital width (95th centile – 25 mm) + 1 mm, third ventricle width (95th centile – 2 mm) + 1 mm
- Doppler flow ACA R.I. >0.85 (Serial increase)

↓

If ventricular width >4 mm +97 centile for age:

- Repeated early lumbar punctures/ventricular taps-controversial

Diuretic drugs to reduce cerebrospinal fluid (CSF) production–no proven role, worse outcome in terms of shunt surgery and death or disability (acetazolamide with furosemide)

- Ventriculoperitoneal shunt after CSF clears and CSF protein level <1.5 g/L

Fig. 4.1: Algorithmic approach to IVH

Chapter

5 Neonatal Apnea

Sriparna Basu, Ashok Kumar

ABSTRACT

Apnea is a common neonatal problem especially in preterm neonates. Apnea of prematurity (AOP) occurs secondary to the physiological immaturity of respiratory control which is often exacerbated by hypoxia, hypercapnia, altered sleep states, gastroesophageal reflux, anemia etc. Standard clinical management includes correction of precipitating causes, methylxanthine therapy, continuous positive airway pressure (CPAP) or mechanical ventilation in extreme cases. Other therapies, such as, kangaroo mother care (KMC), CO_2 inhalation etc. need further evaluation. The major concern is the disturbance of cerebral hemodynamics during the period of apnea which may affect cerebral oxygenation and result in long-term neurodevelopmental sequelae.

Key Words: Apnea, Apnea of prematurity, Continuous positive airway pressure, Neonate, Kangaroo mother care (KMC), Methylxanthine therapy.

INTRODUCTION

Apnea is a common neonatal problem encountered in an NICU. It may occur secondary to an underlying illness or more commonly due to idiopathic apnea of prematurity (AOP) in preterm neonates. In term infants apnea is almost always due to a pathological cause. The major concern associated with neonatal apnea is the disturbance of cerebral hemodynamics which may affect short-term cerebral oxygenation and long-term neurodevelopmental outcome.

CASE SCENARIO

An extremely preterm (27^{+3} weeks) female neonate, weighing 920 gm, was delivered via cesarean section to a 24 years old primigravida mother with placenta previa. The mother received proper antenatal care and 2 doses of betamethasone 24 hours prior to delivery. The baby did not require any delivery room resuscitation. 1 and 5 minutes Apgar scores were 7/10 and 8/10, respectively. She was admitted in NICU for prematurity and low birthweight. She was managed with parenteral nutrition and orogastric feeding with expressed breastmilk. Sepsis screen was negative, metabolic profile and electrolytes were normal.

Contd.

Contd.

She remained well for first 48 hours. On day 3 of life, she developed apnea with desaturation (SpO_2 <80%) and bradycardia (HR <100/min). On examination, she was found to lie in a position with neck flexion, nesting was not done, temperature probe of the warmer was not properly attached leading to maximum heater output causing hyperthermia (surface temperature was measured to be 38.7°C).

The baby was managed with proper positioning with slightly extended neck by shoulder roll, head was kept in midline. Oxygen inhalation was started. Tap water sponging was done to reduce hyperthermia. After initial stabilization, rest of the vitals, mean arterial pressure and systemic examination was found to be normal. She kept on having repeated episodes of apnea with desaturation and bradycardia, which initially responded to physical stimulation but later on required positive pressure ventilation with bag and mask. She was loaded with caffeine and put on CPAP.

Laboratory investigations including hematological, biochemical tests, arterial blood gas (ABG) analysis, USG cranium and 2-D Echocardiography were normal. A diagnosis of apnea of prematurity (AOP) in an extremely preterm low birthweight baby was kept.

CRITICAL CASE ANALYSIS

The risk factors for AOP in this infant were extremely low birthweight (ELBW). Neck flexion and hyperthermia were the initial precipitating factors. Extensive investigations were done to rule out the secondary causes of apnea. Caffeine and CPAP were started as she required positive pressure ventilation with bag and mask.

INTERACTIVE TOPIC DISCUSSION

What is the definition of neonatal apnea?

No respiratory effort, i.e., cessation of respiratory airflow for a period more than 20 seconds or a shorter respiratory pause associated with oxygen desaturation/cyanosis and/or bradycardia in a neonate within first 28 days of life.

How do you define apnea of prematurity (AOP)?

AOP is defined as cessation of respiratory airflow for a period more than 15–20 seconds associated with oxygen desaturation ($SpO_2 \leq 80\%$ for ≥ 4 s)/cyanosis and/or bradycardia (heart rate <2/3 of baseline for ≥ 4 s) in a neonate of gestational age less than 37 weeks. Short breathing pauses for 5 to 10 seconds not accompanied with oxygen desaturation or bradycardia occur frequently in premature infants and are considered normal.

AOP is the most common cause of apnea in preterm neonates occurring due to immaturity of the respiratory centre of the brain. Usual age of onset is 2–7 days of life. Apnea beginning immediately after birth or developing for the first time after 7 days, suggests a pathological cause. AOP usually resolves with postnatal maturity, by 34 to 36 weeks post-menstrual age.

What is apnea of infancy?

Onset of apnea occurring in infants with a gestational age of 37 weeks or more is usually referred as apnea of infancy.

What are the etiologies of neonatal apnea?

Though the most common cause of apnea in neonates is apnea of prematurity, but other secondary causes (Box 5.1) must be ruled out before making the diagnosis of AOP.

Box 5.1: Secondary causes of neonatal apnea

- *Neonatal sepsis* – It is the most common secondary cause of apnea which should always be ruled out.
- *Diseases affecting central nervous system (CNS)* – Intraventricular hemorrhage (IVH), seizures, meningitis, perinatal asphyxia and hypoxic ischemic encephalopathy, neuromuscular disorders, neonatal stroke/infarction, birth trauma, congenital malformations involving CNS.
- *Cardiovascular* – Anemia, hypo/hypertension, patent ductus arteriosus (PDA), congestive heart failure, coarctation, congenital cyanotic heart diseases, hypovolemia.
- *Pulmonary* – Respiratory distress syndrome, pneumonia, transient tachypnea of the newborn, meconium aspiration syndrome or other aspiration pneumonias, pneumothorax, hypoxia, intrinsic/extrinsic mass or lesions causing airway obstruction, upper airway collapse, atelectasis, phrenic nerve paralysis, malformations of chest, pulmonary hemorrhage.
- *Metabolic* – Hypoglycemia, hypocalcemia, hypo/hypernatremia, high ambient temperature, hypo/hyperthermia, hyperammonemia, acidosis, inborn errors of metabolism.
- *Gastrointestinal* – Gastroesophageal reflux (GER), esophagitis, necrotising enterocolitis, intestinal perforation, abdominal distension.
- *Drugs* – Maternal intake of opiates, prostin, phenobarbitone, chloral hydrate or other sedatives, general anesthetics, magnesium sulfate, beta-blockers, narcotic abstinence syndrome, postnatal exposure to sedatives, hypnotics or narcotics.
- *Miscellaneous* – Neck flexion, nasal edema or the presence of a nasogastric feeding tube, vigorous suction of pharynx causing vagal stimulation, painful procedures.

What are the physiological effects of apnea?

- Decrease in arterial oxygen saturation.
- Decrease in heart rate.
- Decrease in cerebral blood flow leading to CNS depression if apnea is severe.
- Increase in venous pressure.
- Decrease in muscle tone.

What is the incidence of AOP?

The incidence of AOP is inversely proportional to the neonate's gestational age and birthweight.

- <10% at gestational age ≥ 34–35 weeks.
- 15% at gestational age 32–33 weeks.
- 50% at gestational age 30–31 weeks.
- Almost all at gestational age <29 weeks and <1000 gm.

What are the types of AOP?

AOP are of three types, central, obstructive and most commonly mixed.

- **Central apnea** (40%) – It is caused by decreased central nervous system stimuli to respiratory muscles. Both the respiratory effort and airflow cease simultaneously resulting in absence of chest wall movement and airflow.
- **Obstructive apnea** (10%) – It is caused by pharyngeal instability and collapse, neck flexion or nasal obstruction. Absence of airflow occurs even in presence of chest wall movement.
- **Mixed apnea** (50%) – A combination of both types of apnea, central apnea is either preceded or followed by obstructed respiratory effort.

What is the pathogenesis of AOP?

AOP is considered to be a developmental disorder that self-resolves with time and neurological maturity. It is more 'physiological' than a 'pathological' immaturity of respiratory control. The common factors involved in the pathogenesis of AOP are discussed below.

- **Transition from low to high oxygen environment at birth** – *In utero* the fetal PaO_2 is 23–27 mm Hg, which changes to a PaO_2 80–100 mm Hg after birth. Immature respiratory pattern because of fewer synaptic connections and poor myelination of the immature brainstem may delay this postnatal adjustment. Moreover, the postnatal rise in PaO_2 may also silences the peripheral chemoreceptors, resulting in delayed onset of spontaneous breathing.
- **Neurotransmitters and apnea** – Enhanced sensitivity to inhibitory neurotransmitters, such as gamma-aminobutyric acid (GABA), adenosine, serotonin, and prostaglandin, is a major cause of poor respiratory control in premature infants.
- **Effect of sleep states and movements** – Premature infants spend a relatively larger proportion of their time in rapid eye movement (REM) sleep, with a relatively smaller amount in wakefulness. Activities of upper airway muscles are reduced markedly during sleep predisposing the upper airway to collapse, especially during inspiration when the upper airway is subjected to airway collapsing forces. REM sleep is associated with paradoxical breathing and unstable oxygen saturation which often lead to apnea. Moreover, motor activities after arousal are also associated with laryngeal closure and apnea.
- **Hypoxic ventilatory depression** – In hypoxic condition after birth, premature infants elicit an initial transient increase in respiratory rate and tidal volume for few minutes, followed by a late, sustained decline in spontaneous breathing lasting for several weeks.
- **Peripheral chemoreceptor stimulation** – Hypocapnia seen after hyperventilation may also lead to apnea in premature infants.
- **Ventilatory response to hypercapnia** – In response to hypercapnia, premature infants increase ventilation by prolonging the expiration, but not increasing breath rate or tidal volume, leading to less minute ventilation. Contradictory movements of respiratory muscles, especially diaphragm, in response to hypercapnia may also play a role in AOP.
- **Responses to laryngeal chemoreflex** – Stimulation of the laryngeal mucosa mediated through superior laryngeal nerve can also lead to apnea, bradycardia, and hypotension in premature infants.
- **Genetic vulnerability** – Recent reports also suggest a possibility of genetic basis of AOP.

What are the differential diagnoses of AOP?

The major differential diagnoses of AOP are **periodic breathing** and **neonatal seizures**. Periodic breathing is defined as three or more periods with no respiratory effort lasting 3 seconds or more in a 20 second period. It is not accompanied with desaturation or bradycardia and is a normal neonatal breathing pattern. Apnea may be an uncommon presentation of a neonatal seizure. The apneic episode is usually associated with tachycardia and other features of the primary disease are present.

How do you monitor a neonate with apnea?

All neonates less than 34 weeks gestation should be routinely monitored for at least the first week of life or until there has been an absence of apneic episodes for at least 7 days. Neonates of >34 weeks gestation should be monitored for apnea when they are sick and clinically unstable. Common monitoring devices are:

(i) **Pulse oximeters** – Used in hospital settings to detect changes in heart rate and/or saturation.

(ii) **Ripple mattress with movement sensors** – Which detect chest/abdominal movements during respiration.

(iii) **Thoracic impedence monitors** – Which detect changes in thoracic impedence that occur with breathing.

Apnea monitors are mainly used for home monitoring by parents with resuscitation training. These devices cannot detect obstructive apnea. Moreover, they may raise alarm falsely with normal periodic breathing.

What measures do you take to reduce the occurrence of AOP?

(i) Positioning – Ensure the neonate's head and neck are positioned in midline and avoid flexion of neck to maintain a patent airway. Infants can be nursed prone as prone positioning improves thoracoabdominal synchrony and stabilize the chest wall without affecting breathing pattern. Other positioning, such as, extension of the neck 15° from the prone position (head elevated tilt position) and a more comfortable three-stair-position that maintains the head and abdomen in a horizontal position was reported to improve apnea, bradycardia, and desaturation.

(ii) Avoid vigorous suctioning of moth and pharynx.

(iii) Avoid hypo/hyperoxia.

(iv) Avoid metabolic disturbances.

(v) Avoid placement of nasogastric tubes in tiny neonates – Orogastric tube placement is preferred.

(vi) Avoid fluctuation of temperature and high environmental temperature.

(vii) Treatment of anemia – Hemoglobin should be maintained above 10 g/dL in neonates experiencing frequent apneic episodes.

What is the treatment protocol for apnea?

Institution of interventions should occur in the order of increasing invasiveness and risk.

1. **Diagnose and treat precipitating causes**

   If apnea is not physiological, investigations need to be done to identify the underlying causes, such as, respiratory diseases, sepsis, hypotension, hypoglycemia, PDA, IVH, GER, anemia, etc. and treat appropriately.
2. **Clear airway:** Suction mouth and nostrils, if visible secretions are present.
3. Tactile stimulation (gentle rubbing of soles of feet or chest wall is usually all, i.e., required for episodes that are mild and intermittent).
4. Initiate a trial of nasal prong air/oxygen airflow.
5. Positive pressure ventilation may be required if spontaneous respiration does not resume with tactile stimulation. If positive pressure ventilation is required to treat apneic episodes, CPAP or mechanical ventilation may be considered.
6. Initiate pharmacotherapy (methylxanthines).
7. Initiate a trial of low-pressure nasal continuous positive airway pressure (CPAP).
8. Initiate mechanical ventilation.

What are the indications for initiation of methylxanthines and/or CPAP?

- Spontaneous resolution of apnea – start methylxanthines if frequent episodes associated with desaturations (SaO_2 <80%) and/or bradycardia (HR <90), one or more per hour over a long period of time such as 12–24 hours.
- Mild to moderate apnea (Associated with desaturations <80% and bradycardia <90) – start methylxanthines if multiple episodes occur more than 6 over a 12-hour period or 12 over a 24-hour period.
- Severe (Prolonged vigorous stimulation or need for bag and mask ventilation with or without oxygen) – start methylxanthines if more than 1 episode in a 24-hour period.

Methylxanthines

The most commonly used methylxanthines are Caffeine (1,3,7-trimethylxanthine) and Theophylline (1,3-dimethylxanthine).

Mechanism of Action – Methylxanthines are powerful CNS stimulants and reduce apnea by multiple mechanisms. They are non-selective antagonists of adenosine receptors. Although both A1 and A2 receptors are involved, a greater role for A2A receptors has been observed. Methylxanthines reduce apnea through blockade of A2A receptors on GABAergic neurons. Methylxanthines also increase CO_2 sensitivity, and neural respiratory drive while decreasing the hypoxic depression of breathing. They also improve diaphragmatic contraction and respiratory muscle function. All these lead to an enhancement of minute ventilation.

Dosages

Caffeine Citrate – 20 mg/mL containing the equivalent of 10 mg/mL of caffeine is available for either IV/per oral (PO) use.

- Loading dose – 20 mg/kg/dose of caffeine citrate IV/PO
- Maintenance dose – 5 mg/kg/day of caffeine citrate given Q6h

- Mean plasma half life – 102 (37–231) h
- Therapeutic level – 8–20 ug/mL
- Toxic level – >30 ug/mL.

If the apnea frequency does not improve 48 hours after the caffeine loading dose, a further loading dose of 20 mg/kg caffeine citrate may be given and the maintenance dose may be increased to 7.5 mg/kg/day and then to 10 mg/kg/day if apnea persists. When reloading with caffeine, the time of last maintenance dose given should always be reviewed. It may be appropriate to reduce the loading dose or to wait for more than 12 hours from the last maintenance dose before reloading.

Several clinical trials have also used a very high initial loading dose of 40 mg/kg caffeine (followed by 20 mg/kg every 24 h) with a standard loading dose of 10 mg/kg (followed by 5 mg/kg every 24 h). The high-dose group showed significant reductions in extubation failure, duration of ventilation, and apnea after extubation compared with the standard low-dose group. There is a word of caution with the high loading dose of 25 mg/kg of caffeine as it reduces cerebral blood flow velocity.

Theophylline – Aminophylline ampoule 250 mg/10 mL is available for IV infusion

Theophylline 50 mg/5 mL (Theoped syrup) is available for oral use.

- Loading dose – 6 mg/kg/dose IV/PO
- Maintenance dose – 6 mg/kg/day divided Q6h/Q8h/Q12h IV/PO
- Mean plasma half life – 30 (12–64) h
- Therapeutic level – 6–12 ug/mL
- Toxic level – >20 ug/mL

Methylxanthines should always be infused slowly over a minimum of 20 minutes. Rapid IV pushes may lead to sudden death from cardiac arrhythmias.

What are the adverse effects of methylxanthine therapy?

Methylxanthines carry some risks of adverse events enumerated in Box 5.2. Toxic levels produce tachycardia, cardiac dysrhythmias, increased energy expenditure, and delayed gastric emptying with feeding intolerance, diuresis, jitteriness and seizures at very high doses. Serum levels should be performed if the infant is showing signs of toxicity or is failing to respond to the increased maintenance dose. Caution should be executed in neonates with seizures.

Box 5.2: Adverse effects of methylxanthine therapy

- Tachycardia, cardiac dysrhythmias
- Increased cardiac output
- Opening up of PDA
- Vomiting
- Excessive diuresis
- Increased cerebral metabolic rate
- Decreased cerebral blood flow
- Hyperglycemia

Contd.

Contd.

- Increased plasma glycerol
- Increased lung glycogen metabolism
- Decrease cholesterol synthesis in glial cells
- Decreased cerebral cell growth and division
- Decreased retinal blood flow.

What methylxanthine compound is preferred?

Systematic reviews of methylxanthine therapy in AOP have shown that both caffeine and theophylline are equally effective in reducing apnea within 2–7 days of starting treatment. But, caffeine is safer and has a wider therapeutic range than theophylline. Moreover, the plasma half-life of caffeine is 102 hours compared to 30 hours for theophylline requires once daily dosing schedule in caffeine. Enteral absorption is more reliable for caffeine. The famous CAP (**C**affeine in **A**pnea of **P**rematurity) trial has shown that caffeine reduces the rate of bronchopulmonary dysplasia, duration of respiratory support and functional neurodevelopmental disabilities at 18 months. The neuroprotective effect was not documented in the same cohort at 5 years.

How to wean a neonate from caffeine?

Caffeine may be stopped abruptly as it has a very long half-life. This is usually done when the infant has reached 32–34 weeks postconceptual age and is no longer have apneas. Cardiac monitoring can be discontinued when the caffeine is stopped, but an apnea monitor should be used for 5 days after stopping caffeine.

Is there any role of caffeine in the prevention of AOP?

Recent evidences do not support the use of prophylactic caffeine for preterm infants at risk of apnea.

What is the role of nasal continuous positive airway pressure (CPAP) and high/low flow nasal cannula (HFNC) in the management of AOP?

Nasal CPAP is effective in reducing apnea in preterm infants, especially in presence of airway obstruction. CPAP maintains airway patency by its splinting effect, increases functional residual capacity during active sleep when there is a reduction in tonic and post-inspiratory activity of the diaphragm resulting in better oxygenation. It also causes alteration of the Hering-Breuer reflex leading to higher lung volumes thereby minimizing inspiratory duration and decreasing airway collapse by prolonging expiratory time. Furthermore, CPAP increases stabilization of the chest wall musculature, decreases activity of the intercostal inspiratory inhibitory reflex, and inhibits feedback through laryngeal mechanoreceptors resulting into more stable respiratory rhythm and less apnea. CPAP is not effective in central apnea.

High/low flow nasal cannula (HFNC): This is especially effective with mixed and obstructive apneas. Both high and low HFNC can be a useful adjunctive therapy in some infants with apnea who are already receiving methylxanthines. High flow produces a distending pressure, especially in the very low birth- weight infants. The magnitude of this distending pressure depends on flow rate, nasal leak and mouth closure. Efficacy is similar to nasal CPAP.

Low flow nasal cannula acts through neural mechanism by stimulation of mechanoreceptors in the nose and the larynx.

When do you start mechanical ventilation in AOP?

MV is started when caffeine and HFNC and CPAP have been tried and there are still significant apneas. It is effective in all types of apneas.

What is the role of doxapram in the prevention of AOP?

Doxapram is a potent non-specific stimulant of the central nervous system, increases tidal volume and minute ventilation. It is rarely used for the management of apnea refractory to methylxanthine therapy, if facilitities for CPAP/mechanical ventilation are not available.

It is not routinely recommended for AOP because its side effects, such as, irritability, seizures, elevated blood pressure, hyperglycemia, gastric retention, increase in cerebral oxygen consumption and a decrease in oxygen delivery mediated by a decrease of cerebral blood flow. Hypertensive episodes may be associated with an increased risk of intraventricular hemorrhage. The side effects occur because of 0.9% benzyl alcohol used as a preservative in injection doxapram. Doxapram infusion is started at 0.5 mg/kg/h and increased gradually to a maximum of 2–2.5 mg/kg/h. The infusion should be continued for a period of 48 hours before weaning. Methylxanthine therapy should be continued during doxapram infusion.

What are the novel/intriguing therapies used for the management AOP?

The following novel/intriguing therapies used for the management of AOP:

1. **Kangaroo mother care (KMC):** Recently, KMC has achieved widespread acceptance for stable infants because of the calming effects on the baby's clinical status and vital signs. Infants receiving KMC had fewer apneic and bradycardic events than those who did not receive KMC.
2. **Sensory stimulations:** Sensory stimulants, including tactile and olfactory stimulation, are useful in the treatment or prevention of AOP by generating excitatory, non-specific neuronal activity in the brainstem center to stimulate respiratory activity.

   Olfactory stimulation has also been used for the treatment of AOP. Pleasant odor, such as vanillin, a stimulus known to affect the olfactory nerve, has been found to elicit increased respiratory drive, whereas unpleasant odors caused decreased respiratory effort, during active sleep when apnea is more common.
3. **CO_2 inhalation:** CO_2 is the physiologic stimulus for breathing in mammals. Apnea occurs when the CO_2 baseline decreases below the apnea threshold. A rise in CO_2 of 1 to 2 mm Hg above the apnea threshold may reduce or abolish apnea. Recently, a randomized controlled trial showed that inhalation of a low 0.8% CO_2 concentration in premature infants is as effective as theophylline in decreasing apnea. This exposure to 0.8% CO_2 also had no effect on cerebral blood flow velocity. Though the effect of long-term exposure is not known.
4. **Exogenous stochastic stimulation:** Low-level exogenous stochastic stimulation has been found to stabilize the breathing pattern in preterm infants. Mechanosensory stimulation was achieved

using actuators embedded within the infant's mattress. The stimulus intensities were subthreshold for causing behavioral arousal or for causing shifts in the power spectrum of EEG activities. An improvement in breathing stability associated with decreased incidence of apneic pauses and a reduction in O_2 destauration was observed.

What are the short-term and long-term consequences of apneas?

Short-term

Prolonged apnea and bradycardia in preterm neonates can decrease the systemic blood pressure and lead to cerebral hypoperfusion, which may contribute to hypoxic-ischemic injury of the immature brain.

Long-term

The long-term consequences of apnea are controversial. Poor neurodevelopmental outcomes may occur due to the possible coexistence of neurological injury in premature infants. A higher frequency and severity of AOP were found to be associated with a higher incidence of unfavorable outcomes or death. Increased number of AOP days was also found to be associated with neurodevelopmental impairment such as cerebral palsy and blindness at 3 years of age.

Is there any association of AOP and sudden infant death syndrome?

The risk of sudden infant death syndrome in premature infants is three times higher than that of full-term infants. The risk factors for sudden infant death syndrome in premature infants are strongly associated with maternal age, tobacco use, meteorological factors, and genetics but not AOP.

What is the prognosis of AOP?

In preterm infants the frequencies of apneic episodes decrease gradually during the first months of postnatal life. The lower the gestational age, the longer the period AOP persists. AOP disappears in most infants by 36–40 weeks post-conceptional age. However, extremely premature infants (24–28 gestational weeks) are at risk for experiencing apnea until the post-menstrual age of 44 weeks.

What precautions do you take during immunization of an infant who had AOP?

Infants with AOP may experience apnea and bradycardia following the first series of immunizations. It is better to immunize these infants before discharge while they are still in NICU. These events are less likely to occur during subsequent immunizations.

CONCLUSIONS

Apnea is a very common complication in premature infants which usually disappears spontaneously with increase in the post-conceptional age. Common interventions for apnea include physical stimulation, pharmacotherapy and respiratory assistance in the form of CPAP or mechanical ventilation.

TAKE HOME MESSAGES

- Apnea is a common complication in premature infants usually occurring after between day 2–7 days of life. One should be vigilant for its occurrence.
- Though apnea in premature neonates may be because of physiological immaturity, secondary causes must be ruled out before making the final diagnosis.
- In neonates with recurrent episodes of apnea, the drug of choice is caffeine, because of its safety margin and once a day dosage interval. Prophylactic caffeine does not have a role.

FURTHER READING

1. Henderson-Smart DJ, De Paoli AG. Methylxanthine treatment for apnoea in preterm infants. *Cochrane Database Syst Rev* 2010; (12):CD000140.
2. Henderson-Smart DJ, Steer PA. Caffeine versus theophylline for apnea in preterm infants. *Cochrane Database Syst Rev* 2010;20;(1):CD000273.
3. Henderson-Smart DJ, De Paoli AG. Prophylactic methylxanthine for prevention of apnoea in preterm infants. *Cochrane Database Syst Rev* 2010;(12):CD000432.
4. Mathew OP. Apnea of prematurity: Pathogenesis and management strategies. *J Perinatol* 2011;31:302–310.
5. Mohammed S, Nour I, Shabaan AE, Shouman B, Abdel-Hady H, Nasef N. High versus low-dose caffeine for apnea of prematurity: A randomized controlled trial. *Eur J Pediatr* 2015; 3 [Epub ahead of print].
6. Schmidt B, Roberts RS, Davis P, Doyle LW, Barrington KJ, Ohlsson A, Solimano A, Tin W. Caffeine for Apnea of Prematurity Trial Group. Long-term effects of caffeine therapy for apnea of prematurity. *N Engl J Med* 2007;357:1893–1902.
7. Schmidt B, Anderson PJ, Doyle LW, Dewey D, Grunau RE, Asztalos EV, *et al.* Survival without disability to age 5 years after neonatal caffeine therapy for apnea of prematurity. *JAMA* 2012;18;307:275–282.
8. Zhao J, Gonzalez F, Mu D. Apnea of prematurity: From cause to treatment. *Eur J Pediatr* 2011;170:1097–1105.

Chapter

6 Cyanosis in the Newborn

Rahul P Bhamkar, Anjali Kulkarni

ABSTRACT

Cyanosis in newborn, though a common presenting feature in various newborn illnesses, poses a significant diagnostic challenge. Cardiorespiratory causes predominate but hematologic, metabolic and neuromuscular disorders also need to be considered. It requires rapid assessment, diagnosis and initiation of therapy. A systematic approach for differentiating various causes of cyanosis helps in planning management.

Supportive treatment should be started as soon as cyanosis is noticed. Prostaglandin E1 infusion should be started as early as possible in ductus dependent cyanotic heart disease. A timely treatment and referral as required can save the life of infant.

This chapter presents the case-based approach for various conditions presenting with cyanosis in newborn.

INTRODUCTION

The term, *cyanosis*, refers to bluish discoloration of skin, nail beds or mucous membrane. The word is derived from the Greek word Kuaneous which means dark blue. Cyanosis depending on the site where it is present can be classified as central or peripheral cyanosis. Acrocyanosis or peripheral cyanosis, when only extremities are affected, is generally a physiologic finding in the newborn. In contrast, central cyanosis which is evident in mucous membrane and tongue indicates presence of potentially serious and life threating ailment and requires immediate evaluation. Cyanosis could be due to various conditions like cardiac, respiratory, central nervous system, hematologic or metabolic. It is important to determine the cause of cyanosis, so that necessary investigations and management can be planned accordingly.

CASE SCENARIO

A newborn male baby delivered by LSCS to G2P1L1 mother by normal vaginal delivery at 38 weeks of gestation. Birth history was unremarkable. Birthweight 3.5 kg. Apgar scores were 8 and 9 at 1 and 5 minutes. His physical examination was normal. Baby was breast feed immediately after birth and

Contd.

Contd.

was kept with mother. At 7 hours of age baby developed tachypnea and cyanosis and was shifted to NICU for further evaluation.

On examination: Baby was alert, normothermic, HR 153/min; RR: 72/min mild intercostal in drawing and nasal flaring present, Central cyanosis present with SpO_2: 83% without oxygen; CRT = 4 sec, peripheral pulses well felt in all four limbs; BP: 65/37 mm Hg. On auscultation, lungs were clear bilaterally and no heart murmur was auscultated.

He was started on oxygen by hood with FiO_2 of 60% but there was no rise in oxygen saturation.

Chest radiograph was done and was normal. ABG was done which showed pH: 7.32, PCO_2: 36, PO_2: 38, HCO_3: 21, oxygen saturation: 70%. Echocardiography done showed D-transposition of great vessels with 5 mm VSD and 3 mm PDA. Prostaglandin E1 infusion was started. Baby was put on mechanical ventilator and shifted to Pediatric cardiac surgical center. An arterial switch procedure was successfully and baby was discharged home 3 weeks later.

CRITICAL CASE ANALYSIS

The full-term baby with uneventful birth history was normal at birth. This makes the respiratory cause of the cyanosis less likely. Similarly, onset of cyanosis and tachypnea is simultaneous in this case. In respiratory cyanosis, generally respiratory distress starts earlier followed by the cyanosis. Although, the respiratory rate is markedly increased, signs of respiratory distress are not that prominent. It is further supported by the auscultatory findings that air entry was bilaterally equal and chest was clear. The time of presentation with cyanosis in a full-term baby, i.e., 7 hours with uneventful birth history points towards cardiac causes of cyanosis as by this time duct may start closing

The cardiac cause is further supported by the hyperoxia test, that in spite of 100% oxygen, oxygen saturation didn't improve which would not happen in respiratory ailments. Chest X-ray ruled out the pulmonary pathology. Also in such cases if oxygen saturation improves by starting of the prostaglandin E1 infusion, it confirms cyanotic heart disease which is ductus dependent. The most common cyanotic heart disease presenting within first 24 hours after birth in newborns is transpositions of great arteries (TGA).

INTERACTIVE TOPIC DISCUSSION

What is cyanosis?

Cyanosis is the bluish discoloration of the skin, mucous membrane or nail bed. Let's first understand the basic physiology behind cyanosis. As we know, oxygen in blood is carried mostly by hemoglobin. Each gram of hemoglobin carries 1.34 ml of oxygen. Only a small amount of oxygen is carried dissolved in plasma, i.e., 0.003 mL of oxygen per 100 ml of plasma. Deoxygenated hemoglobin is dark blue or purple in color which is responsible for producing visible cyanosis.

Cyanosis depends on the absolute concentration of reduced hemoglobin rather than oxygen saturation or ratio of reduced hemoglobin to oxyhemoglobin. Cyanosis becomes apparent when deoxygenated hemoglobin reaches 5 gm per 100 ml. So, severely anemic may escape recognition if the level of deoxyhemoglobin is below the level of detection. Also in newborn because of relative concentration and characteristics of fetal hemoglobin cyanosis will not be observed until PaO_2 falls below 40 mm Hg in contrast to adults where the value is 50 mm Hg.

What are the types of cyanosis?

Cyanosis depending on the site where it is present is classified into central and peripheral cyanosis. Central cyanosis involves the mucous membrane whereas peripheral cyanosis, also called as acrocyanosis, is present only on extremities.

In acrocyanosis PaO_2 is normal, but there is increased oxygen extraction due to sluggish circulation of blood through capillaries. So, there is a large amount of deoxygenated hemoglobin present on the venous side. It is mostly normal finding in the newborn especially when there is vasoconstriction in extremities because of transient hypothermia. Similarly, polycythemic newborn may exhibit cyanosis because peripheral sludging of desaturated red cells. However, sometimes serious causes like sepsis can also lead to peripheral cyanosis due to vasomotor instability or low cardiac output.

What are the different conditions in the newborns leading to cyanosis?

The different conditions causing cyanosis can be classified into three major categories as follows:

A. Airway: Upper and lower airway diseases

B. Breathing: Lung diseases, central depression

C. Cardiac and circulatory problems.

Differentiation into these is the most important step in the diagnosis and treatment of cyanotic newborn. Table 6.1 gives the different conditions causing cyanosis under different categories.

Table 6.1: Different conditions causing cyanosis

A. Airway Diseases	
Upper Airway	Choanal Atresia, Laryngomalacia, Vocal Cord Paralysis.
Lower Airway	Tracheal stenosis, Vascular ring, Subglottic hemangioma, Foreign body.
B. Breathing: Lung Diseases	
Parenchymal	Respiratory distress syndrome, transient tachypnea of newborn, Meconium aspiration syndrome, pneumonia, pulmonary hypoplasia, pulmonary hemorrhage, CCAM, atelectasis.
Extra parenchymal	Congenital diaphragmatic hernia, pneumothorax, pleural effusion, hemothorax.
Hypoventilation (central depression)	Asphyxia, maternal sedation, intraventricular hemorrhage, seizure, meningitis, encephalitis. Phrenic nerve injury, neonatal myasthenia gravis.
C. Cardiac and Circulatory	
Cardiac	5Ts: Tetralogy of Fallot, Tricuspid atresia, Transposition of great arteries, Total anomalous pulmonary venous return, Truncus arteriosus, pulmonary atresia, Ebstein's anomaly, hypoplastic left heart.
Circulation	Persistent pulmonary hypertension of newborn, Sepsis, hypothermia, hypoglycemia, polycythemia, methemoglobinemia.

What is the importance of maternal and birth history?

A thorough maternal and birth history is of utmost important. It gives clues about the etiology of cyanosis in many cases. Tables 6.2 and 6.3 summarize the clues in antenatal and birth history and associated conditions respectively.

Table 6.2: Antenatal history and associated conditions causing cyanosis

Antenatal history	Associated conditions
Gestational diabetes mellitus	TTN, RDS, Hypoglycemia, TGA
Oligohydramnios	Pulmonary hypoplasia
Pregnancy induced hypertension	IUGR, polycythemia, hypoglycemia
Lithium intake	Ebstein's anomaly
Advanced maternal age	Trisomy 21 associated with cyanotic and acyanotic heart diseases

Table 6.3: Birth history and associated conditions causing cyanosis

Birth history	Associated cause of cyanosis
PROM, Fever, GBS	Sepsis
Sedatives/anesthetics	Respiratory depression, apnea
Cesarean section	TTN, PPHN
Preterm infant	RDS
Meconium	MAS (Pneumonia)

What are the key points on physical examination which differentiate cyanosis due to various conditions?

First, determine whether cyanosis is central or peripheral. Peripheral or acrocyanosis is common in newborn and is generally a benign condition. Infant should be checked for hypothermia. Physical examination should be performed under a radiant warmer and when the baby is quiet. Growth characteristics of the baby should be noted whether small or large for gestational age.

If it is central cyanosis, the primary focus should be on determining the degree of the respiratory distress. Its absence will suggest congenital heart disease or methhemoglobinemia. Congenital heart disease will present with tachypnea which is without signs of respiratory distress. Respiratory insufficiency due to pulmonary disease will present with nasal flaring, retractions, grunting. Neurological conditions giving rise to cyanosis will present with hypoventilation or irregular and shallow breathing.

What are the further findings on systemic examination which will narrow down the diagnosis?

Respiratory System

Look for signs of respiratory distress as mentioned above. Upper airway obstruction presents with stridor, supraclavicular and suprasternal retractions, whereas lower airway diseases will present intercostal, subcostal retractions and grunting. On auscultation, absent or poor air entry on either of the side may be due to pneumothorax, pleural effusion or atelectasis. In CDH, in addition to decrease air entry, peristaltic sounds may be heard on auscultation. Crepitation will be heard in pulmonary hemorrhage and pneumonia.

CVS Examination

Assess heart rate, any evidence of murmur. Serious lesions like TGA are not associated with murmur while relatively benign conditions like VSD are associated with loud murmur. Heart sounds should be assessed. Loud and single second heart sound is seen in pulmonary hypertension, TGA and pulmonary atresia.

Abdominal Examination

Scaphoid abdomen will be seen in congenital diaphragmatic hernia whereas distended abdomen can be seen in necrotizing enterocolitis or intestinal obstruction leading to respiratory distress, sepsis which may present with cyanosis. Similarly, absence of bowel sounds indicates paralytic ileus associated with sepsis, peritonitis and gangrenous bowel.

CNS Examination

Hypoventilation leading to cyanosis can occur in CNS conditions like birth asphyxia, intraventricular hemorrhage, maternal sedation, meningitis etc. Phrenic nerve palsy can be associated with Erb's palsy following traumatic vaginal delivery.

How does the timing of presentation matter?

Ductus arteriosus closes 24–48 hours after birth. This is the time during which ductus dependent cyanotic heart diseases manifest in newborns. Therefore, TGA (D-transposition) and truncus arteriosus which are ductus dependent present immediately or within 24 hours after birth. Truncus arteriosus, TAPVC and tetralogy of Fallot which are not ductus dependent present afterwards in the neonatal period.

Respiratory causes like RDS, TTN, congenital pneumonia, MAS, CDH present immediately or within 24 hours after birth whereas sepsis, acquired pneumonia, pneumothorax, pulmonary hemorrhage present later in neonatal period. Similarly, CNS causes like IVH, Meningitis and encephalitis present later in neonatal period.

What are the investigations to differentiate various causes of cyanosis?

Table 6.4 summarizes various investigations giving clue to for the differential diagnosis for cyanosis in newborn. The investigations should be corroborated with the findings in physical examination to reach best possible diagnosis.

Table 6.4: Various investigations suggesting differential diagnosis of cyanosis in newborn

Investigation	Diagnosis
CBC: Increased or decreased, increased CRP	Sepsis
Hematocrit >65%	Polycythemia
Serum glucose	Hypoglycemia
ABG: PaO_2	To confirm central cyanosis
Increased $PaCO_2$	Pulmonary or CNS disorder, heart failure
Decreased pH	Sepsis, circulatory shock, severe hypoxemia
Decreased SaO_2, Normal PaO_2	Methemoglobinemia
Chest X-ray	
Pulmonary pathology	Pnemothorax, pulmonary hypoplasia, diaphragmatic hernia, pulmonary edema, pleural effusion, cystic adenomatoid malformation

Contd...

Contd...

Cardiac Pathology	
Cardiomegaly and vascular congestion	Heart failure
Heart shape: Boot shaped heart	Tetralogy of Fallot
Box shaped heart (massive cardiomegaly)	Ebstein's anamoly
Egg on end appearance	TGA
Snowman's sign (Figure of eight)	TAPVC

What is hyperoxia test?

Hyperoxia test is a tool to differentiate between cyanosis due to respiratory and cardiac condition. It is based on the principal that in absence of fixed cardiac shunt, 100% oxygen will increase the alveolar PO_2 leading to increase in arterial PO_2. In cyanotic congenital heart disease, little or no rise in PaO_2 is expected after breathing 100% oxygen (for 10 minutes). However, this test will not differentiate between pulmonary hypertension and congenital cyanotic heart disease as the findings will be similar in them.

What is importance of 2D Echo and ECG in diagnosing a cyanotic baby?

Echocardiogram is the definitive test in diagnosis of congenital cardiac lesions and pulmonary hypertension. A technician who is trained in performing echocardiogram in newborns and a pediatric cardiologist are required to perform 2D Echo.

ECG has limited value as a diagnostic test. Right ventricular dominance is normal in newborn, which is also a finding in cases of cyanotic congenital heart disease. Left axis deviation with left ventricular dominance is seen in tricuspid atresia or pulmonary atresia with intact ventricular septum. ECG plays a very important role in the diagnosis of arrhythmia.

What is the initial part of management of a cyanotic newborn?

Cyanosis in newborn requires urgent attention and supportive treatment while the diagnosis is underway. Infant should be treated in thermoneutral environment using radiant warmer. If baby is on enteral feeds it should be withheld. Baby should be started on intravenous fluids. Hypoglycemia is common in newborns and in critically ill neonates; therefore, blood sugar should be monitored and treated with intravenous glucose to keep blood sugar above 55 mg/dL. Umbilical venous and arterial line can be placed for monitoring and sampling purposes in babies less than 10 days old.

Monitor airway, breathing and circulation. If there is respiratory distress or apnea or hypoventilation, an airway should be established and assisted ventilation should be started. Oxygen should be used as needed but unnecessary use of oxygen should be avoided especially in preterm infants. Hyperoxia has also shown to increase the oxidative stress and damage lung parenchyma and vascular functions even in term infants. Initiating oxygen therapy with 40–60% oxygen is a good option and then going up or down as per the requirement. If the infant has minimal response to oxygen in terms of saturation, it may be due to cardiac disease. In such cases giving oxygen will in fact worsen the condition as it may promote the duct closure.

Other metabolic activity should also be looked for. Hypocalcemia is often present in critically ill infant and should be corrected based on the ionized serum calcium levels. Blood gases should be monitored and correlated with clinical condition the baby and other findings on blood investigation and X-ray.

When should prostaglandin E1 be started?

As discussed earlier, any cyanotic baby with clear lung field, whose saturation are not improving with oxygen or failed hyperoxia test or who is deteriorating with oxygen and not having any finding or investigation pointing to a specific condition should be suspected to have duct dependent cyanotic heart disease. Such lesions should ideally be confirmed with 2 D Echo, but pending 2D Echo (if facility is not available immediately or baby needs to be transferred to other center) they should be started on Prostglandin E1 infusion to keep the duct patent. PGE1 reopens the closing ductus and prevent it from closing by increasing concentration of intracellular cAMP. Timely use of prostaglandin E can significantly decrease the morbidity and mortality in newborns with cyanotic heart disease.

How should prostaglandin E1 be administered?

Prostaglandin E1 is started as an infusion at 0.05 mcg/kg/min (maximum 0.4 mcg/kg/min) which can be reduced to 0.01–0.02 mcg/kg/min when patient is stable. There is evidence that doses greater than 0.1 mcg/kg/min are not more effective, and may cause an increase in adverse reactions.

What are the precautions to be taken and adverse event associated with prostaglandin E infusion?

Adverse event with Prostaglandin E are generally uncommon. However, about 20% of infants who receive it may have one or more adverse reactions.

Three common side effects are apnea, fever, and flushing. Apnea is an indication for assisted or mechanical ventilation. A decrease in systolic arterial pressure of greater than 20% should be treated by volume expansion with 10 ml/kg of colloid. Hypoglycemia may develop after several hours of treatment.

Infant should be monitored for respiratory rate, temperature, blood pressure and arterial blood gases and pH at the initiation of and intermittently during infusion.

What are condition specific treatment approaches for cyanosis in newborn?

After the cause of cyanosis has been established, treatment should be directed in the specific direction according to the pathology. Covering the detail treatment for each pathology will be out of scope of this chapter. However, Table 6.5 summarizes in brief the specific management according to the underlying condition causing cyanosis.

Table 6.5: Condition-specific management for cyanotic neonate

Condition	Management
Airway diseases	
Upper airway obstruction	Oral airway, Intubation, Tracheostomy
Lower airway obstruction	Bronchoscopy, Surgery
Lung Diseases	
Parenchymal	Ventilation, CPAP (treatment of underlying causes with antibiotics, surfactant, physiotherapy as necessary)
Extra parenchymal	Surgical correction for CDH, drainage of fluid air in case of pneumothorax, pleural effusion, hemothorax
Hypoventilation	Ventilation, antibiotics as necessary

Contd...

Contd...

Circulatory and Cardiac	
Cardiac	Surgical correction of defect, anti-failure drugs
Circulatory	Sildenafil, ventilation, Nitric oxide (PPHN) Partial exchange transfusion (Polycythemia) Antibiotics (Sepsis) Methemoglobinemia (Methylene blue, hyperbaric oxygen)

CONCLUSIONS

Cyanosis in newborn requires urgent assessment, diagnosis and initiation of therapy. Diagnosing the cause of cyanosis can be quite challenging at times. A systematic and rational approach is necessary in such a situation. The combination of detail antenatal and birth history and proper physical examination helps in planning out the diagnosis oriented investigation. Nevertheless, it is also important to provide prompt supportive care to the baby while the diagnosis is underway. Prompt recognition, timely intervention and appropriate referral can save the life of the neonate.

TAKE HOME MESSAGES

- Central cyanosis in newborn requires urgent attention and evaluation.
- Treatment should be started promptly while the diagnosis is underway.
- A through history and complete physical examination is essential.
- Knowledge of the way of presentation of various conditions with cyanosis in newborn and a systematic approach for differentiating various causes helps in planning out the proper investigations.
- Differentiating between respiratory and cardiac causes of cyanosis is possible based on signs and symptoms, which can be later confirmed by investigations.
- For newborns with cyanotic heart disease presenting soon after birth, a timely treatment with Prostaglandin E1 to keep the duct open can be life-saving.

FURTHER READING

1. Eichenwald EC, Weisman LE, Kim MS. *Overview of cyanosis in newborn.* UpToDate 2014. Available at: www.uptodate.com. Accessed on: 2 March 2016.
2. Steinhorn RH. Evaluation and management of the cyanotic neonate. *Clin Pediatr Emerg Med* 2008;9:169–175.
3. Rudolph C, Rudolph A, Lister G, Lewis, Gershon A. *Rudolph's Pediatrics*, 22nd edn. London: McGraw Hill 2011.
4. Sasidharan P. An approach to diagnosis and management of cyanosis in term infant. *Pediatr Clin North Am* 2004;51:999–1021.
5. Vitharani K. Jeyll AM. *An approach to neonatal cyanosis. Available at:* learnpediatrics.com/files/2010/07/Neonatal-Central-Cyanosis. Accessed on: 10 March 2016.

Chapter

7 Respiratory Distress Syndrome

Suraj Gupte, Rita Fernandes

ABSTRACT

Respiratory distress syndrome, earlier termed "hyaline membrane disease", is an important cause of respiratory distress in preterm neonates. Less the gestational age and birthweight, higher is the incidence of RDS. Typically, the neonate presents with respiratory distress within first 6 hours of life. Surfactant deficiency is the root cause. Hence, its replacement reduces needs for initial inspired oxygen and ventilation. Even risk of complications, mortality and mortality is also cut down. Prevention of prematurity is the best safeguard against RDS.

Key Words: Antenatal steroids, Assisted ventilation, Hyaline membrane disease, Low birthweight, Prematurity, Rescue therapy, Respiratory distress syndrome, Surfactant.

INTRODUCTION

Respiratory distress syndrome (RDS), is characterized by increasing respiratory distress within 6 hours of birth. Earlier known as "hyaline membrane disease", it is one of most common and important causes of respiratory distress in preterm infants. Infrequently, it may occur in term infants suffering from the genetic abnormalities of surfactant system.

CASE SCENARIO

This baby was born to a young mother, gravid 2, para 2 (G2P2) by cesarean section at 31 week of gestation. The mother suffered from poorly controlled hypertension. His weight was 1.5 kg. After 2 hours of birth, he developed respiratory distress in the form of tachypnea, nasal flaring, chest, expiratory grunting and cyanosis which worsened despite oxygen therapy. Downe's score was 5. He was, therefore, put on CPAP which also proved ineffective. At this stage, CXR showed classical "whiteout" appearance which supported the clinical diagnosis of RDS. Moreover, the infant had apnea thrice.

Eventually, he was put on assisted ventilation along with administration of intratracheal surfactant on three occasions. He was also given indomethacin for PDA.

Repeat CXR after surfactant therapy showed improved aeration of the lungs bilaterally.

He was discharged after 4 weeks.

CRITICAL CASE APPRAISAL

The risk factors for RDS in this neonate were prematurity (30 weeks), LBW (1.2 kg), lack of administration of antenatal steroids, hypertension in mother and Cesarean section. Onset of increasing respiratory distress with CPAP failing to maintain saturation and classical whiteout radiological picture virtually confirmed the diagnosis of severe RDS.

Specific surfactant therapy on three occasions along with assisted ventilation, indomethacin for PDA and supportive measures proved successful in saving this infant.

INTERACTIVE TOPIC REVIEW

What is RDS?

RDS, a disorder of lung surfactant deficiency, is characterized by increasing respiratory distress (tachypnea, chest retractions and grunting) within 6 hours of life.

What is its incidence?

Incidence of RDS is inversely proportional to gestational age at birth and birthweight. At < 30 weeks gestation, 60% of neonates are likely to develop RDS. Exact incidence, mortality and outcome may be difficult to determine in neonates < 28 weeks since, on account of known structural lung immaturity, they are given prophylactic surfactant at birth. It is difficult to predict how many of them may develop RDS if this therapy is withheld.

What is the modus operandi of development of RDS?

The coating of lung alveoli with surfactant, comprising phospholipids and proteins, prevents alveolar collapse at the end of expiration. In term neonates, surfactant pool size at birth is around 100 mg/kg of phospholipids. This size is reduced to < 25 mg/kg in preterm neonates in whom a tendency for reduced compliance and alveolar collapse at end-expiration occurs. The net outcome is

- Persistent hypoxemia
- Metabolic acidosis
- Myocardial depression
- Hypotension.

What is the major risk factor for RDS?

The front-ranker in risk factors is prematurity and low birthweight.

What are the other antenatal and perinatal factors that too influence the development of RDS?

These include maternal diabetes, perinatal asphyxia, chrioamininitis, nonimmune hydrops, cesarean section, etc.

What are the clinical features?

RDS usually presents within first 6 hours of birth, often right after delivery, with respiratory distress in the form of tachypnea, nasal flaring, chest retractions (sternal, subcostal and intercostals), expiratory grunting and cyanosis. Without oxygen supplementation, the infant fails to maintain saturation.

Any other clinical features?

Pallor resulting from anemia or peripheral vasoconstriction, cardiovascular instability warranting close monitoring of blood pressure, and cyanosis, sometime masked by pallor, from right-to-left shunt.

RDS, may be severe, needing assisted ventilation.

Any complications?

Air leak syndriomes, significant shunting through a PDA, or early signs of BPD.

These complications delay recovery.

How to assess severity of RDS?

A neonate with RDS showing hike in FiO_2 requirement to maintain a saturation of 90–92% in preterm and 94–96% in a term baby RDS is likely to be heading towards severity.

What is the role of scoring system in assessing the severity of RDS?

Though Silverman score is most suited for preterms with RDS, Downes' score is more comprehensive and can be applied to any gestational age and condition.

Scoring is done at every 30–60 minutes interval. Simultaneously, a chart is maintained to determine progression of distress.

A score of >6 is indicative of impending respiratory failure.

What exactly is Silverman scoring system?

Silverman's scoring system is presented in Table 7.1.

Table 7.1: Silverman scoring system for respiratory distress in preterm neonates

Feature		
Score 0	**Score 1**	**Score 2**
Chest movement	Equal respiratory	Lag see-saw respiration
Intercostal retractions	None	Minimal marked
Xiphoid retractions	None	Minimal marked
Nasal flaring	None	Minimal marked
Expiratory grunt	None	Audible with stethoscope Audible without stethoscope

What is Downe's scoring system?

Whereas Silverman's score is applicable to only premature infants, Downe's score can be used even in full-term neonates. Table 7.2 presents the Downe's scoring system.

Table 7.2: Downe's scoring system

RDS Score	0	1	2
Cyanosis	None	Cyanotic in air	Cyanotic in 40% O_2
Retractions	None	Mild	Severe
Grunting	None	Audible with stethoscope	Audible without stethoscope
Air entry-make baby cry and listen to breath sounds while baby cries	Clear	Delayed or decreased	Barely audible
Respiratory rate	60	60–80	80 or apneic episodes

An score of 6 or more is an indication for ventilatory assistance.

What is significance of expiratory grunt?

Expiratory grunt is an early feature of the RDS. It results from partial closure of the glottis during expiration, thereby trapping alveolar air and maintaining functional residual capacity (FRC).

What is significance of apneic spells?

Apneic episodes at this early stage may be due to

- Thermal instability
- Sepsis
- Hypoxemia/respiratory decompensation
- Respiratory failure.

PDA is common association in RDA neonates. Is this murmur audible in the sick baby?

No. PDA murmur is usually heard during the recovery phase of RDS. It at this stage that pulmonary vascular resistance falls below systemic levels, resulting in left-to-right shunt.

What is differential diagnosis of RDS?

Pulmonary conditions include congenital pneumonia, TTN, MAS, PPHN, malformations of lung.

Extrapulmonary conditions include severe anemia, polycythemia, CHD, CNS disorders.

What is role of shake test in diagnosis?

It is a rapid bedside method for identifying surfactant deficiency. It consists in adding 0.5 ml of absolute alcohol in 0.5 mL of gastric aspirate (obtained within 1 hour of birth) in a 4 mL glass test tube which is then vigorously shaken for 15 seconds. After 15 minutes, the mixture is observed for formation of stable foam – an indicator of surfactant presence.

Interpretation is as follows:

- No stable foam: Negative
- Very small bubbles in meniscus extending 1/3rd or less of distance around test tube: 2+
- Single rim of bubbles extending 1/3rd to all around the test tube: 2+
- A rim of bubbles all the way around the test tube and a double row in some areas: 3+
- A double row or more of bubbles: 4+

How to interpret shake test?

Shake test negative or 1+ .... 60% chances of RDS.

Shake test 2, 3 or 4+ .... 5% chance of RDS.

What are radiologiocal changes in Chest X-ray in RDS?

1. Bilateral reticulogranular pattern as a result of scattered atelectasis.
2. Ground glass appearance from confluent reticulogranular shadows.
3. Air bronchogram as a result of translucent air-filled bronchi against airless, solid, atelectatic lung.
4. Complete white out lungs as a result of loss of delineation of heart margins from global atelectasis.
5. Normal or slightly increased heart size.
6. Larger thymic silhouette than in infants of comparable size without RDS.

What are the therapeutic modalities?

1. Appropriate resuscitation
2. Supportive measures
3. Surfactant therapy
4. Ventilation.

The patient should be treated in a humidified incubator. Oxygen flow should be so regulated as to maintain the arterial oxygen concentration between 70 and 90 mmHg. The oxygen should be cut down as soon as possible to minimize the danger of retrolental fibroplasia and/or bronchopulmonary dysplasia. Humidity should be 60–80% in the incubator. The rectal temperature needs to be kept around 36.5 °C.

If the baby continues to be "bad", continuous positive airway pressure (CPAP) by a respirator, a mask or intranasal tube should be given. CPAP avoids need for assisted ventilation in quite a proportion of infants with RDS.

If, despite 100% oxygen or CPAP, the infant shows poor response, assisted ventilation may be resorted to by an expert.

The use of intravenous fluids, especially 1–2% sodium bicarbonate in 5 or 10% dextrose in water, to counter acidosis, is of value. Its dose is 3–5 mEq/kg in 24 hours. It is better if the dose of sodium bicarbonate can be monitored by the pH of the arterial blood. For instance, the dose for a pH of less than 7.00 is 7 mEq/ kg whereas for a pH of 7.25–7.30 it is only 1 mEq/kg.

Broad spectrum antibiotic cover (say ampicillin/cefotaxime plus gentamicin) should be given for underlying/superadded infection.

Indomethacin, 0.2 mg/kg (0, IV) may be given 12 hourly for a total of 3 doses for the associated PDA which can worsen existing hypoxemia.

How about surfactant therapy?

Endotracheal instillation of exogenous surfactant, preferably natural surfactants (from calf) is indicated in VLBW infants needing 30% oxygen and mechanical ventilation (rescue therapy).

The so-called InSurE approach involves intubation, surfactant, and rapid extubation to CPAP.

Table 7.3 gives the commonly used surfactant preparations and their dosage.

Table 7.3: Commonly used surfactant preparations and their dosage

Brand name	Source	Availability (volume)	Concentration (per ml)	Dose	Interval between doses	Max doses
Survanta (Abbot)	Bovine minced	8 ml and 4 ml	1 ml = 25 mg	100 mg/kg = 4 ml/kg	6 hr	2
Curosurf (Nicholas)	Porcine minced	1.5 ml	1 ml = 80 mg	First: 200 mg/kg = 2.5 ml/kg Repeat: 100 mg/kg = 1.25 ml/kg	12 hr	2
Neosurf (Cipla)	Bovine lavage	5 ml and 3 ml	1 ml = 27 mg	135 mg/kg = 5 ml/kg	12 hr	2

It is often said that RDS is best prevented than treated. But how to prevent it?

1. Avoidance of premature deliveries and, thereby prevention of pulmonary immaturity.
2. Antenatal steroid (betamethasone, dexamethasone or glucocorticoid) therapy to all mothers in preterm (<35 weeks) labor.

Any other uses of antenatal steroids?

Over and above RDS, it reduces incidence of intraventricular hemorrhage, necrotizing enterocolitis, patent ductus arteriosus and hemodynamic instability and overall neonatal mortality.

Any preventive role of surfactant?

Surfactant (endotracheal) first dose to symptomatic premature infants soon after birth or during the first few hours of life (early rescue) may be useful in preventing RDS in preterm infants.

What are the Complications of RDS?

These may well be secondary to prematurity or in relation to management.

Pulmonary: Pulmonary interstitial emphysema, pneumothoprax, pulmonary hemorrhage, broncho-pulomonary dysplasia, air-leak syndromes, superadded sepsis/pneumonia, subglottic stenosis.

Extrapulmonary: PDA, intraventricular hemorrhage, ROP.

What can be the sequelae in survivors of RDS?

Survivors suffer from neurologic, pulmonary or ophthalmic sequelae.

What is role of surfactant replacement therapy?

Surfactant replacement reduces

- Initial inspired oxygen and ventilation requirements
- Incidence
- Complications and
- Mortality of respiratory distress syndrome.

What are the liklely complications during management of RDS?

Pulmonary

- Pulmonary hemorrhgage
- Pulmonary emphysema
- Pulmonary pneumothorax
- Nosocomial pneumonia
- Bronchopulomonary dysplasia
- Airleak syndromes
- Suglottic stenosis

Extrapulmonary

- IVH
- PDA
- ROP

Any role of antibiotics?

Yes, initially it is advisable to coadminister antibiotics based on hospital protocol (usually a penicillin plus an aminoglycoside) in view of risk for sepsis and difficulty in differentiating RDS CXR from that of neonatal pneumonia.

Is erythropoetin useful?

At present, it remains debatable if erythropoietin can be useful for preventing anemia in neonates with extremely low birthweight during the acute phase of RDS.

Any role of inhaled nitric oxide?

Inhaled nitric oxide is now accepted treatment for hypoxic respiratory failure in near-term and full-term infants.

It is being proposed as a potential intervention in premature infants at risk for developing BPD and RDS.

What is the prognosis?

Without treatment, RDS carries a bad prognosis.

With appropriate and timely treatment, most infants (80–90%) can be saved. If the baby tides over first 2–5 days, natural remission (heralded by spontaneous diuresis) may occur.

In mild disease (uncomplicated RDS), beginning of recovery is expected after 48 hours and discontinuation of oxygen possible by 7th day. Administration of surfactant in such a baby curtails the course of the condition.

In severe cases, prognosis is bad. However, timely administration of surfactant along with supportive measures saves a large majority of the cases.

What factors influence the prognosis in RDS?

- Extent of prematurity and low birthweight
- ACS therapy
- Timing of surfactant therapy
- Ventilation
- Comorbidities
- Complications

CONCLUSIONS

Respiratory distress syndrome, earlier termed "hyaline membrane disease", is a leading cause of respiratory distress in preterm neonates. As a rule, the neonate presents with respiratory distress within first 6 hours of life, often soon after birth. Replacement therapy with surfactant reduces needs for initial inspired oxygen and ventilation. Even risk of complications, mortality and mortality is reduced. The best safeguard against RDS lies in prevention of prematurity.

TAKE HOME MESSAGES

- RDS is one of the most common and important causes of respiratory distress in preterm infants.
- Incidence of RDS is inversely related to gestational age and birthweight.
- Most infants characteristically present within first 6 hours of birth with respiratory distress.
- Surfactant replacement reduces initial inspired oxygen and ventilation requirements as well as the incidence, complications and mortality of respiratory distress syndrome.
- Despite substantial improvements in the treatment of RDS, prevention remains the best treatment.

FURTHER READING

1. Vishnu Bhat V, Renitha R. Surfactant. In: Gupte S, Gupte SB (eds). *Recent Advances in Pediatrics (Special Vol 21: Neonatal and Pediatric Intensive Care)*. New Delhi: Jaypee 2011:145–158.
2. Dudell GG, Stoll BJ. Respiratory tract disorders. In: Kliegman RM, Behrman RE, Jenson HB, Stanton BF (eds): *Nelson Textbook of Pediatrics*, 18th edn. Philadelphia: Saunders, 2008:731–741.
3. National Neonatology Forum. *Report of National Neonatal Perinatal Database*, New Delhi: National Neonatology Forum, India 2002–2003.
4. Kulkarni A, Sharma H. Respiratory distress syndrome. In: Gupte S, Gupte SB (eds). *Recent Advances in Pediatrics* (*Special Vol 21: Neonatal and Pediatric Intensive Care*). New Delhi: Jaypee 2011:115–144.

Chapter 8

Persistent Pulmonary Hypertension of the Newborn (PPHN)

Nitasha Bagga, Dinesh Chirla

ABSTRACT

Persistent pulmonary hypertension of newborn (PPHN) is a syndrome of failed circulatory adaptation at birth. It is seen in about 2/1000 live born babies. It usually complicates term and near term infants but it can be occasionally seen in preterm infants as well. Most commonly PPHN is secondary to delayed or impaired relaxation of the pulmonary vasculature associated with diverse neonatal pulmonary pathologies, such as meconium aspiration syndrome, congenital diaphragmatic hernia and respiratory distress syndrome. Gentle ventilation strategies, lung recruitment, inhaled nitric oxide and surfactant therapy have improved outcome and reduced the need for ECMO in PPHN. Various modalities of treatment like systemic or inhaled vasodilators like sildenafil, prostaglandin E1, prostacyclin and endothelin antagonists are briefly overviewed in this article.

Key Words: Extracorporeal membrane oxygenator, High frequency ventilation, Nitric oxide, Persistent pulmonary hypertension, Surfactant.

INTRODUCTION

Persistent pulmonary hypertension of the newborn (PPHN) is a syndrome characterized by sustained elevation pulmonary vascular resistance (PVR) and is often associated with normal or low systemic vascular resistance (SVR). This leads to extrapulmonary shunting from right to left across persistent fetal channels – patent ductus arteriosus (PDA) and patent foramen ovale (PFO) leading to labile hypoxemia. This article discusses in detail about most common etiological factors for PPHN, clinical diagnosis and evidence base management of such a neonate including inhaled nitric oxide, high frequency ventilation, surfactant and extracorporeal membrane oxygenator. As this field is rapidly evolving, this article also reviews the promising new treatment approaches.

CASE SCENARIO

A term newborn with birthweight of 2.9 kg delivered by normal vaginal with meconium stained liquor, developed respiratory distress at 1st hour of life and was started on hood box oxygen. Initial CXR was normal. As the oxygen requirement was persistent, was shifted to NICU for the needful. Because of increase in oxygen requirement and work of breathing baby was started on CPAP of 5 and FiO_2 25%. Initial ABG showed pH 7.19, PCo_2 60, PO_2 36, BE 7.1. Subsequently in next 6 hours, PEEP was increased up to 7 and FiO2 to 60%. In view of persistent respiratory distress, hypoxemia and respiratory acidosis, baby was intubated and was started on mechanical ventilation with CMV mode, PIP 20, FiO_2 60%, rates 50, PEEP 7. Baby was well-sedated. As there was no improvement in ABG and clinical condition, inspite of optimising ventilator settings of maximum PIP 27, rates 60, FiO_2 100%, one dose of surfactant was considered. The baby continued to be hypoxic and had had respiratory acidosis.

The baby was started on high frequency ventilation with delta P 30, frequency of 10, FiO_2 100% MAP 13. Repeat CXR showed good recruitment and ABG also showed improvement in respiratory acidosis. But hypoxemia was still persistent with OI of 30. 2D Echo done at this stage showed high right ventricular pressures with TR jet. After confirming the diagnosis of PPHN, Baby was started on IV sildenafil and IV $MgSO_4$. As there was no response inhaled nitric oxide was considered and was started with dose of 20 ppm. Slowly there was a good improvement in PaO_2 and OI came down to 15. Subsequently iNO was weaned off and stopped in next 48 hours. Baby was extubated to hood box oxygen and subsequently to room air. Baby was discharged home on day 10 of life on direct feeds and first follow-up visit was uneventful.

CRITICAL CASE ANALYSIS

PPHN secondary to MAS is considered to be the most common. In the present case when baby presented with respiratory distress and persistent respiratory acidosis, common parenchymal lung causes were considered and all recruitment manoeuvres were tried. As the respiratory distress and hypoxemia were disproportionate to the lung pathology, that was the time when possibility of secondary PPHN was considered and diagnosis was confirmed with 2D Echo.

On conventional ventilation baby had persistent respiratory acidosis. Hence, HFOV was started. The baby responded well to it. Magnesium sulfate reduces pulmonary pressure but can also cause hypotension. Because of the cost and easily availability many of the babies are started on Sildenafil which is selective pulmonary vasodilator. Inhaled nitric oxide is the treatment of choice in PPHN with OI > 20. Baby responded well to various ventilator strategies and vasodilator therapy specifically iNO, $MgSO_4$ and Sildenafil. Although the role of surfactant in PPHN is not proven. However, it was given to the baby considering secondary surfactant deficiency due to MAS.

INTERACTIVE TOPIC DISCUSSION

How should PPHN be defined?

Persistent pulmonary hypertension of the newborn is a syndrome characterized by sustained elevation of pulmonary vascular resistance and is often associated with normal or low systemic vascular resistance.

This leads to extrapulmonary shunting from right to left across the persistent fetal channels – patent ductus arteriosis (PDA) and foramen ovale.

What are the various etiological factors leading to PPHN?

Failure of pulmonary circulation to undergo the normal transition after birth leads to PPHN. Various factors which are associated with PPHN are described in Figure 8.1.

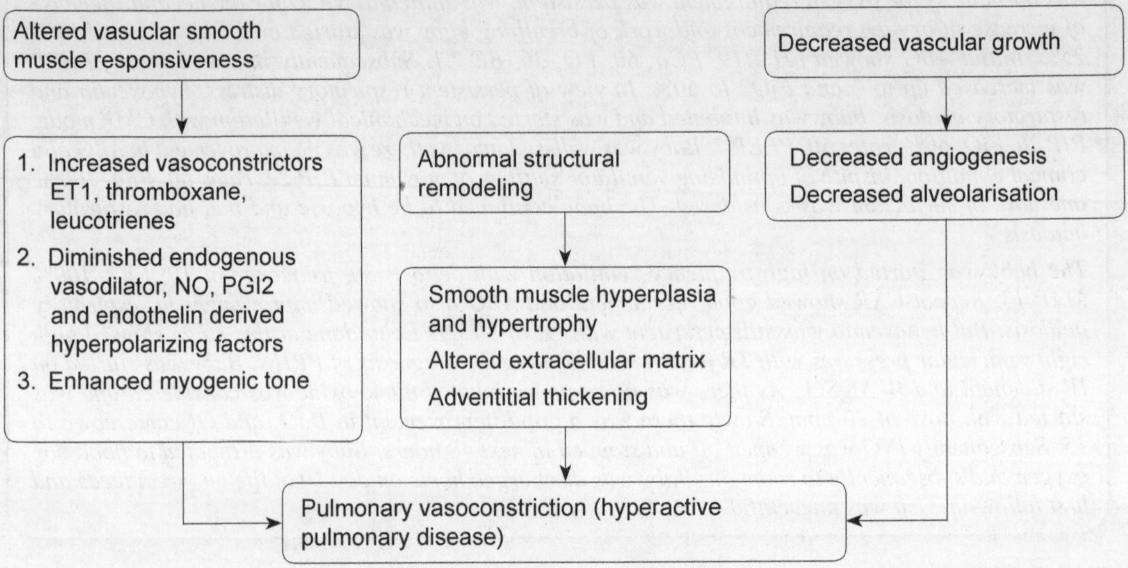

Fig. 8.1: Various factors which are associated with PPHN

Can we classify PPHN depending on the causes?

Yes. The classification is given in Figure 8.2.

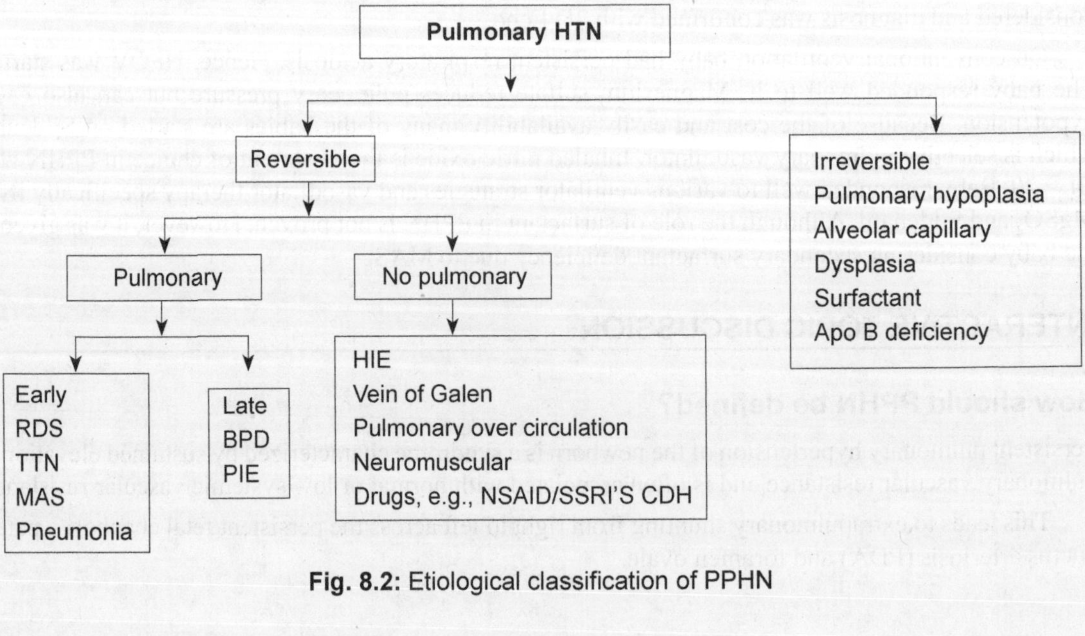

Fig. 8.2: Etiological classification of PPHN

What are the risk factors during perinatal or neonatal period which can actually lead to PPHN?

Risk factors for development of PPHN are listed in Table 8.1.

Table 8.1: Potential risk factors for development of PPHN

1.	Male gender
2.	African or Asian maternal race
3.	Pre-conception maternal overweight
4.	Maternal diabetes
5.	Maternal asthma
6.	Cesarean section
7.	Late preterm and SGA
8.	Chorioamnionitis
9.	Antenatal exposure to SSRI's and NSAID
10.	Hypothermia
11.	Hypocalcemia
12.	Hypomagnesemia
13.	Polycythemia

What are the clinical signs when you start expecting PPHN?

1. PPHN is clinically suspected in near term or term neonates who have labile hypoxemia with variable oxygen saturations in spite of proper oxygenation and lung recruitment therapies.
2. Another clinical clue is hypoxemia disproportionate to the amount respiratory distress.
3. Difference in preductal and post-ductal oxygen saturations of > 20% points towards PPHN.

What are the various ways to confirm diagnosis of PPHN?

1. Initial evaluation includes an ABG and CXR. Hypoxemia disproportionate to the severity of parenchymal disease on chest radiography should suggest idiopathic PPHN. Evidence of underlying parenchymal lung disease, such as RDS and MAS, may be seen on CXR in secondary PPHN.
2. ABG can guide us by measuring preductal and post ductal PaO_2. A difference in arterial PO_2 > 20 mm Hg should be considered suggestive of PPHN.
3. Echocardiography with real time doppler remains the gold standard to confirm the diagnosis. Right to left or bidirectional shunting of blood at level of foramen ovale is classically seen, as well as high pulmonary arterial/right ventricular systolic pressure estimated by Doppler velocity of tricuspid regurgitation jet. The direction of the shunt at atrial or ductal level also provides clues to the management.
4. A blood workup is helpful to identify etiological factors for PPHN. A baseline abnormal WBC, CRP and platelet count indicates towards infection. Blood glucose, calcium and polycythemia are helpful to rule out metabolic causes.

5. Recently, B-type natriuretic peptide (BNP) was proposed as a biomarker in PPHN, especially to asses efficacy of treatment and to predict rebound PPHN. However, its value in practical management of PPHN is presently unclear.

Once the case of PPHN has been diagnosed, what are the management strategies available?

Broad objectives are outlined in Table 8.2.

Table 8.2: Treatment objectives in PPHN

1. Supportive measures
2. Correction of underlying cause
3. Ventilation support: Decreased hypoxemia and hypercapnea
4. Correction of metabolic disorders–Hypocalcemia, Hypoglycemia and Hypomagnesemia
5. Nutritional supports

1. **Supportive measures:** Play important role in successful management PPHN.
   - Maintain normothermia.
   - Maintain normoglycemia.
   - Correction of acidosis.
   - IV nutrition/or if hemodynamically stable entral feeds.
   - Maintaining low noise in NICU.
   - Minimal stimulation along with judicious use of sedation of analgesia with morphine or fentanyl, paralysis is usually avoided.
   - Systemic blood pressures to be maintained at normal values as per gestation.
   - Minimal invasive procedures and minimal handling.
   - Management of electrolyte balance is important especially calcium and magnesium levels.
2. **Treatment of underlying disease:**
   - **Ventilation and oxygenation:** Ventilation is crucial for PPHN treatment since it facilitates alveolar recruitment and lung expansion thus improving V/Q mismatchin.

     Conventional and HFV many be used to reduce V/Q mismatch. In studies comparing effectiveness of HFV with conventional mode of ventilation in infants, neither mode of ventilation was more effective in preventing ECMO.

     But HFO has been advocated to improve lung inflation while potentially decreasing lung injury through volutrauma.

     Combine HFO and iNO therapy is found to be more effective in rescuing infants with PPHN. "Gentle ventilation" strategies with optimal PEEP relatively low PIP and some permissive hypercapnea is now being recommended to ensure adequate lung expansion without causing barotrauma.

3. **ECMO:**

- **Indicators for treatment:**
  (i) Severe respiratory failure irresponsive to conventional treatment.
  (ii) Birthweight > 2 kg.
  (iii) < 7 days of assisted ventilation
  (iv) Reversible pulmonary disease
  (v) Absence of congenital heart disease
  (vi) Absence of IVH/Severe coagulopathy

  1 year outcome for the babies in severe respiratory failure treated with ECMO are comparable to those infants who survived without ECMO. The increasing application of newer therapies such as iNO and HFO and surfactant, over past 10 years has greatly reduced the need of ECMO in babies with PPHN secondary to parenchymal lung disease. Currently, fewer than 5% of neonates who have PPHN receive ECMO.

- **Surfactant:** Exogenous surfactant therapy improved oxygenation and reduced the need for ECMO when PPHN was secondary to parenchymal lung disease such as RDS, Pneumonia, Sepsis or MAS.

  A multicenter trial demonstrated that the benefit was greatest for infants with relatively mild disease and with OI of 15–25. Over the past decade, the list use of surfactant in treating secondary PPHN and respiratory failure has increased and might have contributed to improved effectiveness of iNO and reduced need for ECMO.

- **Vasodilators:**
  (a) *Inhaled nitric oxide:* In 1999, inhaled nitric oxide (iNO) was approved by the FDA for use near term and term infants with PPHN. It has been the mainstay of PPHN treatment. It achieves potent and selective pulmonary vasodilatation without decreasing systemic vascular tone. In the intravascular space, it combines with hemoglobin to form methemoglobin, which prevents systemic vasodilatation (selective effect). iNO reduces V/Q mismatch by entering only ventilated alveoli and redirecting pulmonary arterioles.

  There has been significant debate concerning the optimal starting doses as well as time of initation of iNO therapy. Most randomized clinical trials support a starting dose of 20 ppm. Doses higher that 20 ppm has been associated with more adverse effect like, methemoglobinemia.

  Based on current available evidence, the indication for treatment for iNO would be OI more than 15–25 with echocardiographic evidence of PPHN.

  iNO need to be weaned off gradually, over a period of time to prevent the rebound effect. Inspired oxygen concentration (FiO_2) is first weaned off below 60% and then iNO is weaned off at the rate of 5 ppm every 4 hours. Once iNO dose is 5 ppm, gradual weaning at the rate of 1 ppm q 4th hour is performed.

  Contraindications for iNO are severe congenital anomalies, incompatible for life and congenital heart disease (shunt dependant lesion), e.g., Hypoplastic left heart syndrome and interrupted aortic arch.

  (b) *Systemic vasodilators:* Phosphodiesterase inhibitors.

  - Sildenafil: Sildenafil is a Phosphodiesterase (PDE 5) inhibitor. It can be given oral as well as intravenous route.

Oral dose =1–3 mg/kg every 6 hours

Intravenous dose = loading dose 0.4 mg over 3 hours followed by maintenance dose 0.07 mg/kg/hr.

Sildenafil is recommended to continue till PaO_2 are stabilized and oxygen requirement is weaned off to room air.

- Milrinone: This inotropic vasodilator, commonly use in pediatrics and adults intensive care units, but now is currently licensed for treating PPHN. It inhibits PDE3 and relaxes pulmonary arteries. Infants with PPHN refractory to iNO therapy have responded to IV milrinone. A loading dose of 50 mcg/kg followed by maintenance dose of 0.33–1 mcg/kg/hr is commonly used. As with any systemic vasodilator, hypotension is a clinical concern and blood pressure needs to be closely monitor. Milrinone is usually is a drug of choice in presence of PPHN with left ventricular dysfunction.

Just outline the summary of the management of PPHN.

At the outset when we are managing a case of PPHN, there should be some targets kept in mind which guide us to appropriate treatment and are hence mentioned below:

1. Very first and foremost is baby should well-sedated and good analgesia should be considered (avoid routine paralysis).
2. Gentle Ventilation: Aim is to avoid further injury to lung. There has been lot of debate about how much oxygen saturation is acceptable. As much it is important to correct hypoxemia it is also essential to avoid oxygen free radical injury. Similarly though low CO_2 causes respiratory alkalosis it is at the cost of over-ventilation and compromise of cerebral circulation. The current consensus of acceptable targets are:
   (a) *Target saturations:* Preductal 90–97%
   (b) *Target PaO_2:* Preductal 55–80 mm Hg
   (c) Target $PaCO_2$ 45–60 mm Hg as long as pH is > 7.25.
3. pH > 7.25; Lactate < 3; Urine output >1 ml/kg/hr.
4. Hemodynamic stability is another very important consideration. Mean BP > 35 mm Hg and vassopressors can be considere as if required.
5. Good nutrition by means of total parentral nutrition, normoglycemia and normocalcemia are another goals in management of PPHN.
6. Early surfactant can be considered if dealing with parenchymal lung disease like MAS. 8–9 rib expansion in CXR should be indicator of good lung recruitment.
7. To start with conventional ventilation, PIP <25–28 cm H_2O, PEEP 4–5 cm H_2O and rates of 40.
8. Consider HFO if PIP > 28 cm H_2O is require to maintain $PaCO_2$ < 60.
9. Inhaled nitric oxide is considered if clinically pre-post ductal saturation difference of >5–10% or echocardiographic evidence of PPHN (typically OI > 15–25).

What are the future promising therapies in management of PPHN?

Bosentan: Bosentan, an oral dual endothelin-1 receptor antagonist, may be an option for the treatment of PPHN. This RCT results showed that bosentan was more effective adjuvant treatment for PPHN in neonates than placebo. All infants who received bosentan showed significant improvement in oxygenation at 6 hours after initiation of treatment. Moreover, the duration of mechanical ventilation was significantly decreased compared with placebo group. Bosentan may be a useful adjuvant therapy in neonates with PPHN in centers lacking iNO and ECMO.

Adenosine: Adenosine infusion given IV at 25–50 mg/kg/min was shown to improve oxygenation in babies with PPHN in a randomized placebo-controlled pilot study. There were no systemic hypotension or arrhythmias observed in this study. However, the improvement in oxygenation was not sustained,

Prostacyclin: As the mechanism of action is by increasing cAMP in vascular smoot muscle cells, it may have a role in the treatment of PPHN refractory to iNO. Combination therapy with iNO has also been reported (15). In neonates, higher doses may be required than those conventionally used in older children (>20 ng/kg/min). Systemic vasodilation and hypotension may be problematic, Superoxide dismutase. SOD reverses the impaired vasodilation in PPHN by reducing the production of reactive oxygen species and peroxynitrite formation. In addition, SOD protects the lung from oxidant damage caused by combination of exogenous NO and high inspired O_2 concentration in animal models (16). New studies indicate that superoxide dismutase (SOD) may augment responsiveness to iNO. SOD scavenges converts superoxide radical to hydrogen peroxide, which subsequently is converted to water by the enzyme catalase. Administration of recombinant human superoxide dismutase (rhSOD) has been tested in preterm infants without adverse effects and with trends toward decreased pulmonary morbidity.

Tetrahydrobiopterin (BH4): Tetrahydrobiopterin (BH4) is a vital cofactor for eNOS (nitric oxide synthase) function but also an important intracellular antioxidant. Depletion of BH4, or oxidation of BH4 into dihydrobiopterin (BH2), can uncouple eNOS function and shift eNOS from NO formation into O_2^- formation. NO not only relax arteries but also mediate blood vessel formation (angiogenesis). Method to increase endothelial cell BH4 content might improve eNOS function and help angiogenesis. Its recently demonstrated that sepiapterin, a precursor for BH4, can recouple eNOS and correct the impaired angiogenesis in PPHN pulmonary artery endothelial cells.

L-arginine: L-Arginine is the substrate for eNOS and has been shown to improve eNOS function *in vitro* but fails to show benefit *in vivo*. However, L-citrulline, a precursor of L-arginine, can go into endothelial cells effectively and has been shown to ameliorate the severity of hypoxia induced pulmonary hypertension in animal model.

Milrinone: The efficacy and safety of milrinone in the treatment of PPHN are not known and its use should be restricted within the context of RCTs. Such studies should address a comparison of milrinone with placebo (in clinical situations where iNO is not available) or, in well resourced countries, should compare milrinone with iNO or as an adjunct to iNO compared with iNO alone.

List salient features of important drugs employed in PPHN.

Table 8.3 provides the requisite information.

Table 8.3: Drugs used in the management of PPHN

Therapy	Mechanism of action	Doses	Side effects
Inhaled NO	Increased cGMP levels via stimulation of sGC activity	5–20 ppm through ventilator	Methemoglobinemia, formation of NO_2 and peroxinitrite, inhibition of platelet aggregation
Dipyridamole	Increased cGMP levels via non-specific PDE inhibition IV	0.3–0.6 mg/kg	Systemic vasodilation and hypotension
Sildenafil	Increased cGMP levels via specific PDE-5 inhibition	PO 0.5–2 mg/kg/ dose every 6 hours IV 0.4 mg/kg over 3 hours loading f/b infusion 1.6 mg/kg/d	Hypotension especially with NO, impaired retinal vascular growth, thrombocytopenia is a relative contraindication
Milrinone	Increased cAMP levels via specific PDE-3 inhibition	0.33–0.99 µg/kg/min IV infusion	Systemic hypotension, Intraventricular hemorrhage (IVH)
Prostacyclin (PGI2)	Increased cAMP levels via adenylate cyclase enzyme	5–40 ng/kg/min IV infusion	Hypotension
Iloprost	Increased cAMP levels via adenylate cyclase enzyme	20 µg/kg/dose every 90 min inhalation	None reported
Beraprost sodium	Increased cAMP levels via adenylate cyclase enzyme	0.5–1.0 µg/kg/dose 12 hourly	Watery diarrhea, flushing, Headache
Magnesium sulphate	Modulates vascular contraction by affecting calcium influx thereby inhibits SMC depolarization and promotes vasodilation	IV 200 mg/kg loading over 20 min f/b 20–150 mg/kg/h infusion	Bradycardia, hypotension, respiratory depression
Adenosine	Release of endogenous NO, stimulation of K+-ATP channels, and decreased calcium influx	30–90 µg/kg/min IV infusion	
Bosentan	Increased cGMP levels via ET-1 receptor antagonism	PO 1 mg/kg/dose 12 hourly	Systemic hypotension

CONCLUSIONS

Echocardiography with real-time Doppler flow imaging is the gold standard for the diagnosis of PPHN which usually presents with respiratory distress along with cyanosis, often in spite of adequate ventilation and needs high index of suspicion. The overall approach in management of PPHN should focus on restoring the cardiopulmonary adaptation while avoiding lung injury and adverse effects on systemic perfusion. Prolonged exposure to 100% oxygen and aggressive ventilation can be avoided by judicious application of newer therapies, such as iNO, surfactant replacement, an inotropic support. Combined iNO and HFOV therapy was found to be more effective in rescuing infants with severe PPHN.

TAKE HOME MESSAGES

- PPHN represents a failure of the unique adaptations that occur at birth in the pulmonary circulation.
- High index of clinical suspicion is required for diagnosis in babies without risk factors. Echocardiography with real-time Doppler flow imaging is gold standard for the diagnosis of PPHN.
- Overall approach in management of PPHN should focus on restoring the cardiopulmonary adaptation while avoiding lung injury and adverse effects on systemic perfusion. Prolonged exposure to 100% oxygen and aggressive ventilation can be avoided by judicious application of newer therapies, such as iNO, surfactant replacement, an inotropic support.
- Combined iNO and HFOV therapy is more effective in rescuing infants with severe PPHN, probably by improving intrapulmonary shunt which favors release of NO in the area of action.
- iNo Prompt not only causes improvement of oxygenation indices but also spares the need for (ECMO).
- Sildenafil is a potent and highly selective inhibitor of PDE5 that produces pulmonary vasodilation.

FURTHER READING

1. Hernández-Díaz S, vanMarter LJ, Werler MM, Louik C, Mitchell AA. Risk factors for persistent pulmonary hypertension of the newborn. *Pediatrics* 2007;120: e272–282.
2. Winovitch KC, PadillaL, Ghamsary M, Lagrew DC, Wing DA. Persistent pulmonary hypertension of the newborn following elective caesarean delivery at term. *J Matern Fetal Neonatal Med* 2011;24:1398–1402.
3. Vijlbrief DC, Benders MJ, Kemperman H, van Bel F, deVries WB. B-typenatriuretic peptide and rebound during treatment for persistent pulmonary hypertension. *J Pediatr* 2012;160:111–115.
4. Carlo WA, Beoglos A, Chatburn RL, Walsh MC, Martin RJ. High-frequency jet-ventilation in neonatal pulmonary hypertension. *Am J Dis Child* 1989;143:233–238.
5. Walsh BK, Gentile MA, Grenier BM. Orienting new respiratory therapists into the neonatal/pediatric environment: A survey of educators and managers. *Respir Care* 2011;56:1122–1129.
6. Dhillon R. The management of neonatal pulmonary hypertension, *Arch Dis Child Fetal Neonatal Ed* 2012; 97: F223–228.

Chapter

9 Meconium Aspiration Syndrome

Utpal Kant Singh, Suraj Gupte, Rita Fernandes, James Nelson

ABSTRACT

Meconium aspiration syndrome (MAS) is defined as respiratory distress in an infant born through meconium staining of amniotic fluid (MSAF) in whom the other causes of distress have been ruled out.

The mechanisms of respiratory distress in MAS include mechanical obstruction, chemical injury and surfactant dysfunction. In addition, two major complications, i.e., PPHN and air leak syndrome may contribute to the respiratory distress. A "hyperoxia" test is useful to differentiate PPHN from other parenchymal lung disorders.

The principles of treatment of MAS include maintenance of adequate oxygenation and a "gentle" ventilation approach. If CV is not successful, conversion to HFV is recommended. Supportive therapies, including inotropic support, fluid and electrolyte balance and sedation are critical components of the management of MAS. Inhaled NO is the therapy of choice for PPHN.

Key Words: Air-leak syndromes, Amniotic fluid, Fetal hypoxia, Hyperoxia test, Inhaled NO, Meconium, Meconium aspiration syndrome, Meconium staining of amniotic fluid (MSAF), Persistent pulmonary hypertension of the newborn (PPHN).

INTRODUCTION

Normally, meconium is passed within the first 2 days of birth. However, intrauterine distress can cause early passage of meconium, resulting in meconium staining of amniotic fluid (MSAF). This staining of amniotic fluid can range from greenish-tinged amniotic fluid to thick and viscous fluid, often described as resembling pea soup. There is a stronger association of MSAF with fetal hypoxia when a "non-reassuring" pattern is seen on fetal heart monitoring.

Meconium aspiration occurs when the neonate aspirates meconium and amniotic fluid into its lungs *in utero* or during the delivery process.

CASE SCENARIO

A female baby born at 41 weeks of gestation to a mother suffering from poor controlled hypertension by cesarean section (because of fetal distress) presented with respiratory distress, cyanosis, grunting, nasal flaring, tachypnea (respiratory rate 78/min) and retractions. Heart rate was 150/min. Chest was barrel-shaped. Skin appeared stained yellow with evidence of peeling.

On auscultation, diffuse crepitations and rhonchi were heard.

Her weight was only 2.3 kg in spite of her gestation age of 41 weeks.

Diagnosis: *Neonatal respiratory distress in a SGA neonate MAS with PPHN.*

Treatment: *CPAP failed to improve her condition. However, she responded to assisted ventilation for 48 hours. She continued to need oxygen for almost another month.*

CRITICAL CASE ANALYSIS

Maternal hypertension, SGA, fetal distress, etc. present in the case under review is factors that predispose to MAS. The cause of respiratory distress in this infant was, therefore, quite obvious. The fact that the neonate didn't respond to 40% oxygen therapy at all and had to be subjected to assisted ventilation points to the severity of MAS in this case. It is noteworthy that in spite of recovery from acute MAS, the baby continued to need oxygen for about a month thereafter. This is expected in a case of severe MAS.

INTERACTIVE TOPIC REVIEW

What is meconium?

It is a sterile, viscous, tar-like material present in the intestines of the growing fetus. Lanugo, cholesterol, intestinal epithelial cells, mucus, intestinal secretions, enzymes such as phospholipases, bile salts, drug metabolites and amniotic fluid are its constituents.

Passage of meconium in a fetus occurs early in gestation and then ceases by 20 weeks. This coincides with maturation of the gastrointestinal tract and innervation of the anal sphincter.

How often does the meconium staining of amniotic fluid occur?

Some 13% of all deliveries have meconium staing of amniotic fluid (MSAF).

What is meconium aspiration syndrome?

Out of the neonates with MSAF, about 6% aspirate meconium into the lungs in utero, during delivery or soon after birth followed by respiratory distress.

Meconium aspiration syndrome (MAS) is defined as respiratory distress in an infant born with MSAF in whom the other causes of distress have been ruled out.

How to classify MAS?

MAS can be classified by severity (Table 9.1).

Table 9.1: Classification of MAS

Classification	Comments
Mild	Requiring ≤ 40% O_2 for ≤ 48 hours
Moderate	Requiring >40% O_2 for >48 hours
Severe	Requiring assisted ventilation for >48 hours; often associated with persistent pulmonary hypertension in the newborn (PPHN).

What are risk factors predisposing to MAS?

These are hypoxia, placental insufficiency, pre-eclampsia and maternal hypertension, oligohydramnios and maternal use of cocaine.

The risk of developing MAS in an infant born through MSAF increases with heavy MSAF, nulliparity, postmature gestational age, fetal heart rate abnormalities (especially tachycardia without accelerations), presence of meconium below the vocal cords, cesarean section and low Apgar scores. Low umbilical artery pH can be a predictor of overall morbidity in such infants.

What is its pathophysiology?

Neuronal stimulation of a mature gastrointestinal tract is responsible for MAS. Vagal stimulation occurs in response to cord or head compression at the time of fetal distress. There is an increase in circulating catecholamines that stimulates release of placental corticotrophin-releasing factor (CRF). The CRF activation at the level of myenteric plexus triggers release of acetylcholine and increases colonic smooth muscle motility. It also causes relaxation of the anal sphincter that allows passage of meconium into the amniotic fluid.

Normal fetal respiration causes movement of fluid from fetal lungs to the amniotic fluid. In instances of distress, compromised placental circulation or hypoxia, gasping is initiated by the fetus. This results in inhalation of amniotic fluid with meconium into the fetal lungs.

MAS cause respiratory distress in the infant after delivery, by several mechanisms. The initial presentation of MAS is primarily as a result of mechanical airway obstruction by thick meconium. However, there are other mechanisms of injury as well. These include atelectasis, air trapping, chemical injury/pneumonitis, surfactant dysfunction and PPHN.

1. ***Mechanical airway obstruction:*** Thick meconium causes varying amount of obstruction in the alveoli. If the obstruction is complete, it results in atelectasis and collapse of the alveoli. If the obstruction is partial/incomplete, it causes a 'ball-valve' effect and results in air trapping. This occurs because the airway diameter is reduced during expiration. The trapped air causes hyperinflation of the alveoli which may rupture and cause air leak syndromes like pneumothorax, pneumomediastinum or pneumopericardium.
2. ***Chemical injury/pneumonitis:*** Meconium induces inflammation via its chemotactic properties. The presence of meconium in the alveoli triggers a local increase in activated neutrophil count and in plasma proteins, while preventing the neutrophil oxidative burst. It activates the complement cascade and increases the cytokine release. There is specifically an upregulation of interleukin-8 (IL-8) and tumor necrosis factor-alpha (TNF-α). Meconium also causes apoptotic cell death of the airway epithelial cells.

3. ***Surfactant dysfunction:*** Meconium causes surfactant dysfunction by two mechanisms, direct inhibition of surfactant as indicated by *in vitro* studies and acquired surfactant dysfunction by causing inflammation. Meconium increases the viscosity and the surface spreading rate of pulmonary surfactant. The degree of inhibition or dysfunction is proportional to the amount of meconium aspirated or present in the lungs. Presence of the debris of meconium causes an inflammatory cascade that inactivates endogenous surfactant and causes a decrease in its local concentration.
4. ***PPHN:*** Mechanism for development of PPHN in MAS is not entirely understood but there are several proposed pathways. The presence of meconium may induce PPHN via release of vasoactive substances, induction of hypoxia and by release of inflammatory cytokines. Endothelins and prostaglandins are vasoconstrictors which are released after aspiration of meconium. These substances cause acidosis and hypoxia by constricting the umbilical vessels (if meconium aspiration has occurred *in utero*), which in turn results in injury to the pulmonary vascular bed. The hypoxic injury can lead to abnormal muscularization of distal pulmonary vasculature. Presence of meconium has been shown to trigger complement activation, release of TNF-α and platelet activating factor. These may contribute further to the inflammation seen in the alveoli and resulting increase in pulmonary vascular resistance. Significant muscularization of the pulmonary arterioles indicates that ongoing fetal stress or chronic intrauterine hypoxemia may be an important contributor to the infant's pulmonary symptoms.

What are the Clinical features of MAS?

MSAF neonate may be either vigorous or depressed from hypoxia at birth. Common manifestations include:

- Cyanosis, grunting, nasal flaring, tachypnea and retractions.
- Barrel-shaped chest secondary to air trapping.
- Yellow or green staining of nails, umbilical cord and skin.
- On auscultation, rales and rhonchi may be heard.

Respiratory distress develops in the first few hours of birth and persists for several weeks. Left untreated, it may worsen, ending up in respiratory failure.

What is differential diagnosis?

The following conditions fall in the differentials:

- Sepsis.
- Pneumonia.
- Respiratory distress syndrome (RDS).
- Persistent pulmonary hypertension of the newborn (PPHN).
- Transient tachypnea of the newborn.
- Congenital diaphragmatic hernia; and
- Transposition of the great arteries.

How to reach the I diagnosis of MAS?

Diagnosis is primarily clinical. A neonate with MSAF and respiratory distress with no obvious cause must be suspected to have MAS.

CXR shows overinflated lungs and segmental atelkectasais, hetrogenous opacities, flat diaphragm, retrosternal lucency, bilateral pneumonia and signs of airleak syndromes. Cardiomegaly may also be observed.

What special investigations are needed?

1. Pulse oximetry helps record the level of hypoxemia seen in the newborn. A difference between pre-ductal and post-ductal saturation of >10% indicates shunting via the patent ductus arteriosus (PDA).
2. Arterial blood gas may reflect one or more of the following:
   (a) Low PaO_2 secondary to V/Q mismatch.
   (b) High base deficit reflective of metabolic acidosis secondary to the perinatal stress.
   (c) Respiratory acidosis or alkalosis, depending on the severity of the disease.
   (d) "Hyperoxia test" may be needed to differentiate PPHN from other parenchymal lung disorders. Place the infant under the oxyhood in 100% oxygen (or if being ventilated, increase the FiO_2 to 1.0) for 10 minutes. Obtain an arterial blood gas.
      - PaO_2 >100 mm Hg is seen in parenchymal lung disease.
      - PaO_2 50–100 mm Hg is seen in parenchymal lung disease or cardiovascular disease.
      - PaO_2 of <50 mm Hg is seen in fixed right to left shunt cyanotic heart disease or PPHN.
3. Differential cyanosis is seen in newborn PPHN where pre-ductal (right arm) oxygen saturation is higher than the post-ductal (right leg) saturation by at least 10%.
4. An echocardiogram is used to identify PPHN and measure the severity of pulmonary hypertension. It will also detect shunting through the PDA or patent foramen ovale (PFO).
5. Complete blood count (CBC) may be significant for polycythemia as a result of intrauterine stress.
6. A blood culture is usually sent, prior to starting antibiotics.

What is the differential diagnosis?

The following differentials should be kept in mind:

1. Transient tachypnea of the newborn.
2. Spontaneopus pneumothorax.
3. Persistent pulmonary hypertension of the newborn.
4. Lung malformations.
5. Cardiac disease.

What is the antepartum management?

Antepartum: Given the association of MSAF with the potential development of MAS, attempts have been made to dilute the meconium by doing amnioinfusion. In clinical settings with standard peripartum surveillance, the evidence does not support the use of amnioinfusion for MSAF. In settings with limited peripartum surveillance, where complications of MSAF are common, amnioinfusion appears to reduce the risk of MAS.

While there is controversy about the increased incidence of chorioamnionitis and/or endometritis with MSAF, use of intrapartum antibiotics may be advisable.

What is the peripartum management?

Peripartum: Current guidelines do not recommend intrapartum suctioning of all infants born through MSAF, as it does not seem to impact on the incidence of MAS. Attempts to prevent aspiration of meconium by using procedures, e.g., cricoid pressure or chest compression are potentially hazardous, and are not recommended.

Delivery through MSAF is considered a high-risk situation for a neonate; hence at least 2 personnel skilled in neonatal resuscitation should be on hand to attend such deliveries. In the event that an infant born through MSAF is not "vigorous", he/she should be immediately handed over to the neonatal resuscitation team for further management.

What is the postpartum management?

Principles of treatment include:

1. Maintenance of oxygenation.
2. Maintenance of adequate ventilation; and
3. Prevention of air leaks.

   A. **Vigorous Infant:** If the infant is "vigorous" (defined as having strong respiratory efforts, good muscle tone and a heart rate of >100 beats/minute), the usual routine of the neonatal resuscitation algorithm should be followed: Clearing the mouth and nose of secretions and drying the infant.

      While at low risk, the child should continue to be observed for any signs of MAS. Most symptomatic infants will show signs of respiratory distress within the first 12 hours of life.

   B. **Depressed Infant:** If the infant appears "depressed", tracheal intubation and suctioning of the meconium, under direct visualization, is recommended. Prophylactic gastric lavage or routine chest physiotherapy do not improve outcomes in MAS and hence, are not recommended.

Appropriate oxygenation (pre- and post-ductal saturations > 90%; PaO_2 > 80 mm Hg) can be achieved by delivering oxygen by head box. If the FiO_2 requirement is >0.6, nasal continuous positive pressure (NCPAP) may be attempted. Caution needs to be taken when administering NCPAP in infants with MAS, as there is an increased risk of air leaks under such circumstances. If blood gas analysis shows evidence of hypercapnia ($PaCO_2$ > 60 mm Hg) and acidosis (pH < 7.25) along with hypoxemia (PaO_2 < 50 mm Hg), or the child is apneic, despite the above efforts, mechanical ventilation should be instituted.

What should be the supportive therapy?

Supportive therapy includes usually restricting fluids on the first day to 60 cc/kg. Inotropic support may be achieved by using dopamine or dobutamine. Glucose should be maintained in the euglycemic range.

After blood cultures are sent, infants with MAS are usually started on antibiotics, as per the local NICU preference, pending culture results. Most infants with MAS need to be sedated – the drugs of choice are morphine or fentanyl, given as a continuous infusion. Some infants may need to be paralyzed, using vercuronium.

What should be the next step if adequate ventilation and/or oxygenation are not being achieved with the above measures?

Next approach should be to convert the ventilator support to high frequency ventilation (HFV). Some may also prefer to convert from CV to HFV, if air leaks occur. The two common modalities of HFV include high frequency oscillatory ventilation (HFOV) and high frequency jet ventilation (HFJV). While detailed descriptions of the use of HFV is outside the scope of this chapter, the guidelines for the blood gases and saturations remain the same as in CV.

Any role of surfactant?

Me conium is known to inactivate surfactant. Hence, exogenous surfactant replacement therapy has been used as a therapy for MAS.

Surfactant administration may reduce the severity of respiratory illness and decrease the number of infants with progressive respiratory failure requiring support with extracorporeal membrane oxygenation (ECMO).

Mention Complications

- The most common complications of MAS are the air leak syndromes like pneumothorax and pneumomediastinum.
- PPHN is a serious complication of MAS and may increase the morbidity and mortality associated with MAS.

Is there any relationship between MAS and sepsis?

No, there is no association of MAS with risk of septicemia.

What are the long-term adverse effects?

1. Alveolar hyperinflation and airway hyper-reactivity to exercise.
2. Neurodevelopmental outcomes.
3. ECMO–treated patients: Low IQ.
4. Cord pH and 2 hour arterial pH <7.20: Sizures.
5. iNO–treated patients: Cerebral palsy, neurodevelopment disability, vision impairment and hearing loss.

What are the preventive measures?

1. Fetal heart monitoring and surveillance may assist in decision making for delivery of the infant.
2. Amnioinfusion may be useful only in the setting where fetal surveillance is not available.

3. Intubation and suction of the trachea after the delivery only if the newborn is depressed (minimal respiratory effort, poor muscle tone, heart rate <100/minute).
4. Prevention of the major complications of MAS, i.e., air leaks and PPHN, by maintenance of oxygenation and judicious ventilation.

What is the mortality?

Without ventilator support, mortality is extremely high in severe MAS.

With ventilator support, it can be reduced to 30–40%.

CONCLUSIONS

Respiratory distress in MAS is due to mechanical obstruction, chemical injury, surfactant dysfunction. and two major complications (PPHN and air leak syndrome). Maintenance of adequate oxygenation and a "gentle" ventilation approach, cardioversion, conversion to HFV plus inotropic support, fluid and electrolyte balance and sedation are the major therapeutic modalities.

TAKE HOME MESSAGES

- Risk factors for MAS include maternal hypertension, toxemia, small-for-gestational age neonate, fetal distress, postmaturity and Cesarean section.
- Mechanisms of respiratory distress in MAS include mechanical obstruction, chemical injury, surfactant dysfunction, and complications such as PPHN and air leak syndrome.
- "Hyperoxia" test is useful to differentiate PPHN from other parenchymal lung disorders.
- Principles of treatment of MAS include maintenance of adequate oxygenation and a "gentle" ventilation approach. If CV is not successful, conversion to HFV is recommended.
- Supportive therapies include inotropic support, fluid and electrolyte balance and sedation.
- When PPHN complicates MAS, inhaled NO is the therapy of choice.

FURTHER READING

1. Basu S, Kumar A, Bhatia BD, Satya K, Singh TB. Role of steroids on the clinical course and outcome of meconium aspiration syndrome: A randomized controlled trial. *J Trop Pediatr* 2007;53:331–337.
2. Malhotra Y, Bhandari V. Meconium aspiration syndrome. In: Gupte S, Gupte SB (eds). *Recent Advances in Pediatrics (Special Vol 21: Neonatal and Pediatric Intensive Care)*. New Delhi: Jaypee 2011:115–144.
3. Okazaki K, Kondo M, Kato M, Kakinuma R, Nishida A, Noda M, Taniguchi K, Kimura H. Serum cytokine and chemokine profiles in neonates with meconium aspiration syndrome. *Pediatrics* 2008;121:e748–753.
4. Salvesen B, Fung M, Saugstad OD, Mollnes TE. Role of complement and CD14 in meconium-induced cytokine formation. *Pediatrics* 2008;121:e496–505.
5. Short BL. Extracorporeal membrane oxygenation: Use in meconium aspiration syndrome. *J Perinatol* 2008; 28 (Suppl 3):S79–83.

Chapter

10 Pulmonary Hemorrhage in the Neonates

P Preetham, Dinesh Chirla

ABSTRACT

Pulmonary hemorrhage is seen in 3–12% of very low birthweight (VLBW) babies. Severe hemorrhage is fatal in 50% of these babies. Risk factors for the occurrence of PH are intra-partum asphyxia, infection, persistent ductus arteriosus, need for resuscitation in the delivery room, low gestational age (GA) and birthweight, use of surfactant therapy, and lack of antenatal corticosteroid use. Presentation is sudden and diagnosis is clinical with presence of blood from the trachea and associated hypoxemia and increased ventilatory requirements.

The aim of treatment is to control the bleeding and maintain oxygenation. Treatment is supportive only with appropriate volume, inotropes and blood products. High PEEP and high frequency ventilation can improve the oxygenation.

High fatality rates are seen in VLBW babies which can be as high as 50–75%.

Key Words: Increased ventilator requirement, Inotropes, Lung diseases, Pulmonary hemorrhage, Surfactant, Very low birthweight.

INTRODUCTION

Severe pulmonary hemorrhage (PH) is a life-threatening event that sometimes occurs in very low birthweight (VLBW) infants with a prevalence rates of 3–12% and carry a mortality risk as high as 50%. The following are reported as risk factors for the occurrence of PH: intrapartum asphyxia, infection, persistent ductus arteriosus, need for resuscitation in the delivery room, low gestational age (GA) and birthweight, use of surfactant therapy, and lack of antenatal corticosteroid use. Pulmonary hemorrhage is defined pathologically as the presence of extravasated erythrocytes in the pulmonary alveoli, septa or both. Clinically, it is depicted by bloodstained frothy secretions, exuding or aspirated from the trachea. Rapid deterioration of ventilatory function, progressive hypoxia and hypercarbia with associated respiratory acidosis are noted in affected infants. The presence of hemoglobin, red cell membrane lipids, and serum proteins can increase the surface tension resulting from surfactant dysfunction and cause secondary RDS.

CASE SCENARIOS

Case 1

Baby KS was a VLBW male infant born at 27 weeks' gestation. The pregnancy was complicated by premature rupture of membranes and mother was monitored for sepsis. She had received a course of antenatal steroids in the week before delivery. Delivery was by emergency cesarean section on account of fetal bradycardia and breech presentation. Apgar scores were 6 and 7 at 1 and 5 minutes, respectively. Umbilical arterial blood gases were normal. Birthweight was 845 gm; he was small-for-gestational age (SGA).

Early in the hospital course, he received two doses of surfactant for RDS and required moderate ventilatory support. He was on vasopressors for hypotension and was treated with a course of indomethacin for closure of a clinically significant patent ductus arteriosus (PDA) on the fourth and fifth days of life. He had evidence of sepsis on the 3rd day of life with leukopenia and thrombocytopenia for which he was treated with appropriate broad-spectrum antibiotics.

He was extubated to CPAP on the fourth day and on the sixth day he developed increased respiratory distress with desaturation. He started to have bleeding from the nose and developed bradycardia. While intubating his trachea was found to be full of fresh bloo. Hence, the neonate was diagnosed to have pulmonary hemorrhage (PH). He became anemic and hypotensive which were treated with inotropes and blood products.

Investigations at the time of pH: *CBP: Hb 8 gm/dl, WBC: 22,100, Platelet count: 33,000/cumm. PT: 24 sec, INR: 1.9 and APTT: 60 sec. SE: S. Na 144, S. Potassium: 4.2, S. Chloride:101.*

Treatment: *He required blood products in the form of FFP and PRBC and platelets to correct his coagulation parameters, low Hb and low platelets. He had a high oxygen requirement of 85% with a high PIP and PEEP of 6. Bleeding got reduced. However, as the oxygen requirement continued to be high, he was given one more dose of surfactant after which his oxygen requirements decreased. He could be extubated after 48 hours.*

Outcome: *He was on CPAP for the next 3 days, was weaned to oxygen and to room air over the next 7 days and was discharged at 34 weeks post-menstrual age (PMA).*

Case 2

This was a female baby delivered at term to a primigravid mother by emergency LSCS indication being fetal bradycardia and meconium stained amniotic fluid. She was 2 kg at birth and Apgar scores were 3, 5 and 7 at 1, 5 and 10 minutes. Cord ABG showed severe respiratory and metabolic acidosis with pH of 6.92. He had to be intubated and ventilated in view of poor respiratory efforts. She was gradually weaned on the ventilator and had minimal ventilator requirements by 48 hours of life, however, she developed sudden desaturation and bleed through the endotracheal tube. She continued to bleed and had low oxygen saturations in spite of 100% oxygen and a PEEP of 7–8 cm.

Treatment: *She was placed on a high frequency oscillator (HFOV) with MAP of 14 cm , Frequency of 10 , after which the bleeding decreased and the oxygenation improved. Coagulation parameters were deranged suggesting DIC which were corrected by FFP, platelet rich plasma and PRBC.*

Outcome: *She was extubated after 72 hours and was discharged home on day 10 of life.*

CRITICAL CASE APPRAISAL

The history of a VLBW neonate developing a pulmonary hemorrhage in the first week of life is very well-known. The diagnosis of PH is clinical only with the presence of bloody tracheal aspirates and subsequent deterioration in respiratory parameters. PH can be seen secondary to reopening of PDA and a large shunt across the ductus. One other reason for PH can also be trauma to the tracheobronchial tree and the other differential diagnosis is pulmonary edema.

- Treatment is supportive and no definite protocol exists.
- High PEEP helps in splinting the alveoli and preventing further bleeds.
- Few studies have demonstrated the benefit of surfactant in reducing the oxygen requirements in neonates with PH.

INTERACTIVE CASE DISCUSSION

How common is PH?

Prior to the surfactant cra PH occurred as a terminal event in SGA and asphyxiated neonates. After the introduction of surfactant it is commonly noted in babies with respiratory distress syndrome (RDS). Depending on the birthweight and the criteria used to diagnose PH it is seen in 5–12% of VLBW babies.

What are the common predisposing factors for PH?

In the presurfactant era perinatal risk factors which contributed to PH included intra-partum asphyxia, breech delivery, cesarean section for pre-eclampsia, multiple gestations, LBW, IUGR and male sex. Correlates of PH after the introduction of surfactant have been severity of RDS, type of surfactant and its timing of administration, maternal anmtibiotic therapy and presence of PDA. Increased pulmonary blood flow and ductal shunting may contribute to pulmonary hemorrhage in PDA with studies showing that increased size of the ductus was associated with increased risk of PH.

The role of coagulation abnormalities is "unclear", although secondary disseminated intravascular coagulation is not uncommon. Prophylactic treatment with synthetic surfactant increased the risk of pulmonary hemorrhage, meta-analysis showing a RR of 3.28 (95% CI 1.50–7.16). Surfactant therapy has also been demonstrated to cause in vitro cytotoxicity, leading to impaired membrane integrity at the level of the alveolar capillary membrane. The degree of cytotoxicity differs for different surfactants and different dosages.

What is the pathophysiology of PH?

PH is considered to be pulmonary edema secondary to stress failure of alveolar capillaries associated with lung over distension, inadequate protective surface tension and fragility of the pulmonary capillary wall. It is postulated that after surfactant therapy pulmonary vascular resistance decreases and there is an increase in the left to right shunting coupled with increase in compliance which causes PH. Massive pulmonary hemorrhage may result from severe pulmonary edema, one of the causes of which is reduced intravascular oncotic pressure associated with fluid overload. These activities may be initiated at the two-cell interface of the alveolar capillary membrane barrier, with PH occurring as a result of disruption of membrane integrity at this interface.

How is PH diagnosed?

It is a clinical diagnosis with presence of bloodstained frothy secretions, exuding from the trachea with deterioration of ventilatory function, hypoxia and hypercarbia and the hematocrit of the secretions from the trachea is around 10%.

What is the treatment for PH?

Management of pulmonary hemorrhage is to improve oxygenation and ventilation by increasing the FIO_2, increasing positive end expiratory pressure, and changing other ventilatory parameters. Fluid resuscitation with blood or albumin is performed if indicated. Treatment is supportive only and involves marinating BP, optimizing fluid and coagulation parameters. Epinephrine spraying through the ET has been found to be beneficial in some neonates with PH.

What is the role of recombinant factor VII?

Use of recombinanat factor VIIa has shown a positive effect on the course of acute life-threatening pulmonary hemorrhage in few preterm infants without occurrence of adverse events, but caution should be exercised in babies having a preexisting IVH where progression can happen.

What is the role of surfactant?

The presence of hemoglobin, red cell membrane lipids, and serum protein increased surface tension and inactivated the surfactant, resulting in secondary RDS. Because of these factors use of surfactant in pulmonary hemorrhage induced RDS was found to be beneficial in a lot of studies to improve oxygenation and secondary RDS developing because of PH. Exogenous surfactant replacement can reverse this process even in the continued presence of inhibitor molecules and thus has potential utility in the therapy of PH in preterm infants. Lower birthweight and lower gestational age are significantly associated with having a good response to exogenous surfactant after PH. A shorter interval between the onset of pulmonary hemorrhage and surfactant administration showed an immediate response to the surfactant, followed by no increase in ventilator index.

What should be the ventilatory strategies in PH?

Excessive blood flow to the lungs because of PDA result in increased hydrostatic pressure and increased lung fluid filtration in the pulmonary microvasculature (measured as lymph flow), which led to deterioration of pulmonary function. High PEEP can be used to optimize the recruitment, oxygenation as well as to drive the alveolar fluid in to the interstitial spaces. To control pulmonary hemorrhage, mean airway pressure (Paw) can be increased and patients can be put in a prone position to improve oxygenation.

Is HFOV helpful?

There are studies which show that HFOV is helpful to provide better oxygenation and better outcome. "Open-lung strategy" employed during HFOV, with high CDP (continuous distending pressure), rapidly recruits and maintains lung volume in diffuse alveolar disease. In lung hemorrhage the usage of high CDP tamponades the transudation of hemorrhagic edema and cells from engorged capillaries, and decreases blood flow from ruptured vessels by increasing intrathoracic pressure and reducing pulmonary blood flow.

What is the prognosis of PH?

PH carries a mortality of 50–75% based on the severity. Of those who develop moderate or severe pulmonary hemorrhage, 46% are likely to die and 60% of the survivors are likely to develop CLD. There is also a greater incidence of major neurodevelopmental handicap in those who survive pulmonary hemorrhage.

How can PH be prevented?

PH can be prevented by avoiding trauma while suctioning, better sedation and optimizing the coagulation parameters and strictly monitoring fluid balance. During week 1, prophylactic indomethacin reduced the risk for serious pulmonary hemorrhage by 35%. Prophylactic indomethacin reduces the rate of early serious pulmonary hemorrhage, mainly through its action on patent ductus arteriosus. Hemocoagulase Reptilase, prepared and designed from venom of Brazilian snake Bothrops prophylactically used in sick neonates at an increased risk of PH was found to be beneficial in one study. Endotracheal hemocoagulase (0.25 KU) every 4–6 hourly in addition to ventilation in neonates at high risk for PH administration of hemocoagulase, when given through the endotracheal tube, is effective against pulmonary hemorrhage in mechanically ventilated neonates. None of the interventions are recommended routinely till we get more evidence.

CONCLUSIONS

PH is common in neonates with IUGR and birth asphyxia and is commonly seen in the 1st week of life. High PEEP is known to improve the oxygenation by lung recruitment and also helps to redistribute water into the interstitial space. HFOV can be tried in neonates having persistent hypoxia and continuing bleeding. Mortality can be as high as 50–75% in babies with PH. Surfactant with high PEEP and HFOV can be tried for a better outcome.

TAKE HOME MESSAGES

- PH is common in neonates with IUGR and birth asphyxia, commonly seen in the 1st week of life.
- High PEEP is known to improve the oxygenation by lung recruitment and also helps to redistribute water into the interstitial space.
- HFOV can be tried in neonates having persistent hypoxia and continuing bleeding.
- Though fatal in >50% of cases, PH can be managed by supportive care and optimizing ventilation

FURTHER READING

1. Ferreira CH, Carmona F, Martinez FE. Prevalence, risk factors and outcomes associated with pulmonary hemorrhage in newborns. *J Pediatr (Rio J)* 2014;90:316–322.
2. Gleason C, Juul S. *Avery's Diseases of the Newborn*, 9th edn. Philadelphia: Saunders 2011.
3. Rennie JM, Roberton NR. *Textbook of Neonatology*, 5th edn. London: Churchill Livingstone, 2012.
4. Zahr, Abou R, Ashfaq A, Marron-Corwin M. Neonatal pulmonary hemorrhage. *NeoReviews* 2012: e302–e306.
5. Yen T A, Wang C C, Hsieh, W S, Chou H C, Chen, C Y, Tsao, P N. Short-term outcome of pulmonary hemorrhage in very-low-birth-weight preterm infants. *Pediatr Neonatol* 2013;54:330–334.

Chapter

11

Necrotizing Enterocolitis

Sriparna Basu, Ashok Kumar

ABSTRACT

Necrotizing enterocolitis (NEC) is a devastating acquired disease which predominately affects premature and low birthweight infants. It is characterized by various degrees of mucosal or transmural necrosis of the intestine. The exact pathogenesis remains illusive, but prematurity, formula feeding, infections and intestinal hypoxia-ischemia have been shown to be the major pathways of intestinal injury. If not detected and treated early NEC can lead to widespread bowel necrosis, sepsis, and death. Awareness of the risk factors for NEC, early trophic feeding with breast milk and administration of probiotics has been shown to reduce the incidence of NEC.

Key Words: Bowel necrosis, Formula feeding, Intestinal hypoxia-ischemia, Intestinal injury, Low birthweight neonate, Necrotizing enterocolitis, Premature neonate, Prevention, Probiotics, Risk factors.

INTRODUCTION

Necrotizing enterocolitis (NEC) is the most frequent gastrointestinal emergency in preterm neonates with a frequency ranges from 7–11% in very low birthweight infants (birthweight <1500 gm). Incidence and mortality is inversely proportional to birthweight and gestational age, however, 10% of NEC may occur in full-term infants. There is no consistent association between gender and rates of NEC. However, male VLBW infants have a higher mortality. An estimated 20–40% of infants with NEC undergo surgery. The overall survival rate is 75% but mortality varies considerably according to birthweight (10–44% in infants <1,500 gm, 0–20% in infants >2,500 gm).

CASE SCENARIO

A preterm, intrauterine growth restricted (29^{+4} weeks) male neonate, weighing 900 gm, was delivered normally to a 24-year-old primigravida mother with rheumatic heart disease and premature onset of labor. The mother had not received any betamethasone prior to delivery. She got was hospitalized with congestive cardiac failure.

Contd...

Contd...

The baby cried immediately after birth and was apparently normal on examination. Attendants took the baby home and tried to feed him with cow's milk with a cotton wick. On 4th day of life, the baby developed poor feeding, lethargy, abdominal distention and passage of blood mixed stool. He was seen by local doctor on the next day and referred to hospital.

On examination, the baby was hypothermic with respiratory distress; abdomen was tense, distended and erythematous with a right lower quadrant tenderness. A palpable bluish discoloration was present over the scrotum. Bowel sounds were absent. Capillary refill time was 5 seconds.

Blood glucose was 25 mg/dL, arterial blood gas and electrolyte analysis showed acidosis, and hyponatremia. Complete blood count showed a hemoglobin of 11.2 gm/dL, total leucocyte count of 4400/mm^3 and platelet count was 22,000/mm^3. X-ray abdomen done in erect posture showed pneumoperitonium.

A diagnosis of necrotizing enterocolitis (NEC) Stage IIIb in an extremely low birthweight baby was made.

After stabilization of vitals and management of shock, he was put on total parenteral nutrition (TPN), IV antibiotics, platelet transfusion and other supportive measures.

Surgical referral was taken and the baby was taken for exploratory laparotomy.

CRITICAL CASE ANALYSIS

The risk factors for NEC in this infant were extremely low birthweight (ELBW), intrauterine growth restriction (IUGR), unhygienic feeding practice with cow's milk and lack of breastfeeding. Tense distended abdomen with bluish discoloration over the scrotum and absent bowel sounds pointed towards intestinal perforation. The classical triad of acidosis, hyponatremia and thrombocytopedia and pneumoperitonium further supported the diagnosis and confirmed the need for surgical intervention.

INTERACTIVE TOPIC DISCUSSION

What is the etiology of NEC?

The exact etiology of NEC is unknown. NEC has not been reported in a fetus, suggesting that postnatal factors are the likely contributors to its etiology. Serious intestinal injury following a combination of vascular, mucosal, toxic and other insults in a relatively immature gut is probably the contributing factor. A genetic predisposition may also play a role. Reported epidemic clusters point towards an infective etiology. Studies have documented isolation of bacterial, fungal and viral pathogens, though negative cultures are also documented. Colonization of the gut by pathological organisms, such as *Escherichia coli*, *Klebsiella*, *Salmonella* spp., *Staphylococcus epidermidis* etc. as well as spread of apparently harmless commensals through the damaged intestinal mucosa has been demonstrated.

What is the pathogenesis of NEC?

Major risk factors for NEC are prematurity, formula feeding; bacterial colonization and hypoxia-ischemia which have been demonstrated to increase the risk of mucosal and epithelial injury. Recent studies suggest that gut microbiome and genetic composition of individuals can also be important risk factors predisposing to NEC.

(i) **Prematurity and Impaired Host Defense:** The most important risk factor of NEC is prematurity which is associated with poor intestinal motility, digestion, absorption, and circulatory regulation predisposing the preterm infant to the risk of intestinal injury. Moreover, lack of physical barrier, impaired immunologic host defense, including intraepithelial lymphocytes and secretory IgA and deficiency of biochemical factors such as lactoferrin, epidermal growth factor, heparin binding epidermal growth factor, transforming growth factor, insulin-like growth factor, oligosaccharides, and polyunsaturated fatty acids (PUFA) make preterm neonates vulnerable to NEC.

(ii) **Formula Feeding:** Early introduction and rapid advancement of enteral feeding with formula, is the next most important risk factor for NEC. It often leads to gastric over distention and compromise of splanchnic circulation. Increased osmolarity, bacterial colonization and substrate fermentation are other important factors to cause mucosal injury. On the other hand, initiation of trophic feeding with breast milk has been found to be protective.

(iii) **Bacterial Colonization:** Bacterial colonization also plays a key role in the initiation of intestinal injury in premature gut. In healthy breastfed neonates intestines are colonized with anerobic bacterial spp. such as *Bifidobacterium* and *Lactobacillus* within 1 week of age. Normal maternal-infant physical interaction during feeding helps in the development of normal intestinal colonization, which protects against the pathologic microflora in breast-fed infants. Preterm hospitalized infants, separated from the mother have less species diversity and fewer or absent anerobes. This imbalance promotes pathological proliferation, binding and invasion of otherwise nonpathogenic intestinal bacteria, and reduces the anti-inflammatory effects and mucosal defense from probiotic organisms. Moreover, contamination or colonization of the feeding tubes has been demonstrated to contribute to the development of NEC. Commonly isolated bacteria are *Clostridium* sp., *Escherichia coli*, *Klebsiella* sp., *Staphylococcus epidermidis*, and *Enterobacter*.

(iv) **Intestinal Ischemia-Hypoxia:** Intestinal ischemia was reported as an important risk factor for NEC which is often characterized by full thickness ischemic necrosis with scanty neutrophils and a predominant lymphocytic infiltration in earlier studies. Nowadays, it is believed that ischemia disturbs the balance in the microvascular tone related to the production of vascular regulators such as nitric oxide and endothelin, which initiate the pathogenical cascade of NEC. Furthermore, patent ductus arteriosus, another risk factor for NEC, results in intestinal hypoperfusion by diastolic steal phenomenon; especially those treated with indomethacin may show focal intestinal necrosis.

(v) **Other Factors:** Several studies have suggested that blood transfusion may be a risk factor in inducing gut injury in preterm infants known as transfusion associated NEC (TANEC), especially those on enteral feeding. H_2 receptor blockers which are inhibitors of gastric acid, increase the gastric pH, which may enhance pathogenic bacterial growth and increase the risk of NEC. As a genetic predisposition, the loss of the HB-EGF-like growth factor gene, essential for preservation of gut barrier function, was also proposed to be a risk factor. Early use of postnatal steroids may cause intestinal perforation, independent of enteral feeding. However, the use of umbilical artery or venous catheters does not increase the risk of NEC.

What is the pathophysiology of NEC?

Current evidence suggests that the interaction of the epithelial barrier and innate immunity, together with the inflammatory response, play the vital role in the development of NEC in very preterm infants. Damage to the intestinal mucosal barrier, from enteral feeding, bacterial colonization and intestinal ischemia, in presence of an inadequate host defense and repair mechanism, results in the activation of the inflammatory cascade of intestinal injury and NEC.

In premature infants, intestinal mucosa is damaged by a variety of conditions, including hypoxia, infection, microcirculatory dysfunction and lack of feeding and the natural healing of the epithelium with mature enterocyte migration and proliferation is inhibited allowing the translocation of pathogens from the intestinal lumen to the mucosa.

Innate immunity has been demonstrated to regulate the epithelial barrier in NEC. The specific Toll-like receptors (TLRs), especially TLR4 are important components of the innate immune system located on the epithelial surface, playing a major role in the pathogenesis of NEC. TLR4 is activated by bacterial products, e.g., lipopolysaccharides and other innate immune components. The activation of TLR4 signaling in the intestinal epithelium inhibits enterocyte migration leading to enterocyte apoptosis along with damage to the gut barrier, bacterial translocation; intestinal inflammation; and a systemic inflammatory response through the activation of proinflammatory cytokines and chemokines, such as, IL-1, IL-6, IL-8, and IL-18, platelet-activating factor (PAF), leukotrienes, thromboxanes, free oxygen radicals and nuclear factor kappa B (NFκB).

Several researchers have proposed that vascular endothelial cells also play a major role in inflammatory cascade and acts as an immunomodulator. Endothelin-1 (ET-1) and endothelial nitric oxide (eNO) are involved in the pathogenesis of NEC. ET-1 is a potent vasoconstrictor and eNO is a potent vasodilator. An imbalance between vasoconstriction and vasodilatation properties of the endothelin often leads to the ischemia of the affected tissue causing NEC.

How do you describe the pathology of NEC?

NEC commonly affects the terminal ileum followed by colon and other segments of the small intestine. On gross examination, the intestines appear congested, discolored and thickened due to edema and in advanced cases gas-filled cysts may be visible in intestinal walls which may progress to appear dark, gray and gangrenous and may perforate. Pneumatosis intestinalis, the formation of gas bubbles within the intestinal wall is a characteristic finding seen in most patients with NEC, resulting from fermentation and gas production by bacteria. The intestinal wall perforates when the disease is severe with transmural involvement.

Histopathological examination shows microvascular thrombi, submucosal gas-filled cysts (intestinal pneumatosis), vascular congestion, edema, necrosis and loss of villi and a variable degree of inflammatory infiltrate in the mucosal and submucosal areas. Late changes are characterized by coagulation necrosis with hemorrhage and gangrenous bowel wall susceptible to perforation.

What are the risk factors for NEC?

NEC occurs more commonly in preterm infants, the smallest and most premature infants are the most vulnerable ones. Full-term and late preterm infants may also develop the disease in presence of risk factors. Risk factors at different gestational ages are summarized in Table 11.1.

Table 11.1: Risk factors for NEC

Risk factors for preterm infants
• Birthweight < 1000 gm
• Unstandardized approach to feeding, formula feeding, bovine breast milk fortifier
• Chorioamnionitis

Contd...

Contd...

- Perinatal asphyxia
- Sepsis episodes
- Use of broad spectrum antibiotics, e.g., cefotaxime
- Mechanical ventilation
- Use of H_2 blockers, glucocorticoids and indomethacin
- Patent ductus arteriosus (PDA)
- Respiratory distress syndrome
- Umbilical arterial catheter
- Transfusions
- HIV-positive mother
- Maternal drug abuse.

Risk factors for late preterm and full-term infants

- Cyanotic congenital heart disease
- Polycythemia
- Intrauterine growth restriction
- Formula feeding
- Maternal hypertensive disease
- Umbilical catheters
- Perinatal asphyxia
- Sepsis
- Mechanical ventilation
- Exchange transfusion
- HIV-positive mother
- Maternal drug abuse.

What are the clinical features of NEC?

Onset of the disease usually occurs 3–10 days after birth. Age at presentation is inversely related to gestational age at birth, that is, full-term infants with NEC present earlier. Clinical signs and symptoms are non-specific and are sometimes indistinguishable from those of sepsis. Common clinical features include feeding intolerance and increased prefeed residuals, temperature instability, apnea and bradycardia, hypotension, abdominal wall erythema, abdominal distention, emesis, blood in the stool (hematochezia), absent bowel sounds and abdominal tenderness. Less commonly, when the stomach is involved, NEC can also present as hematemesis or hemorrhagic gastric aspirate. During the advanced stage of NEC, the abdomen may appear shiny, distended and erythematous. The infant may assume a frog leg position and is becomes hyporesponsive. On gentle palpation, the abdomen may feel firm, tense, and occasionally a right lower quadrant tender mass may be palpable. In presence of bowel perforation, the abdomen may appear blue or discolored. In male infants, erythema or bluish discoloration of the scrotum may appear if peritoneal fluid from perforated bowel herniates into the scrotum.

Very premature infants may not manifest tenderness and guarding unless NEC is advanced and are less likely to present with pneumatosis intestinalis but more likely to develop pneumoperitoneum. Therefore, a high index of suspicion is required in these infants to establish a diagnosis of NEC, if multiple subtle signs appear that produce a deviation from baseline clinical status. NEC can also present with hematochezia without any other initial signs, especially when NEC involves the distal colon. If the jejunum and terminal ileum are the predominant sites of NEC, then emesis, increased gastric residuals, and/or abdominal distension are the more likely initial presenting signs.

Systemic signs of NEC include lethargy, hypotension, pallor, apnea and bradycardia, worsening of respiratory function, temperature instability, tachycardia, hypo or hyperglycemia. Abnormal laboratory tests include anemia, left shift of neutrophils, neutropenia, and a triad of thrombocytopenia, metabolic acidosis, and hyponatremia. Concurrent bacteremia and sepsis occurs in 40–60% of NEC. Gram-negative sepsis is more common.

Discuss the staging of NEC.

Staging of NEC depending on the disease severity was suggested by Bell *et al.* which was later modified by Walsh and Kliegman. Table 11.2 lists the staging along with clinical, laboratory and radiological features.

Table 11.2: Staging of NEC

Stage	Clinical features	Laboratory features	Radiological features
Ia	Temperature instability, apnea, bradycardia, decreased SpO_2, increased gastric residuals, abdominal distension, stool-occult blood positive	Unremarkable	Unremarkable
Ib	Same as above	Same as above + hematochezia	Unremarkable
IIa	Features of Stage I + decreased or absent bowel sound, guarding of abdominal wall	Mild metabolic acidosis, mild thrombocytopenia	Fixed dilated bowel loops or 'sentinel loop sign', pneumatosis intestinalis
IIb	Features of Stage I and IIa + absent bowel sounds, marked guarding, abdominal wall discoloration or cellulitis, palpable right lower quadrant mass	Metabolic acidosis, thrombocytopenia, hyponatremia	Features of IIA + portal venous gas shadows presenting as 'football sign'
IIIa	Features of Stage I and II + hypotension and disseminated intravascular coagulation	Respiratory acidosis, metabolic acidosis, neutropenia, increased CRP, PT/PTT/INR and D-dimer assays	Features of Stage II + ascites
IIIb	Same as above	Same as above	Features of Stage II and IIIa + pneumoperitoneum

In some patients, pneumatosis intestinalis, portal venous gas and pneumoperitoneum are seen in advanced stage of NEC with gut necrosis or 'NEC totalis' indicative of poor prognosis. Pneumoperitoneum represents bowel perforation and is a surgical emergency.

What are the laboratory and radiological investigations to make the diagnosis of NEC?

- Complete blood count – though non-specific, severe or persistent thrombocytopenia and neutropenia indicate severe disease.

- Sepsis screen and blood culture – may give a clue for antibiotic therapy. Serial C-reactive protein may be useful, with persistently high levels with complications.
- Blood glucose and electrolytes, blood gas, baseline biochemistry and coagulation profile should be done for management.
- Diagnosis is confirmed by abdominal X-ray in supine and in lateral decubitus. Serial abdominal films are often necessary.
- Abdominal ultrasound scanning may also be useful in identifying portal air, perforation and ascites.
- Other imaging techniques being developed include contrast radiography, portal vein ultrasonography, MRI and radionuclide scanning.

What are the biomarkers used to make the diagnosis of NEC?

Early diagnosis and differentiation of NEC from neonatal sepsis and other inflammatory conditions remain a major challenge to the neonatologists, as the clinical management with regard to antibiotic coverage, duration of bowel rest and parenteral nutrition requirements is substantially different in the two conditions. A panel of biomarkers has been proposed that can facilitate early diagnosis and predict the severity or prognosis of NEC. Currently available biomarkers can be classified into three categories: (i) non-specific biomarkers, (ii) enhanced non-specific biomarkers, and (iii) gut-specific biomarkers.

Non-specific biomarkers: These are the mediators of the inflammatory cascade and can be broadly subdivided into three major groups, acute phase reactants and other proteins, cytokines and chemokines, and cell surface antigens. The most widely used acute phase reactant for identifying neonatal sepsis and NEC is C-reactive protein (CRP). CRP is not effective for early diagnosis but serial CRP levels are useful for monitoring of the disease progression and guiding treatment. Other useful acute phase proteins are serum amyloid A (SAA) and apolipoprotein CII (ApoSAA score) which can identify all cases of neonatal sepsis and NEC early, at the time of initial screening.

Other proteins, including procalcitonin, anaphylatoxin (C5a), arginine, endotoxins, platelet-activating factor and related lipids, e-selectin, S100A8/A9, and various GI hormones, e.g., gastrin and neurotensin have also been suggested as useful indicators for either early diagnosis and prognosis but their usefulness have not been validated by larger studies.

Cytokines and chemokines can complement acute phase reactants in predicting the severity of illness and prognosis. Proinflammatory cytokines, e.g., interleukin (IL)-6 and tumor necrosis factor (TNF)-α, and chemokines, e.g., IL-8, interferon-γ inducible protein-10 (IP-10), regulated upon activation of normal T-cell expression and secretion (RANTES), are early biomarkers for diagnosing neonatal sepsis and NEC but their levels tend to fall within 24 hours of appropriate treatment. The sequential use of IL-10, an anti-inflammatory cytokine along with IL-6 and RANTES can accurately prognosticate the development of disseminated intravascular coagulation at the onset of clinical presentation with 100% sensitivity and 97% specificity.

Cell surface antigens, e.g., natural killer cell CD69, neutrophil CD64, and CD11b are important early inflammatory biomarkers in preterm infants, as these are expressed within minutes of cell contact with bacteria or their products and the antigen expression persists for more than 24 hours. Since 0.05 ml of whole blood sample is required for flow cytometry, cell surface antigens are ideal for surveillance and early diagnosis of NEC in high-risk infants.

Enhanced Non-specific Biomarkers of NEC: This category comprises non-specific biomarkers of inflammation isolated from stool, indicating increased intestinal mucosal permeability and/or disruption of mucosal integrity. The most studied biomarker in this category is calprotectin which has been proposed as an early diagnostic or surveillance biomarker for diagnosing intestinal inflammation and NEC. Calprotectin is a heterodimeric peptide secreted by neutrophils and macrophages and is highly resilient to bacterial degradation. There is wide variation of calprotectin concentrations in meconium and fecal matter, of neonates of different gestational and postnatal age. The recommended optimum cut-off level for identification of NEC ranges from 200 to 2000 mg/gm in different studies.

Other agents include fecal S100A12 (calgranulin C), a proinflammatory protein, which is also released in large quantity into the bowel lumen by neutrophils and monocytes following GI mucosal inflammation. Fecal S100A12 is reported to be significantly elevated 4-10 days before and up to 2 weeks after disease onset in preterm NEC patients compared with healthy controls.

The enhanced non-specific biomarkers have several limitations to be used as routine biomarkers for predicting and diagnosing NEC. Since the stool specimen is a solid medium, excreted proteins in the bowel lumen are not homogeneously dispersed throughout the entire fecal medium and there is wide variation in protein concentrations between stool samples since focal segments of the GI tract is affected in NEC.

Gut-specific Biomarkers of NEC: Specific biomarkers for GI mucosal injury and/or NEC which can differentiate neonatal sepsis from NEC, are the proteins that are either exclusively or predominantly produced by epithelial or goblet cells, lining the lumen of the GI tract. This category includes intestinal fatty acid binding protein (I-FABP), liver fatty acid binding protein (L-FABP), claudin-3, and trefoil factor-3 (TFF-3). These gut barrier proteins are released in large quantities of into the bloodstream in presence of severe inflammation of the intestinal mucosa by damaged intestinal tissues and epithelial cells.

Measurement of their concentrations in serum or urine is supposed to allow early diagnosis of NEC and assessment of the severity of intestinal damage. The urinary markers are useful in differentiating severe NEC with extensive intestinal involvement from milder focal segmental disease and function as important adjunctive indicators to plan surgery in critically ill NEC infants.

Emerging Biomarkers of NEC

Other emerging classes of potential predictors or biomarkers include mediators of oxidative stress, micro-RNA (miRNA), and volatile organic compounds (VOCs).

How do you manage a case of NEC?

Infants who develop NEC should be transferred to a level III NICU with readily available surgical facility. Treatment outlines for NEC include:

- Bowel rest.
- Gastric decompression by nasogastric or orogastric tube.
- Supportive management – intravenous fluids to correct hypovolemia, maintain perfusion and compensate for third space losses, correction of hypotension by vasopressor.
- Respiratory support by CPAP or mechanical ventilation.

- Correction of metabolic acidosis and electrolyte imbalance – hyponatremia and hyperkalemia.
- Nutritional management by total parenteral nutrition (TPN) with early and adequate protein supplementation is needed (3.5–4 gm/kg/day) to maintain positive nitrogen balance and to allow repair of injured tissue. Other nutritional supplements which have been tried to decrease the incidence of NEC include L-arginine and zinc supplementation. L-arginine supplementation leads to the formation of endothelial nitric oxide which is an important regulator of vascular perfusion and increases gut perfusion. Zinc is to be helpful in the maintenance of the epithelial barrier function and induction of adequate immune responses in experimental models.
- Strict implementation of infection control measures is critical. After obtaining culture of blood and urine, prompt initiation of treatment with appropriate broad spectrum antibiotics based on the sensitivity of locally prevalent pathogens in the individual NICU is vital. If surgical intervention is performed, peritoneal fluid and intestinal tissue should be sent for gram stain, culture and sensitivity. The utility of a stool culture is questioned because fecal matter has many bacterial species. Usual antibiotic regimens include ampicillin (or a cephalosporin) and gentamicin (or other aminoglycoside). Addition of a third antibiotic to provide anerobic coverage (e.g., clindamycin or metronidazole) is indicated when there is evidence of peritonitis or bowel perforation. IV antibiotics are continued for a minimum period of 10–14 days. Antifungals may be added in neonates who received broad spectrum antibiotics, not responding to antibacterial drugs and once perforation is suspected or confirmed. Antibiotics should be modified as per blood culture report and clinical response of the neonate.
- Inflammation of the intestine and peritoneum is painful. Attention to pain control and minimal handling are integral parts of management.
- Blood component therapy if required, however, restrictive strategies are to be followed. Unnecessary transfusions may precipitate NEC.
- Frequent clinical monitoring of vitals, perfusion and urine output.
- Laboratory and radiological assessments are conducted at regular intervals to determine the progress of the disease as neonates with NEC can rapidly deteriorate as sepsis becomes overwhelming.
- Indications for surgical consultation – abdominal wall cellulitis, fixed dilated bowel, tender abdominal mass, clinical deterioration not responsive to medical management, perforated/necrotic bowel is suspected. Identification of a pneumoperitoneum due to bowel perforation and the presence of necrotic bowel are two absolute indications for surgical intervention.

Stage-wise management of NEC is summarized in Table 11.3.

Table 11.3: Stage-wise management of NEC

Stage	Management
Ia	Assess the neonate more frequently in presence of risk factors, such as, prematurity, perinatal asphyxia, on CPAP or mechanical ventilation, sepsis, PDA etc. Hold feeds if green tinged, increase feeds cautiously, check prefeed abdominal girths.
Ib	Above + send investigations and consider adding antibiotics which can be discontinued after 2 days if sepsis screen and blood cultures are normal.

Contd...

Contd...

IIa	Above + keep the neonate NPO, gastric decompression, X-ray abdomen 6–8 hourly in left lateral decubitus, surgical consultation.
IIb	Same as above + supportive treatment.
IIIa	Same as above + insure adequate coverage for gram-negative bacteria and anerobes.
IIIb	Above + emergency surgery.

What preventive measures can be taken for the occurrence of NEC?

Several measures are taken to prevent the occurrence of NEC in NICU. Among all the measures implementation of feeding guidelines and use of human milk feeding alone is reported to reduce the NEC incidence in half. Awareness of potential risk factors, such as intrauterine growth restriction, use of formula feeds, sepsis, hemodynamically significant PDA treated with indomethacin, H_2 blocker therapy, use of ibuprofen instead of indomethacin to close a PDA, restriction in fluid intake, without compromising hydration and nutrition also help in reducing the risk of NEC.

The commonly taken risk reduction strategies are summarized below:

1. **Single Course of Antenatal Corticosteroids:** Most of the authors have recommended that mothers should receive a single course of antenatal corticosteroids if preterm delivery is expected which will reduce the incidence of NEC.
2. **Early and Preferential Use of Breast Milk:** Standardized feeding guidelines with conservative volumes (20–25 ml/kg per day) to start with helps in prevention of NEC. Studies have shown that infants fed with breast milk develop NEC 6–10 times less often than those fed with formula exclusively and 3 times less often if they receive a mixture of breast milk and formula. Enteral feeding with human milk induces intestinal maturation and healing. The beneficial effects of human milk is provided by macrophages, lymphocytes, secretory IgA, lysozymes, lactoferrin, oligosaccharides, nucleotides, cytokines, polyunsaturated fatty acids (PUFA), growth factors, and different enzymes which increases host immunity, provides mucosal protection and reduces inflammation. Breast milk also contains several growth factors such as recombinant epidermal growth factors (EGF), erythropoietin, erythropoietin-like growth factor, granulocyte colony-stimulating factor (CSF) and cytokines, which play critical roles in normal intestinal development and repair following GI mucosal injury.
3. **Modification of Gut Microbiota Composition by Use of Probiotics and Prebiotics:** Several studies have shown the efficacy and safety of prophylactic enteral probiotic administration in the prevention of NEC in very low birthweight infants. Most of the studies have used *Lactobacillus* alone or in combination with *Bifidobacterium*. Probiotic colonization is found to improve overall GI health, prevent proinflammatory signaling and disease progression by increasing mucosal barrier function and by up-regulating the immune system, reduce mucosal colonization of potential pathogens and alter the key components of intestinal inflammation.

   A recent Cochrane Database Systematic Review and meta-analysis concluded that enteral supplementation of probiotics significantly reduced the incidence of severe NEC (stage II or more) and mortality in preterm infants weighing <1,500 gm at birth. However, there are currently insufficient data with regard to the benefits and potential adverse effects in the most at risk infants, namely those weighing <1,000 gm at birth.

Another proposed preventive strategy is to supplement with prebiotics to enhance the growth of potentially beneficial intestinal microbes such as *Bifidobacterium*. Common prebiotic agents include the oligosaccharides inulin, galactose, fructose, lactulose, and combinations of these nutrients. While the theoretical benefit has been reviewed, little information is currently available to support the benefit from their use in the prevention of NEC.

4. **Modulation of Inflammatory (TLR4) Signal:** In animal experiments, celastrol, a novel cell permeable triterpenoid antioxidant, has been used as an upregulator of Heat shock protein (Hsp70) which is an inhibitor of TLR4 signal in the intestinal mucosa. Celastrol reduces enterocyte apoptosis and attenuate the severity of NEC. More studies are required for the establishment of these therapeutic options in human for the prevention and treatment of NEC.

   Lipopolysaccharide is one of the most powerful proinflammatory bacterial virulence factors, which induces TLR signaling. LPS-binding protein (LBP), secreted by enterocytes in response to inflammatory stimuli, neutralize LPS and prevent an exaggerated inflammatory response. Drugs targeting LPB are also emerging as a novel therapeutic strategy to facilitate gut healing in NEC.

5. **Fecal Transplantation:** Fecal transplantation by direct transfer of fecal material from a healthy donor to a recipient's upper or lower intestinal tract is being considered as a novel perspective to manipulate intestinal microflora. It has proven effective in the treatment of refractory colitis by *Clostridium difficile* and in some cases of inflammatory bowel disease. However, no data are currently available for neonates with NEC.

6. **New Surgical Techniques:** Several surgical techniques, such as small bowel transplantation, enteroplasty, tissue engineering techniques are coming up as unique, novel strategy for intestinal failure after severe NEC.

What is the differential diagnosis of NEC?

The common differential diagnosis of NEC include sepsis, hemorrhagic disease of the newborn, stress ulcer, volvulus/malrotation, intussusception, pseudomembranous colitis, meconium ileus, gastro-esophageal reflux, focal intestinal perforation and medical conditions, such as congenital heart diseases, metabolic or respiratory acidosis, apnea or prematurity, enteroviral infection, omphalitis, meningitis and urinary tract infection.

What is the outcome?

The overall mortality rate of NEC is 20–40% and varies with the severity and extent of intestinal involvement. Mortality is inversely related to postmenstrual age and weight at birth.

What are the complications associated with NEC?

Complications of NEC include intestinal strictures, enterocolic and enterocutaneous fistula, intra-abdominal abscess, stoma-related complications, perforation, cholestasis and acquired short bowel syndrome after surgery. Intestinal and liver failure can also occur. Strictures usually occur 3–8 weeks after the acute episode but can also be delayed after several months. The most common site of stricture development is colon but ileum or jeujenum may also be involved. Diffuse pneumatosis increases the risk of strictures. Other complications include sepsis and shock, DIC, neurodevelopmental, motor, sensory, and cognitive delay.

CONCLUSIONS

Necrotizing enterocolitis is the most common cause of gastrointestinal-related morbidity and mortality and the most common reason for emergent GI surgery in newborns. Its onset is often sudden and the smallest, most premature infants are the most vulnerable ones. While the pathogenesis of NEC remains incompletely understood, it is well-established that the risk of disease is increased by the administration of infant formula and decreased by the administration of breast milk. Awareness of NEC risk factors and adopting practices to reduce NEC risk, including human milk feeding and probiotics have been shown to reduce the incidence of NEC.

TAKE HOME MESSAGES

- Necrotizing enterocolitis (NEC) is a multifactorial disorder that primarily affects premature infants.
- By developing and adhering to early and exclusive use of human milk in premature infants, use of probiotics, judicious antibiotic use, instituting blood transfusion protocols, the occurrence of NEC may be reduced.
- Awareness of NEC risk factors and timely intervention are the main factors to improve the outcome.

FURTHER READING

1. Terrin G, Scipione A, De Curtis M. Update in pathogenesis and prospective in treatment of necrotizing enterocolitis. *Biomed Res Int* 2014;2014:543765.
2. Stewart CJ, Marrs EC, Magorrian S, Nelson A, Lanyon C, Perry JD, *et al*. The preterm gut microbiota: changes associated with necrotizing enterocolitis and infection. *Acta Paediatr* 2012;101:1121–1127.
3. Ng EW, Poon TC, Lam HS, Cheung HM, Ma TP, Chan KY, *et al*. Gutassociated biomarkers L-FABP, I-FABP, and TFF3 and LIT score for diagnosis of surgical necrotizing enterocolitis in preterm infants. *Ann Surg* 2013; 258:1111–1118.
4. Neu J. Neonatal necrotizing enterocolitis: an update. *Acta Paediatr Suppl* 2005;94:100–105.
5. Sullivan S, Schanler RJ, Kim JH, Patel AL, Trawoger R, Kiechl-Kohlendorfer U, *et al*. An exclusively human milk-based diet is associated with a lower rate of necrotizing enterocolitis than a diet of human milk and bovine milk-based products. *J Pediatr* 2010;156:562–567.
6. AlFaleh K, Anabrees J. Probiotics for prevention of necrotizing enterocolitis in preterm infants. *Cochrane Database Syst Rev* 2014; CD005496.

Chapter

12 Neonatal Hyperbilirubinemia

Anita Singh, Anup Thakur

ABSTRACT

Neonatal jaundice is a common clinical condition requiring medical attention. Standard treatment guidelines for phototherapy and exchange transfusion are available. At increased levels, bilirubin may be neurotoxic. In this chapter, metabolism of bilirubin, mechanism of bilirubin toxicity, features of bilirubin-induced neurological dysfunction (BIND) and standard treatment guidelines are discussed.

Key Words: Acute bilirubin encephalopathy, Bilirubin-induced neurological dysfunction (BIND), Brainstem-evoked response audiometry (BERA), Hyperbilirubinemia, Kernicterus, Neonatal jaundice.

INTRODUCTION

Bilirubin is an active product of heme catabolism and has propensity to deposit in skin and mucus membrane leading to yellowish discoloration which is identified as jaundice or icterus. Almost 60% of term and 80% of preterm babies develop jaundice and a significant proportion of them may require treatment. Most jaundice is benign, but because of the potential toxicity of bilirubin, newborn infants must be monitored to identify those who might develop severe hyperbilirubinemia and acute bilirubin encephalopathy or kernicterus.

CASE SCENARIO

A 35 weeks baby, appropriate for gestational age presented on day 5 of life with jaundice, inadequate feeding, infrequent urination and weight loss of 18%. There was no setting of ABO/Rh incompatibility. Baby was active and there were no abnormalities of cry or tone. Total serum bilirubin was 20.2 mg/dL. G6PD enzyme assay was normal.

Baby was started on intensive phototherapy along with supervised feeding and input/output monitoring. Over next 24 hours, serum bilirubin decreased to 14 mg/dL. Baby started accepting breastfeeding well. At 48 hours of admission serum bilirubin was 11.5 mg/dL and baby regained birthweight. Baby was discharged after 60 hours of admission. Mother was counseled about breastfeeding. Brainstem evoked response audiometry (BERA) done at 1 month of age was normal. Baby was neurologically normal on follow-up.

CRITICAL CASE ANALYSIS

This is a case of neonatal hyperbilirubinemia in a late preterm infant (defined as gestation between 34–36 weeks and 6 days) due to inadequate feeding resulting in excessive weight loss. Late preterm babies are at increased risk of hyperbilirubinemia because of prematurity, poor feeding and immature liver enzyme function. These babies should be actively monitored and followed for hyperbilirubinemia. Blood group incompatibility and evidence of hemolysis should be checked in all cases of hyperbilirubinemia requiring intensive phototherapy and exchange transfusion.

Bilirubin is toxic to brain and cochlea, so these babies should be examined for neonatal encephalopathy at the time of admission. BERA should be done in follow-up.

This baby responded to intensive phototherapy and escaped bilirubin induced neurological dysfunction.

INTERACTIVE TOPIC DISCUSSION

Discuss bilirubin metabolism.

Bilirubin is produced and eliminated from the body throughout the life. Ongoing lysis of red blood cells occurs at increased rate in neonates leading to production of heme (iron protoporphyrin) and globin. Heme is converted to biliverdin due to action of enzyme heme oxygenase. Bilirubin is produced from biliverdin after reduction by biliverdin reductase. Unconjugated bilirubin is transported to the liver bound to albumin. In the liver conjugation of bilirubin occurs by UDP-glucouronyl transferase 1A1 (UGT1A1). Bilirubin is excreted then in the bile to intestine.

Why are neonates at increased risk for jaundice?

Neonates are at increased risk of jaundice due to following reasons:

- Increased red cell mass and decreased half life of red blood cells leading to increased production of bilirubin.
- Impaired conjugation of bilirubin due to immaturity of liver enzymes.
- Impaired excretion of bilirubin from liver.
- Increased bilirubin absorption from intestine as a part of enterohepatic circulation.

Discuss the mechanism of bilirubin toxicity.

At increased level there is significant risk of bilirubin toxicity to brain and auditory pathway. Unconjugated bilirubin, which is not bound to albumin (also referred to as “free” or unbound bilirubin), can enter the brain and cause cell death by apoptosis (programmed cell death) and/or necrosis. It enters the central nervous system in higher concentration as it overwhelms the buffering capacity of blood and tissues or due to alteration in binding capacity of albumin and other proteins. Increased permeability could be secondary to disruption of blood brain barrier.

Postulated mechanisms of neuronal toxicity of bilirubin:

- Passage through lipid components of cell membrane and organelles like mitochondria and interfering with cellular respiration.
- Binding to specific membrane, organelle or cytoplasm proteins and inhibiting there functions.

- Damage and direct interference with function of DNA.
- Neuronal excitotoxicity.
- Increased intracellular calcium level.

What is bilirubin induced neurological dysfunction? What are its types?

The term *bilirubin induced neurological dysfunction (BIND)* denotes the clinical effects of neurotoxicity caused due to hyperbilirubinemia. It can be either acute or chronic.

- **Acute bilirubin encephalopathy** can be transient and reversible. It evolves through following stages:
  - *Stage 1*: Lethargy, poor feeding, hypotonia, vomiting, high pitched cry, diminished moro reflex.
  - *Stage 2*: Fever, irritability, opisthotonus, seizure, rigidity, retrocollis, oculogyric crisis, paralysis upward gaze, crossed extension of legs.
  - *Stage 3*: Hypertonia with marked retrocollis and opisthotonos, stupor, coma, and a shrill cry.
- **Chronic bilirubin encephalopathy** is state of chronic bilirubin induced neurological dysfunction. It represents a tetrad of athetoid cerebral palsy, auditory dysfunction, upward gaze palsy and dental enamel dysplasia. Neuropathological finding of chronic bilirubin neurotoxicity is known as kernicterus which is yellow staining of basal ganglia especially the globus pallidus and subthalamic nucleus.

What is bilirubin induced neurological dysfunction (BIND) score?

Bilirubin induced neurological dysfunction (BIND) score has been described for neurological monitoring and assessment of severity of babies with acute bilirubin encephalopathy (Table 12.1).

Table 12.1: Bilirubin-induced neurological dysfunction (BIND) score

Severity	Score	Mental status	Date/Time	Date/Time	Date/Time
None	0	Normal			
Mild	1	Sleepy, poor feeding			
Moderate	2	Lethargic, Irritable			
Severe	3	Semicoma, Seizures, Coma			
Severity	**Score**	**Muscle tone**			
None	0	Normal			
Mild	1	Neck Stiffness, Mild hyper-/hypotonia			
Moderate	2	Arching neck, retrocolis, Arching trunk			
Severe	3	Bowing of trunk Opisthotonus			
Severity	**Score**	**Cry pattern**			

Contd...

Contd...

None	0	Normal
Mild	1	High pitched
Moderate	2	Shrill
Severe	3	Inconsolable
Total BIND score		
Nurse/MD signature		
Score of 7–9: Represent severe acute bilirubin encephalopathy; urgent interventions are recommended to possibly minimize further brain injury. **Scores of 4–6:** Represent moderate acute bilirubin encephalopathy and is likely to be reversible with urgent bilirubin reduction. **Scores of 1–3:** Represent mild acute bilirubin encephalopathy and are usually reversible with urgent bilirubin reduction strategies. An abnormal ABR or "referred" automated ABR would be indicative of BIND would be suggestive of moderate to severe ABE.		

How can we measure bilirubin by non-invasive technique?

A reliable non-invasive technique for estimation of bilirubin is Transcutaneous bilirubinometry. High correlation between cutaneous bilirubin and TSB form the basis of Transcutaneous Bilirubinometry. These meters work by directing light into the skin of the neonate and measuring the intensity of specific wavelength that is returned. The meter analyzes the spectrum of optical signal reflected from the neonate's subcutaneous tissues. These optical signals are converted to electrical signal by a photocell and are analyzed by a microprocessor to generate a bilirubin value.

Transcutaneous bilirubin (TcB) determination is a useful screening tool and provides accurate result within 2–3 mg/dL of TSB for level less than 15 mg/dL. There is limitation of its use in babies who are on phototherapy. In addition, the ability of transcutaneous instruments to provide accurate measurements in different racial groups requires additional study.

How can we predict the possibility of significant hyperbilirubinemia in a baby before discharge?

1. **Predischarge TSB/TcB:** Possibility of significant hyperbilirubinemia in a neonate before discharge can be predicted on the basis of predischarge TSB/TcB plotted on hour specific normogram given by Bhutani *et al.* This normogram has been constructed in the form of percentile curves (40th, 75th and 95th) (Fig. 12.1). High, upper intermediate, lower intermediate and low-risk categories have been described on the normogram. Babies in high, upper intermediate, lower intermediate and low-risk categories have 39.5, 12.9, 2.26 and 0% risk of developing significant hyperbilirubinemia.
2. **Risk Factors:** Clinical risk factors most predictive of significant hyperbilirubinemia are lower gestational age, exclusive breastfeeding, presence of jaundice requiring phototherapy in previous sibling and predischarge total serum bilirubin.
3. **End Tidal Carbon Monoxide Concentration (ETCOc):** An elevated ETCOc level may be indicative of ongoing hemolysis. Bhutani, *et al.* constructed an age-in-hours-specific ETCOc normogram which may be used in neonates to determine the threshold of increased bilirubin production.

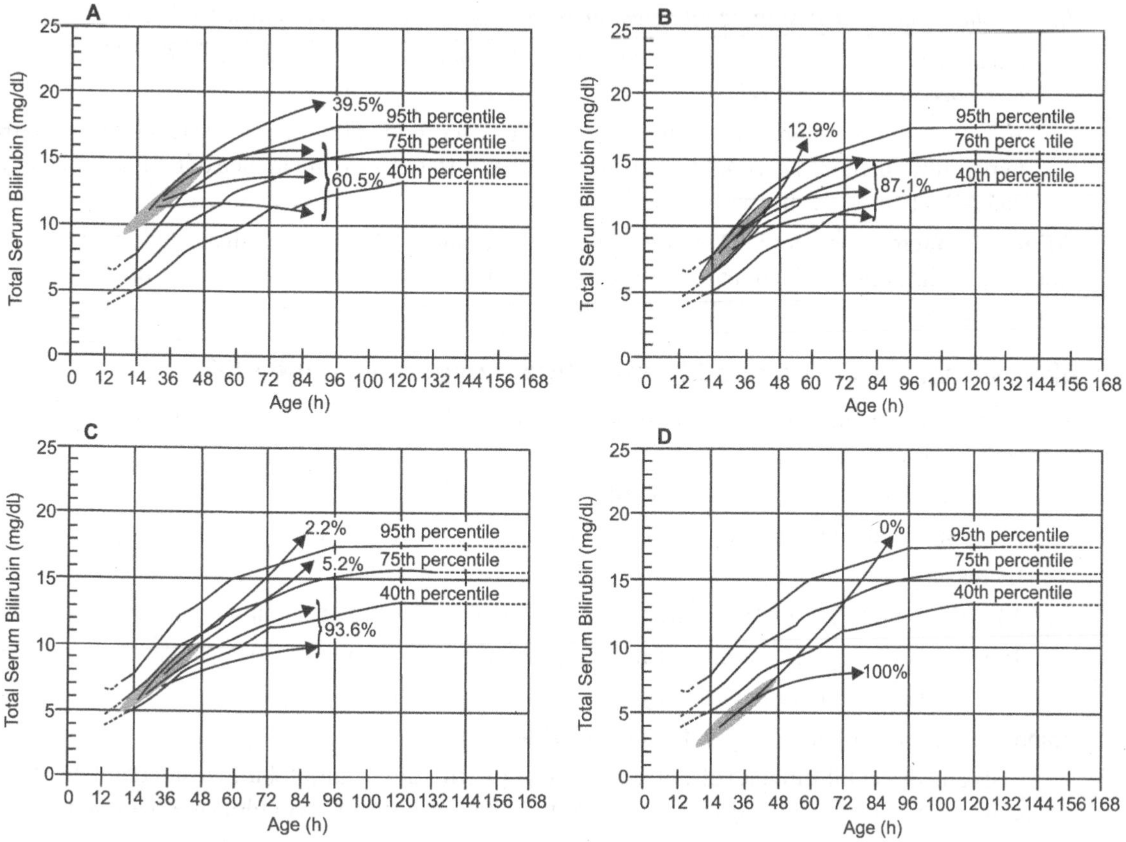

Fig. 12.1: Nomogram for designation of hyperbilirubinemia risk based on hour-specific bilirubin value (Adapted from Bhutani V, Johnson L, Sivieri EM, *et al.*: Predictive ability of a predischarge hour-specific serum bilirubin for subsequent significant hyperbilirubinemia in healthy term and near-term newborns, *Pediatrics* 1999;103:6–14.

Discuss the risk factors for unconjugated hyperbilirubinemia.

- Following are the **major risk factors** for unconjugated hyperbilirubinemia
    1. *Predischarge Total serum bilirubin (TSB) or Transcutaneous bilirubin (Tcb) in high risk zone* (Fig. 12.1).
    2. *Jaundice observed in first 24 hours*: Newborn with overt jaundice in first 24 hours of life are more likely to require treatment with phototherapy.
    3. Blood group incompatibility with positive direct agglutination test (DAT) or known hemolytic disease like G6PD deficiency.
    4. *Late prematurity*: Late preterm gestation is at 8-fold high risk of developing a TSB of ≥20 mg/dL mainly due to lower UGT1A1 enzyme activity and slower maturation as compared to their term counterparts.
    5. *Previous sibling receiving phototherapy*: This could be due to shared environmental and genetic factor or recurrent Rh and ABO hemolytic disease.

6. *Cephalhematoma or significant bruising* as extravasated RBCs has shortened half-life.
7. *Exclusive breastfeeding, particularly if nursing is not going well and weight loss is excessive (>12 percent of birthweight).*
8. *East Asian race:* Neonates of East Asian ethnicity has odds ratio of 3.1 for developing severe hyperbilirubinemia. This could be due to potential differences in incidence of G6PD deficiency and ABO hemolytic disease.

- **Minor risk factors** include: TSB in a high intermediate range (>75th and ≤95th percentile for age-in-hours), jaundice observed before discharge, macrosomic infant of a diabetic mother, polycythemia, male gender and maternal age ≥25 years.

In what situations do we need to investigate hyperbilirubinemia?

- Laboratory investigation for hyperbilirubinemia should be considered when total serum bilirubin concentrations are:
  - 4 mg/dl (68 mmol/l) or greater in cord blood,
  - Increasing at a rate of 0.5 mg/dL (9 mmol/l) or greater per hour over a 4 to 8-hour period,
  - Increasing at a rate of 5 mg/dL (86 mmol/l) or greater per day,
  - 13 to 15 mg/dL (222 to 257 mmol/l) or greater in full-term infants at any time,
  - 10 mg/dL (171 mmol/l) or greater in premature neonates at any time, or
  - When clinical jaundice persists beyond 10 to 14 days of life.
- Laboratory evaluation in a baby with jaundice should include
  - TSB and direct bilirubin levels, blood type (ABO, Rh), direct antiglobulin test, complete blood cell count with differential and smear for red cell morphology, reticulocyte count and serum albumin
  - G6PD enzyme assay if suggested by ethnic or geographic origin or if poor response to phototherapy. Urine for reducing substances–to rule out galactosemia.
  - If history and/or presentation suggest sepsis, blood culture, urine culture, cerebrospinal fluid for protein, glucose, cell count, and culture should be performed.

Discuss the management of neonatal hyperbilirubinemia.

A practice guideline has been given by American Academy of Pediatrics (AAP) for management of neonatal hyperbilirubinemia for babies more than 35 weeks of gestation. Cut-off for intensive phototherapy and exchange transfusion is shown in Figures 12.2 and 12.3. Isoimmune hemolytic disease, G6PD deficiency, asphyxia, significant lethargy, temperature instability, sepsis and hypoalbuminemia (<3 gm/dL) have been identified as risk factors which increases the risk of BIND and in presence of these risk factors the threshold for intervention should be at lower risk line than for the gestation specified category.

How do we decide the cut-offs for phototherapy and exchange transfusion in preterm babies?

Preterm babies have higher prevalence of hyperbilirubinemia and the course is more protracted due to several physiologic differences. For low birthweight babies cut-offs for phototherapy and exchange transfusion were given by Maisel (Table 12.2). In 2010, National Institute of Health and Clinical

Excellence (NICE) guidelines for neonatal jaundice for both term and preterm babies were introduced. These guidelines are useful in deciding gestation specific cut-offs for phototherapy and exchange (available at www.nice.org.uk/CG98). An example of such graph showing cut-off for phototherapy and exchange transfusion is shown in Figure 12.4.

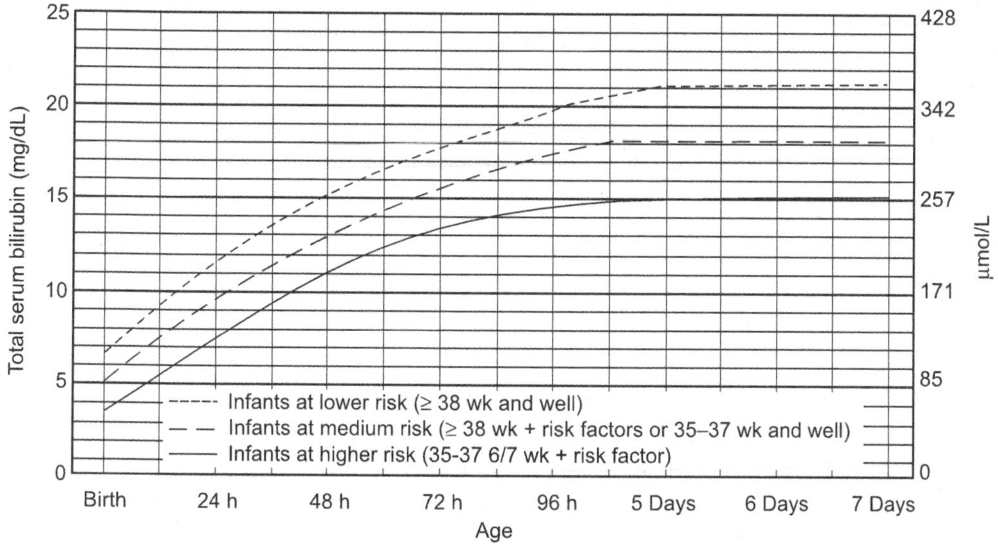

Fig. 12.2: Guidelines for phototherapy in neonates > 35 weeks of gestation

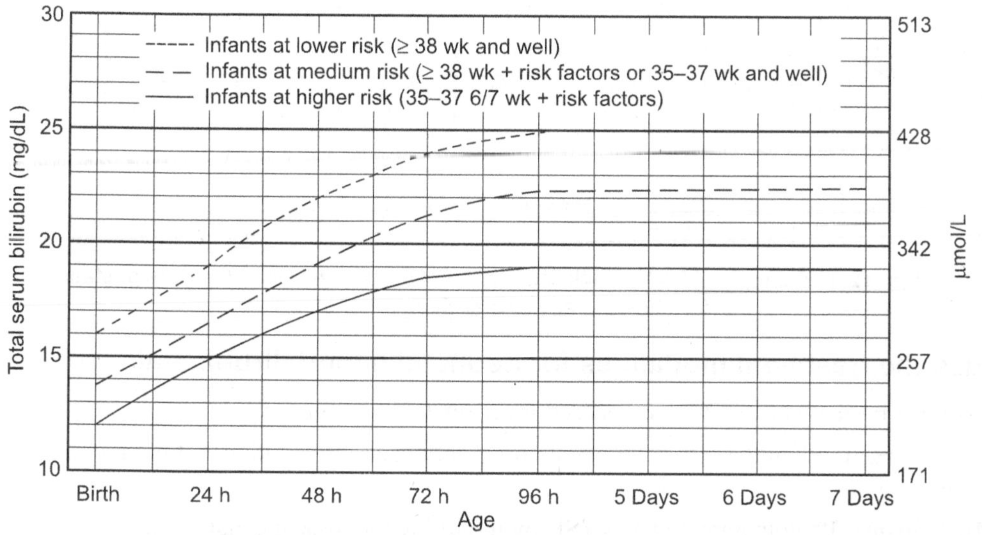

Fig. 12.3: Guidelines for exchange transfusion in babies >35 weeks of gestation

Table 12.2: Guidelines for phototherapy and exchange in low birthweight babies*

	Total bilirubin level [mg/dL(μmol/L)]	
	Phototherapy	**Exchange transfusion**
<1500 gm	5–8 (85–140)	13–16 (220–275)
1500–1999	8–12 (140–200)	16–18 (275–300)
2000–2499	11–14 (190–240)	18–20 (300–340)

*From Maisels

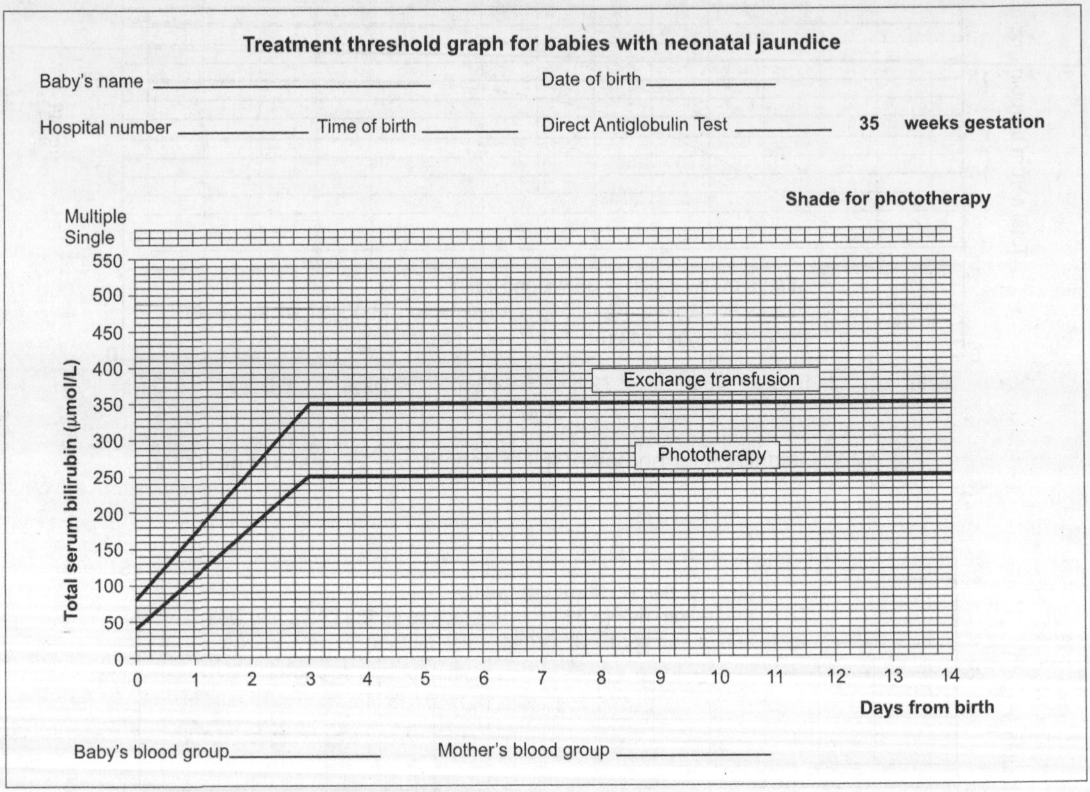

Fig. 12.4: Example of NICE Guidelines for cutoffs in a baby with 35 weeks gestation for phototherapy and exchange transfusion

Discuss the treatment modalities for neonatal hyperbilirubinemia.

There are two basic treatment modalities used for neonatal hyperbilirubinemia.

Phototherapy: Phototherapy is the most commonly used intervention to treat and prevent severe hyperbilirubinemia.

- **Mechanisms:** Phototherapy reduces TSB by the following three mechanisms:
  (i) **Structural isomerization to lumirubin:** Phototherapy converts bilirubin into lumirubin via structural isomerization, i.e., not reversible. Lumirubin, being more soluble substance than bilirubin, is excreted without conjugation into bile and urine.

(ii) **Photoisomerization to a less toxic bilirubin isomer:** Phototherapy converts the stable 4Z,15Z bilirubin isomer to the 4Z,15E isomer, which is more polar and less toxic than the 4Z,15Z form. Unlike structural isomerization to lumirubin, photoisomerization is reversible.

(iii) **Photo-oxidation to polar molecules:** Photo-oxidation reactions convert bilirubin to colorless, polar compounds that are excreted primarily in the urine. This is a slow process and accounts for a small proportion of bilirubin elimination.

- **Technique:** The dose of phototherapy, known as irradiance (measured in microW/cm^2/nm), determines its efficacy. Irradiance depends upon the type of the light used, distance between the light and infant, and the exposed surface area of the infant. Irradiance usually is expressed for a certain wavelength band (spectral irradiance). In *conventional phototherapy,* the irradiance is typically 6–12 microW/cm^2 of body surface area exposed per nm of wavelength (425–475 nm). *Intensive phototherapy* implies irradiance in the blue-green spectrum (wavelengths of approximately 430–490 nm) of at least 30 μW/cm^2 per nm (measured at the infant's skin directly below the center of the phototherapy unit) and delivered to as much of the infant's surface area as possible.
- **Guidelines to provide effective phototherapy:** A technical report from the American Academy of Pediatrics (AAP) summarized the key features to consider for providing effective phototherapy.
  - Emission of light in the blue-to-green range (460–490 nm).
  - Phototherapy light placed at a distance of 10–30 cm from the infant's body depending on the manufacturer's recommendation.
  - Irradiance of at least 30 microW/cm^2/nm.
  - Ability to illuminate maximal body surface area.
  - Demonstration of a decrease in TB during the first 4–6 hours of exposure.

1. **Exchange Transfusion:** Exchange transfusion is used to remove bilirubin from the circulation when intensive phototherapy fails or in infants with signs of bilirubin-induced neurologic dysfunction (BIND). If the TSB is at a level at which exchange transfusion is recommended (Fig. 12.3) or if the TSB level is 25 mg/dL or higher at any time, the infant should be admitted immediately and blood sample should be sent for cross match and blood arrangement for exchange transfusion. Exchange should be done by trained personnel under supervision of a neonatologist in Neonatal Intensive Care unit which is equipped with monitoring and resuscitation facility. Exchange should be done with Rh and ABO compatible blood with baby from CMV negative donor and preferably irradiated.

How to decide when to stop phototherapy?

There is no standard guideline for stopping phototherapy. It depends on age at onset of jaundice and cause of jaundice. In general phototherapy started during birth hospitalization is stopped when TSB is less than the level at which phototherapy was started. For babies who are re-admitted with maximum TSB level of 18 mg/dL or higher, phototherapy can be discontinued once level is below 13–14 mg/dL.

What are the indications of checking rebound bilirubin?

Indications of checking rebound bilirubin within 24 hours after discharge is recommended in the following situations:

- Hemolytic jaundice.
- When phototherapy is initiated early and discontinued before the infant is 3–4 days old.
- Preterm babies.
- Re-admission for hyperbilirubinemia (optional).

Babies need not to stay in hospital to check for rebound bilirubin.

What is the role of intravenous immunoglobulin?

Intravenous immunoglobulin has been shown to reduce the need of exchange transfusion in babies with Rh and ABO hemolytic disease. IVIG (dose 0.5–1 gm/kg over 2 hours) is recommended in infants with isoimmune hemolytic disease if the total serum or plasma bilirubin (TB) is rising despite intensive phototherapy or is within 2 or 3 mg/dL (34–51 μmol/L) of the threshold for exchange transfusion. The dose may be repeated in 12 hours if necessary. The mechanism is uncertain, but IVIG is thought to inhibit hemolysis by blocking antibody receptors on red blood cells.

CONCLUSIONS

Neonatal hyperbilirubinemia is common clinical condition and can be easily managed with intensive phototherapy. Few babies will require exchange transfusion. Bilirubin can be neurotoxic at higher level but early prediction with serum/transcutaneous bilirubin and risk factor based approach will identify the babies at risk and prevent bilirubin induced neurological dysfunction.

TAKE HOME MESSAGES

- Neonatal hyperbilirubinemia is very common neonatal problem requiring medical attention.
- Bilirubin can cause significant neurological dysfunction at higher concentration.
- Predischarge TSB/TcB assessment along with risk factor evaluation should be done in all babies.
- Phototherapy is the most commonly used intervention to treat and prevent severe hyperbilirubinemia. It is a safe and effective method to reduce the toxicity of bilirubin and increase its elimination.
- Exchange transfusions should be done in infants who exhibit clinical findings of bilirubin-induced neurologic dysfunction (BIND) or as per standard AAP guideline thresholds.

FURTHER READING

1. American Academy of Pediatrics, Subcommittee on Hyperbilirubinemia. Clinical practice guideline: Management of hyperbilirubinemia in the newborn infant 35 or more weeks of gestation. *Pediatrics* 2004;114:1297–1316.
2. Bhutani VK, Johnson L, Sivieri EM. Predictive ability of a predischarge hour-specific serum bilirubin for subsequent significant hyperbilirubinemia in healthy term and near-term newborns. *Pediatrics* 1999; 103:6–14.
3. Maisels MJ. Jaundice. In: Avery GB, Fletcher MA, MacDonald MG (eds): *Neonatology: Pathophysiology and Management of the Newborn*, 5th edn. Philadelphia: Lippincott Williams and Wilkins 1999:765–819.
4. Watchko JF. Kernicterus and the molecular mechanisms of bilirubin-induced CNS injury in newborns. *Neuromolec Med* 2006;8:513–529.

Chapter

13 Neonatal Sepsis

Sriparna Basu, Ashok Kumar

ABSTRACT

Despite the advances in neonatal care, neonatal sepsis remains a serious and potentially life-threatening disease globally. The signs and symptoms are often subtle and non-specific being clinically indistinguishable from various non-infectious conditions. If diagnosed early and managed with good supportive care and antibiotics, it is possible to save most cases of neonatal sepsis. The current practice of starting empirical antibiotic therapy in all neonates results in adverse drug effects, nosocomial complications, and emergence of resistant strains. Accurate and quick diagnosis is essential for both protecting the infant from the consequences of the bacterial invasion and preventing damages deriving from the unnecessary use of antibiotics. Proper antenatal care, maintenance of asepsis during delivery, promotion of breastfeeding, decreased interventions and health care hygiene are the best management strategies to reduce the incidence of neonatal sepsis and its sequelae.

Key Words: Clinical features, Diagnosis, Etiology, Neonatal sepsis, Nosocomal complications, Management, Prevention, Resistant strains.

INTRODUCTION

Neonatal sepsis is one of the most common causes of neonatal morbidity and mortality and is recognized as a global health challenge. Though most of the developing countries have witnessed a substantial decline in under-5 mortality, neonatal mortality has remained relatively constant, with an estimated 3.6 million annual neonatal deaths worldwide, accounting for about 40% of under-5 mortality. Over 90% of these deaths occur in the developing countries of Asia and Africa and the most common cause is suspected infections. Each year, approximately 1 million deaths occurring in the neonatal period are caused by sepsis, accounting for approximately 25% of global neonatal deaths and 10% of under-5 mortality.

Despite recent advances in the management of neonatal sepsis, including use of an array of sophisticated biomarkers to diagnose sepsis and use of potent antibiotics, timely identification continues to be a challenge in the management of high-risk neonates. Presentation with subtle and non-specific clinical signs and symptoms either delay the diagnosis and initiation of therapy or leads to over diagnosis and unnecessary use of antibiotics resulting in emergence of drug resistance.

CASE SCENARIO

A 2200 gm term low birthweight male newborn was delivered via normal spontaneous vaginal delivery to a 25-year-old G1P0 syphilis/TORCH/HIV non-reactive, hepatitis B surface antigen negative mother with early preeclampsia. Rupture of membranes occurred 36 hours prided temperature was 39.2 °C on two occasions). She did not receive any intrapartum antibiotic prophylaxis. The baby did not require any delivery room resuscitation. 1 and 5 min Apgar scores were 8/10 and 9/10, respectively. He was handed over to the mother from labor room for breastfeeding. At 4 hours of life the attendants brought the baby to NICU for rapid breathing and poor sucking efforts.

On examination, the vital signs of the baby were T: 37, HR: 140, RR: 74, capillary refill time <3 s, and oxygen saturation of 90–94% in room air. The color of the infant was pink with persistent grunting, retractions, and lethargy. Her fontanel was soft and flat. Heart examination was normal. Bilateral air entry into chest was equal. Abdomen was soft and without any palpable masses. Neurological examination showed normal tone and a weak, intermittent cry.

Laboratory investigations showed CBC with WBC: 3,200, 22% bands, Hb: 15, Hct: 43, platelets: 168,000, blood glucose 52. The chest X-ray was rotated with bilateral diffuse infiltrates and a normal cardiac silhouette. Arterial blood gas (ABG) analysis showed a pH 7.31, PCO_2 43, PO_2 54, BE-4. CSF examination showed 20 WBCs, 1% neutrophils, 17% lymphocytes, 82% monocytes, glucose 39 against blood glucose of 54 mg/dL, protein 103, gram stain shows no organisms. Serum electrolytes were normal. Blood culture report was available after 48 hours and was sterile.

A diagnosis of early-onset sepsis with intrauterine pneumonia in a term low birthweight baby was kept and the infant was managed accordingly.

CRITICAL CASE ANALYSIS

The risk factors for sepsis in this infant were low birthweight, prolonged rupture of membrane, and maternal fever without any intrapartum antibiotic prophylaxis. Though the initial *in utero* to *ex utero* transition was normal, the baby developed respiratory distress with X-ray features suggestive of intrauterine pneumonia. Positive sepsis screen further confirmed the case. Lumbar puncture and CSF examination was done to rule out meningitis as he had alteration of tone and weak cry. It is common for the blood culture to be sterile as the culture positivity rate is 30–40%. Other investigations, such as ABG, blood glucose, serum electrolytes were done to guide the need for respiratory assistance and supportive care.

INTERACTIVE TOPIC REVIEW

What is the definition of neonatal sepsis?

Neonatal sepsis is classically defined as a clinical syndrome characterized by signs and symptoms of infection with or without accompanying bacteremia in the first 28 days of life. It includes various systemic infections of the newborn, such as septicemia, meningitis, pneumonia, osteo-articular infections, urinary tract infections, endophthalmitis etc.

What are the diagnostic criteria for neonatal sepsis?

In 2005, the International Pediatric Sepsis Consensus Conference defined sepsis as a "systemic inflammatory response syndrome (SIRS) in the presence of or as a result of suspected or proven infection".

A SIRS is considered present if at least two of the following four criteria are observed, one of the two being abnormal temperature or leukocyte count:

- Core temperature of > 38.5°C or < 36°C.
- Tachycardia, or bradycardia for children younger than 1 year old.
- Mean respiratory rate of more than 2 standard deviations above normal for age or mechanical ventilation for an acute process not related to underlying neuromuscular disease or the need for general anesthesia.
- Leukocyte count elevated or depressed for age (not secondary to chemotherapy-induced leukopenia) or more than 10% immature neutrophils.

These diagnostic criteria were developed to improve the diagnosis of pediatric sepsis, from newborns to adolescents up to 18 years of age, though the validitiy of these criteria has not been well proven in neonatal sepsis.

Recent researches have shown that monitoring of heart rate characteristics (HRC) may be an early indicator of clinical instability in neonates with sepsis. In a recent study, neonates with culture-proven sepsis had a statistically higher HRC during the 24 hours preceding the septic episode, compared to healthy controls which suggest that HRC is able to serve as an early warning sign of impending clinical instability. Reduced variability and transient decelerations in heart rate may also be seen.

How do you classify neonatal sepsis?

Neonatal sepsis has been classified into early onset sepsis (EOS) and late onset sepsis (LOS). Early-onset neonatal sepsis (EOS) has been variably defined based on the age at onset, with bacteremia or bacterial meningitis occurring at ≤3 days in preterm infants hospitalized in the neonatal intensive care units (NICU) (American Academy of Pediatrics definition) to ≤7 days in term infants (Centers for Disease Control definition based on epidemiology studies). Early onset neonatal infections of viral or fungal etiology may also occur at <7 days of life and must be distinguished from bacterial sepsis.

Late onset sepsis (LOS) is bacteremia or bacterial meningitis occurring after 72 hours in NICU infants and 7 days of life in term infants (variably defined as occurring up to the age of <90 or 120 days).

This classification is helpful to guide the antibiotic therapy as it implies differences in the presumed mode of transmission and predominant organisms. Typically, EOS is considered maternally-acquired, usually from the maternal genital tract before or during delivery, and LOS is generally regarded to originate from the care-giving environment – either a health care or community setting. As a result, EOS and LOS are associated with different sets of pathogens.

In developed countries the cumulative incidence of EOS is 0.98 per 1000 live births. However, the incidence increases with decreasing birthweight. Very-low-birthweight (VLBW, <1500 gm birth-weight) infants have a cumulative incidence of EOS of 11 per 1000 live births. Of those who survive >3 days, 21% will have an episode of LOS.

What are the risk factors for neonatal sepsis?

The risk factors for early onset sepsis include:

- Very low birthweight (<1500 gm), prematurity (<35 weeks of gestation)
- Premature rupture of membranes
- Chorioamnionitis*
- Prolonged rupture of membranes (>24 hours)
- Foul smelling liquor
- Multiple (≥3) per vaginum examinations in 24 hours
- Intrapatum maternal fever (>37.8°C)
- Difficult or prolonged labor (≥24 hours)
- Multiple gestation.

* Chorioamnionitis is defined as intrapartum maternal fever (temperature >37.8°C between onset of labor to delivery) with two or more of the following: Fetal tachycardia, uterine tenderness, prolonged (>24 h) rupture of membrane, malodorous vaginal discharge, or maternal blood leucocytosis (>15,000 leucocytes/µL).

Late onset sepsis is caused by the organisms thriving in the external environment of the home or the hospital. The infection is often transmitted through the hands of the care-providers. The associated factors of late onset sepsis include:

- Very low birthweight, prematurity
- Poor maintenance of asepsis in neonatal unit including improper hand washing techniques
- Lack of breastfeeding
- Delayed enteral feeding
- Prolonged hospitalization
- Poor hygiene
- Frequent handling
- Superficial infections (pyoderma, umbilical sepsis, ophthalmia neonatorum)
- Disruption of skin integrity with needle pricks and use of intravenous fluids
- Prolonged indwelling catheter use
- Invasive procedures
- Ventilator associated pneumonia
- Prolonged antibiotics (use of broad-spectrum antibiotics predispose the infants to fulgal sepsis).

What are the common etiological agents of EOS and LOS?

EOS: The leading cause of EOS is gram-negative enteric bacilli including Escherichia coli and Klebsiella pneumoniae. Other etiological agents include Pseudomonas aeruginosa, Enterobacter, Listeria, Acinetobacter baumannii, Citrobacter, Staphylococcus aureus, Enterococcus etc. Group B Streptoccous (GBS), the leading cause of EOS in developed countries is isolated less commonly in India.

LOS: Common organisms include Staph aureus, Coagulase-negative Staph (CONS), Enterococcus, E. coli, Klebsiella, and Pseudomonas). Fungal infections by different species of Candida, such as C. albicans, C. parapsilosis, C. tropicalis, C. glabrata etc. are common causes of LOS in very low birth weight infants.

What are the signs and symptoms of sepsis?

The signs and symptoms of neonatal sepsis are non-specific and may be highly variable (Table 13.1). A high index of suspicion is required for early diagnosis especially in a tiny preterm neonate. Mothers are usually very perceptive about the subtle changes in the behavior and activity of their neonates and their concerns of "just not looking right" should not be ignored. Common presenting feature of EOS is intra-uterine pneumonia and common presenting features of LOS lethargy and poor feeding. Meningitis is more common with LOS. Neonatal sepsis can also be complicated by metastatic foci of infection, disseminated intravascular coagulation, congestive heart failure, refractory shock and sclerema. Common signs and symptoms of sepsis include hypo/hyperthermia, respiratory distress/apnea, tachycardia, refusal to feed, feeding intolerance, lethargy or irritability, poor/high pitched cry, altered sensorium, hypo/hypertonia, seizures, bulging fontanel, hypotension/poor perfusion, capillary refill time over 3 seconds, bleeding episodes, diarrhea/vomiting, abdominal distention, hepatosplenomegaly, poor weight gain, unexplained jaundice, renal failure (suspected in presence of unexplained weight gain, oliguria, increase blood urea and serum creatinine) etc. In cases of doubt, careful observation along with meticulous examination, and sepsis workup should be done to exclude sepsis. Irritability or high-pitched crying, fever, seizures, blank look, neck retraction or bulging anterior fontanel are highly suggestive of meningitis.

Sclerema is characterized by hardening of the skin that gets bound down to the underlying muscle and bone, hindering respiration and feeding. Skin biopsy shows thickening of the trabeculae supporting the subcutaneous adipose tissue and a sparse inflammatory infiltrate of lymphocytes, histiocytes and multinucleate giant cells. It has a high case fatality rate. Management consists of appropriate antibiotics and supportive management.

Table 13.1: Signs and symptoms of sepsis

General

- Lethargy, poor cry, refusal to suck
- Brady/tachycardia
- Hypothermia or fever (less common)
- Poor perfusion, prolonged capillary refill time
- Metabolic acidosis
- Hypo/hyperglycemia
- Hypotonia, absent neonatal reflexes.

Specific features related to various systems

- **Respiratory:** Respiratory distress, apnea or gasping respiration
- **CNS:** Bulging anterior fontanel, vacant stare, high-pitched cry, excess irritability, stupor/coma, seizures, neck retraction
- **Cardiac:** Hypotension, poor perfusion, shock

Contd...

Contd...

- **Gastrointestinal:** Feed intolerance, vomiting, abdominal distension, paralytic ileus, diarrhea, necrotizing enterocolitis (NEC)
- **Hepatic:** Hepatomegaly, neonatal hyperbilirubinemia
- **Renal:** Acute renal failure
- **Hematological:** Bleeding, petechiae, purpura
- **Skin changes:** Multiple pustules, abscess, sclerema, mottling, umbilical redness and discharge.

How do you diagnose neonatal sepsis?

Making an early, accurate, and rapid diagnosis of neonatal sepsis remains a major diagnostic challenge to the neonatologists. It is difficult to get an ideal diagnostic biomarker for neonatal sepsis which will be excellent in statistical validity, the levels will change early in the disease course and remain altered for a prolonged period of time, to optimize clinical management, monitor disease progress, and guide antimicrobial treatment. Isolation of microorganisms from blood, CSF, urine, pleural fluid or other body fluids is diagnostic of sepsis. Though blood culture is the gold standard, the positivity varies from 30–40% even in best centers. False negative results may arise from insufficient or missing living bacteria in the sample resulting from low specimen volume, transient bacteremia, administration of antibiotics prior to sampling, intrapartum antibiotics to the mother etc. Blood culture should be sent prior to the starting of antibiotics in clinically suspected cases. Inoculation of at least 1 mL of blood is necessary for adequate and appropriate growth. The ideal ratio of blood to culture medium should be 1:10. It also takes at least 48 hours to get the initial culture report in conventional blood culture techniques. A proper aseptic technique should be followed while collecting blood to avoid contamination.

There are a variety of tests which provide indirect evidence for sepsis and are helpful for screening of neonates with sepsis.

- Total leukocyte count (TLC) below 5000/μL.
- An absolute neutrophil count (ANC) of <1800/μL. In neonates neutropenia is more predictive of neonatal sepsis than neutrophilia.
- Immature neutrophils (Band cells + myelocytes + metamyelocytes) to total neutrophils ratio (1TR) >0.20.
- Micro-ESR > 15 mm during first hour.
- Thrombocytopenia (platelet count <150000/μL).
- C-reactive protein (CRP): A CRP value of >10 mg/L is taken as positive.

Among these parameters, a battery of 5 tests including leukopenia, neutropenia, I/T ratio, micro ESR and CRP are often used to rule out sepsis when clinical suspicion of sepsis is high and/or one or more risk factors of sepsis are present. It is commonly known as **"sepsis screen"**. Sepsis screen is considered positive, when two or more tests are positive. Two consecutive negative sepsis screen can reasonably rule out sepsis and antibiotics can be stopped if already started. If the quantitative CRP alone is highly positive or any two parameters of the sepsis screen are positive, a blood culture must be drawn and empirical antibiotics must be started in a symptomatic neonate.

CSF Examination for Diagnosing Meningitis

Lumbar puncture (LP) and CSF examination must be performed in all neonates with suspected LOS and in cases of EOS with suspected meningitis preferably before the starting of antibiotics. Apart from culture and gram stain, other commonly evaluated parameters are total WBC count/µL, percentage neutrophil count, glucose and protein. It should be remembered that a normal newborn may have 0–32 cells and 120–170 mg/dL of protein in CSF. In preterm infants cut-off values of CSF suggestive of meningitis may be in higher side. The WBC cell count must be performed within 30 minutes of drawing CSF. CSF WBC and glucose rapidly fall with time, giving spurious results. LP can be deferred until clinical stabilization is achieved. The cellular and biochemical abnormalities in the CSF with bacterial meningitis persist for up to 3 days. Gram-positive bacteria clear in 36 hours of appropriate therapy whereas gram-negative bacteria may take up to 5 days to get sterilized.

Other Investigations

Other investigations should be done according to the presenting symptoms. Chest X-ray is done in cases of respiratory distress or apnea. Abdominal X-ray should be done for diagnosis of necrotizing enterocolitis. Some investigations are also necessary for supportive management, such as blood glucose, electrolytes, liver function and renal function tests, arterial blood gas analysis, ultrasonography of abdomen and cranium, echocardiography and color Doppler, magnetic resonance imaging of brain etc.

What are the biomarkers used to diagnose neonatal sepsis?

The biomarkers which are currently in use are summarized below:

A. Acute-Phase Reactants

CRP and procalcitonin are the two most commonly used acute-phase reactants in neonatal sepsis. Serum amyloid A is used less frequently.

C-reactive Protein

CRP is produced in liver and the levels start rising within 6 to 8 hours of infection and peak at 24 hours. Inflammation induced by sepsis triggers the release of IL-6, which stimulates an increase in CRP concentrations. The most commonly used cut-off of CRP is 10 mg/L. An increasing CRP level is a better predictor than an individual value. Two normal CRP reports (8–24 hours after birth and 24 hours later) provide strong evidence against bacterial sepsis and antibiotics can be safely discontinued. Serial CRP levels in combination with the absolute and TLC and I/T ratio has been widely used as a negative predictor of sepsis 24–48 hours after the onset of symptoms. CRP is also a reliable marker to monitor progress or guide the duration of antibiotic treatment. It should be remembered that a variety of non-infectious neonatal conditions such as meconium aspiration syndrome, perinatal asphyxia, hemolysis, exposure to glucocorticoids, tissue injury, or surgery can also increase CRP concentrations.

Procalcitonin

Procalcitonin is the peptide prohormone of calcitonin and is an acute phase reactant, associated with the immunomodulation and vascular response of systemic inflammatory response syndrome (SIRS). It is produced by monocytes and hepatocytes. Unlike CRP, it is an early marker of infection, the concentrations increase early within 2–4 hours, after an exposure to a bacterial pathogen during the acute stage of sepsis. Levels peak at 6–8 hours and remain elevated for the next 24 hours, with a half-life of 24–30 hours. Moreover, procalcitonin responses and its concentrations are not affected by the gestational age. The diagnostic utility of PCT in EOS is high, and is useful for the clinicians for the diagnostic workup of a neonate. Moreover, compared to tumor necrosis factor alpha (TNF-α) and interleukin (IL)-6, serum procalcitonin remains high making it more useful in predicting the severity of infection and response to treatment. A positive PCT level is >2.5 ng/mL.

However, reliability of procalcitonin as a single biomarker of neonatal infection is limited by its non-specific elevations in healthy neonates over the first 48 hours of life and in other non-infective conditions such as intracranial hemorrhage, birth asphyxia, and neonatal hypoxemic conditions. When combined with CRP, the diagnostic utility of procalcitonin is high.

Serum Amyloid A

Serum amyloid A (SAA) is an apolipoprotein produced in the liver and is an early acute phase reactant released as a response to infection and injury. SAA is derived from a variety of other tissues such as endothelial cells, monocytes, and smooth muscle cells and regulated by cytokines IL-1, IL-6 and TNF-α. It is a reliable screening marker throughout the first 24 hours after the onset of infection, when compared to other biomarkers such as CRP and IL-6. Serum levels of SAA show greater accuracy in the early suspicion of sepsis and are inversely associated with neonatal mortality and infection, enhancing their reliability and potential to prognosticate mortality in the early phase of an acute infection. Serum levels of SAA have a wide range, which increase with age. SAA levels may be affected by hepatic function and host nutritional status, which may limit usefulness in late neonatal sepsis where hepatic dysfunction and nutritional status may be decreased.

B. Cytokines

Cytokines are cellular signaling proteins that play a crucial role in modulating the host immunological response to infection. As functionally classified, cytokines may be proinflammatory, multiple function and anti-inflammatory. Pro-inflammatory cytokines include interferon-gamma, TNF-α, inducible protein -10 (IP-10), and IL-2, IL-6, IL-8, IL-12, and IL-17. Multiple function inflammatory cytokines include IL-1β, monocyte chemoattractant protein (MCP-1), soluble CD40 ligand (sCD40L) and growth factors, IL-3, granulocyte-colony stimulating factors and their secondary mediators, nitric oxide, thromboxanes, leukotrienes, platelet-activating factor, prostaglandins, and complements. Anti-inflammatory cytokines include IL-4, IL-10, tumor necrosis factor soluble receptor, IL-1 receptor alpha, and transforming growth factor beta 2 (TGF- β2). The evolution of disease and clinical symptoms during neonatal sepsis such as SIRS, disseminated intravascular coagulation (DIC), septic shock, multiple organ dysfunction syndrome, and complement activated response syndrome is dependent upon a complex and delicate balance between the pro-inflammatory, anti-inflammatory, and multiple function cytokines based on their final effect on the immune system, as a result of the activation of the coagulation and complement cascade and the production of prostaglandins, leukotrienes, proteases, and oxidants.

Blood levels of cytokines change rapidly in the setting of neonatal sepsis even before the newborn develops signs or symptoms of sepsis and the rise of acute phase reactants. Several cytokines like interleukin-1β (IL-Iβ), interleukin-6 (IL-6), interleukin-8 (IL-8), interleukin-2 soluble receptor (SIL2R), and tumor necrosis factor-α (TNF-α) have been studied most commonly. As the cytokines do not cross placental barrier, their elevations in umbilical cord blood suggest the possibility of predicting the development of EOS. Later on, cytokine analysis is also useful in predicting LOS.

IL-6

IL-6 is considered an early and sensitive marker of neonatal infection. IL-6 concentrations rise before that of CRP in response to exposure to bacterial endotoxins and a consistent increase in umbilical cord blood IL-6 is documented in newborns with EOS. However, the half-life of IL-6 is short and the levels fall to undetectable values quickly with treatment. The diagnostic accuracy can be further improved by combining IL-6 and CRP in first 48 hours of presumed clinical sepsis.

TNF-α

TNF-α has a very similar kinetics to IL-6. The concentrations of TNF-α are shown to be significantly higher in infected compared to non-infected neonates in multiple studies.

IL-8

IL-8 is produced by monocytes, macrophages, and endothelial cells as a result of infection and has kinetics similar to IL-6. It helps in the activation and chemotaxis of neutrophils. It not only serves as a marker for sepsis but the increase in concentration is also associated with severity of infection.

C. Cell Surface Markers

Circulating inflammatory cells, including, neutrophils, lymphocytes, monocytes, and natural killer cells express cell surface antigens, after activation by microbial products, that can be detected by flow cytometric technology and used as diagnostic markers for sepsis. Several cell surface antigens such as CD11b, CD14, CD64, CD32, CD16, CD69, and sCD163 have been identified to be promising in the detection of congenital sepsis, as well as early and late onset neonatal sepsis. Among them, neutrophil CD64 and CD11b appear to be promising markers for the diagnosis of both EOS and LOS. CD64 is a high affinity Fc receptor for immunoglobulin G that increases expression in response to infection. Neutrophil CD64 is a highly sensitive marker for neonatal sepsis with a sensitivity of 80%, a specificity of 79%, and a cut-off value of 4.02. CD11b is a subunit of the β2 integrin adhesion molecule, normally expressed at a very low concentration on the surface of non-activated neutrophils. There is a 2 to 4-fold increase in neutrophil CD11b expression in infants with blood culture positive sepsis.

D. Granulocyte Colony-Stimulating Factor

Granulocyte colony-stimulating factor (GCSF), a mediator produced by bone marrow, facilitates proliferation and differentiation of neutrophils, and has been proposed to be a reliable infection marker for early diagnosis of neonatal sepsis. A concentration $\geq$ 200 pg/mL has a sensitivity of 95%, and negative predictive value 99% for predicting early onset neonatal bacterial and fungal infections.

Other recent biomarkers of interest that are being explored include pentraxin 3 (PTX3), angiopoietins, suPAR, and soluble triggering receptor expressed on myeloid cells-1 (sTREM-1).

E. Molecular Genetics

Emerging molecular techniques have revolutionized the diagnostic approach to neonatal sepsis. These techniques use multiplex platforms that can measure different markers such as protein, deoxyribonucleic acid (DNA), ribonucleic acid (RNA), 16 S rRNA and miRNA using technologies such as fluorescence in situ hybridization (FISH) and quantitative polymerase chain reaction (qPCR).

qPCR is a rapid test that can be used to detect bacterial DNA in body fluids of the host suspected of having an infection. PCR is based on the fact that the bacteria specific 16S rRNA gene is highly conserved in all bacterial genomes, and so it can be a useful marker for identification of bacteria in clinical samples. FISH can significantly reduce the time required to identify organisms isolated in culture. The use of the probe-based specific qPCR can reduce diagnostic time, help in identifying bacterial species, and improve specificity and positive predictive value. Amplification targeting of 16S rRNA gene is a potentially valuable clinical tool in samples with low copy numbers of bacterial DNA, as this gene is present in 1 to more than 10 copies in all bacterial genomes. The gene also has a number of divergent regions nested within it, so PCR can be targeted for species-specific detection of bacteria in clinical samples. PCR is reported to be a very sensitive (100%), and rapid method for detecting potential pathogens in amniotic fluid and adverse neonatal outcomes. Early exclusion of bacterial infection could help to reduce overuse of antibiotics.

However, during analysis it is necessary to remove small amounts of inherent residual DNA present in the reagents, which may be coamplified, resulting in false positivity. Methods for the removal of potential background contaminations include long wave UV light gamma irradiation DNAse, restriction endonuclease digestion, ultra filtration, and low DNA polymerases. Moreover, detection by PCR does not yield the antimicrobial sensitivity pattern of the pathogen. Real time PCR combined with DNA Micro Array technology may allow not only identification of the organism but also the antimicrobial sensitivity pattern, which is so critical to clinical care.

F. Omics Technology (Genomics, Proteomics, Metabolomics)

Current advances in "omics" research present new opportunities to provide rapid information related to expression of a large number of proteins or functioning metabolites characteristic for neonatal sepsis. These available technologies unify multiple levels of information, such as, genomic, proteomic, and metabolomics to form a more complete understanding of of host physiology and sepsis. Genomics technology helps to identify the genes that demonstrate altered regulation during infection. Proteomic and metabolomics profiling technologies provide insight into the functional expression of proteins or metabolites present in a biological sample. Proteomic processing technology involves separation of proteins based on intrinsic properties such as molecular weight, isoelectric point, or affinity to metals or antibodies. Metabolomics is a dynamic and functional technology which uses spectrometric techniques such as nuclear magnetic resonance and mass spectrometry to provide a window to gene and environmental interactions in neonatal sepsis in a variety of samples blood, urine, saliva or tissue.

What precisely is the statistical validity of sepsis screen and other adjunctive tests?

Table 13.2 provides the said information.

Table 13.2: Statistical validity of sepsis screen and other adjunctive tests of neonatal sepsis

Test	Sensitivity	Specificity	LR^+	LR^-
Total WBC count	44	92	5.5	0.60
Absolute neutrophil count (ANC)	84	34	5.0	0.74
I:T ratio	54.6	73.7	2.07	0.61
CRP	70–93	78–94	3.18–15.5	0.07
Thrombocytopenia	22	99	2.72	0.78

Contd...

Contd...

Any 2 + ve of: ITR > 0.2 TLC < 5000/cumm CRP > 8 mg/L ESR > 15 mm/1st h Haptoglobulin >25 mg/dL	93	88	7.8	0.08
Any 2 + ve of: TLC < 5000/cumm ITR > 0.2 CRP > 1 mg/dL	100	83	5.9	0
Procalcitonin	92	97	6.9	0.19
Interleukin-6	87	93	12.42	0.14
Interleukin-8	91	93	13	0.10
Tumor necrotic factor-α	75	88	6.25	0.28

How do you manage neonatal sepsis?

Though the mainstay of management of sepsis is appropriate antibiotic therapy, attention should also be given to basic supportive care of a sick neonate. The infant should be nursed in a thermoneutral environment to avoid hypothermia or hyperthermia. Oxygen saturation should be maintained in the range 90–94%, and CPAP/mechanical ventilation should be initiated, if required. The infant should be regularly monitored for hypoglycemia/hyperglycemia. Colloids and inotropes are used for maintaining normal blood pressure and tissue perfusion. Nutrition should be maintained by parenteral nutrition. Enteral feeding should be initiated as soon as the baby is hemodynamically stable. Injection vitamin K, packed cells, fresh frozen plasma and platelet transfusion should be used appropriately for the management of anemia and bleeding diathesis. Other organ dysfunctions, such as acute kidney injury, cholestasis etc. should be managed appropriately. Unconjugated hyperbilirubinemia, if present, should be managed with phototherapy and/or exchange transfusion as per standard guidelines.

Antibiotic Treatment

Commonly used antibiotics to treat neonatal sepsis include beta-lactams such as ampicillin, cloxacillin, and cefotaxime; extended-spectrum beta-lactams such as piperacillin-tazobactam; and the carbapenem meropenem. These are bactericidal agents and act by inhibition of the synthesis of the peptidoglycan layer of the bacterial cell wall. Additional antimicrobial classes used for neonatal sepsis include the glycopeptide vancomycin and aminoglycosides. Vancomycin acts through a time-dependent killing process, by inhibiting key peptide subunits from being incorporated into the peptidoglycan bacterial cell wall layer, thus inhibiting cell wall synthesis and is bactericidal for gram-positive organisms. Aminoglycosides bind to the bacterial 30S ribosomal subunit, thus inhibiting protein synthesis. They exert a concentration-dependent killing effect that could be bacteriostatic or bactericidal. Both glycopeptide and aminoglycoside require therapeutic drug monitoring to achieve the correct dose and limit toxicity, mainly ototoxicity and nephrotoxicity.

Management of neonatal fungal infections includes the use of polyenes such as amphotericin B and liposomal amphotericin B, azoles such as fluconazole, and the echinocandins, including caspofungin and micafungin. The polyenes bind to the fungal cell membrane component ergosterol, forming a transmembrane channel that causes leakage of key ions, leading to fungal cell death. Fluconazole inhibits the fungal cytochrome P450 enzyme, thus preventing the conversion of lanosterol to ergosterol, which is essential to the fungal cell membrane; it is primarily a fungistatic agent. Echinocandins act on the fungal cell wall by noncompetitive inhibition of the enzyme (1,3)-D-glucan synthase and can be both fungistatic and fungicidal.

Empirical Antibiotic Therapy

The appropriate empirical antibiotic selection is based on the likely etiologic pathogens based on epidemiologic surveillance. Once blood and, CSF and/or urine samples (collected on clinical suspicion of meningitis and UTI, especially in LOS) are obtained, the combination of ampicillin or cloxacillin and gentamicin is the most appropriate coverage for the common organisms which predominate as etiologic pathogens. If there is concern of meningitis and while awaiting final cultures and susceptibilities, cefotaxime may be added as an agent empirically in stead of aminoglycosides, as CSF penetration of amnoglycosed is poor.. The highly protein-bound agent ceftriaxone is not recommended for neonates with concerns of meningitis due to the risk of acute bilirubin encephalopathy from displacement of free bilirubin from albumin by the drug. It has also been rarely associated with biliary sludging, pseudolithiasis, nephrolithiasis, and pulmonary impairment due to precipitation with calcium ions in neonates with both elevated and normal serum calcium concentrations. In presence of positive culture reports, the further antibiotics therapy should be based on the sensitivity reports. The doses of commonly used empirical antimicrobials in neonatal sepsis are summarized in Table 13.3.

In suspected sepsis by extended-spectrum beta-lactamase (ESBL) producers, such as nosocomial *E. coli* and *Klebsiella pneumoniae* infections, beta-lactam antibiotics, including penicillins, cephalosporins, monobactam aztreonam and most of the aminoglycosides are ineffective, as most ESBL producers demonstrate resistance against these antimicrobials.

Table 13.3: Intravenous antibiotic therapy for neonatal sepsis

Antibiotics in neonatal sepsis	Each dose
Inj Ampicillin (50 mg/kg/dose)	12 hrly (<7 days), 8 hrly (>7 days)
OR	
Inj cloxacillin (50 mg/kg/ dose)	12 hrly (<7 days), 8 hrly (>7 days)
AND	
Inj Gentamicin (5 mg/kg/dose)	24 hrly
OR	
Inj Amikacin (15 mg/kg/dose)	24 hrly

Contd...

Contd...

Antibiotics in meningitis	Each dose
Inj Ampicillin (100 mg/kg/dose)	12 hrly (<7 days), 8 hrly (>7 days)
AND	
Inj cefotaxime (50 mg/kg/ dose)	12 hrly (<7 days), 8 hrly (>7 days)
OR	
Inj cefotaxime (50 mg/kg/ dose)	12 hrly (<7 days), 8 hrly (>7 days)
AND	
Inj Gentamicin (2.5 mg/kg/dose)	12 hrly (<7 days), 8 hrly (>7 days)

How do you optimize the response to therapy and duration of treatment?

In culture positive cases: In most cases infants respond to treatment clinically in the first 24–48 hours of effective antibiotic treatment. Within 72 hours, TLC trends toward normal, I:T ratio improves, and the level of CRP tends to normalize. At 72 hours, repeat blood, CSF, and urine cultures are usually become negative. The treatment duration for culture-proven sepsis varies from at least 10–14 days based on the organism, and in presence of meningitis, the duration should be 21 days or more. Antimicrobial courses may be prolonged if there are complications, such as brain abscesses, osteomyelitis, or endocarditis.

In culture negative cases: In many cases, an etiologic agent is not identified in cultures and antibiotics are started empirically on the basis of clinical suspicion. In these cases, continuation of empirical antimicrobial therapy with ongoing monitoring of the infant is warranted. Often, an empirical 10-day course of antimicrobial therapy is completed. Serial TLC and CRP measurements may help evaluate clinical severity and/or response to empirical treatment which should decline with treatment. The choice of antimicrobial regimen should be based initially on epidemiologic empirical coverage and on clinical response. When cultures drawn prior to initiation of antimicrobial therapy remain negative and the neonate is otherwise well appearing, discontinuation of antimicrobial therapy at 48 hours is recommended. Strong suspicion should be given to the possibility of viral infections, such as HSV, in the setting of a severely ill neonate with negative cultures.

What is the role of adjuvant immunotherapy in neonatal sepsis?

Immunotherapy is often used as an adjuvant for the prevention and treatment of neonatal sepsis. An array of products has been evaluated including intravenous immunoglobulin, myeloid colony stimulating factors, probiotics, glutamine supplementation, recombinant human protein C, and lactoferrin. However, for most of these therapies tested to date, clinical trials have failed to demonstrate a significant effect in neonatal outcomes.

Immunoglobulins

Newborn infants, particularly very low birthweight or preterm neonates, are deficient in IgG, which binds to cell surface receptors, provides opsonic activity, activates complement fixation, promotes antibody dependent cytotoxicity, improves neutrophil phagocytosis and enhance the release of stored neutrophils. Intravenous immunoglobulin (IVIG) is, therefore, a theoretically attractive strategy, with multiple mechanisms of action. However, the recent famous International Neonatal Immunotherapy Study (INIS) using non-specific intravenous immunoglobulin therapy for suspected or proven neonatal sepsis in an international, placebo controlled, multicenter randomised trial, failed to document any beneficial effect of IVIG.

Pentoxifylline

In animal models of sepsis, pentoxifylline, a phosphodiesterase inhibitor, is found to inhibit production of TNF, preserve micro-vascular blood flow, prevent circulatory failure and intestinal vaso-constriction and improves survival. Cochrane Database Syst Rev 2015 from six small studies suggests that the use of pentoxifylline as an adjunct to antibiotics in neonatal sepsis decreases mortality without any adverse effects. Large well-designed multicenter trials are needed to confirm or refute the effectiveness of pentoxifylline in reducing mortality and adverse outcomes in neonates with suspected or confirmed neonatal sepsis and NEC.

Cytokines

Other adjunctive strategies for prophylaxis or treatment of neonatal sepsis include use of the recombinant cytokines Granulocyte Colony Stimulating Factor (G-CSF) or Granulocyte-Macrophage Colony Stimulating Factor (GM-CSF) to prevent neutropenia. However, no systematic reviews of RCTs of these agents are yet available. In RCTs of G-CSF therapy, a trend to reduced mortality was observed which was not statistically significant.

Lactoferrin

Lactoferrin, a normal component of human colostrum and milk, is used in clinical trials to enhance host defense in sepsis and necrotizing enterocolitis (NEC) in preterm neonates. As per Cochrane Database Syst Rev 2015, moderate to low quality evidence suggests that oral lactoferrin prophylaxis with or without probiotics, decreases late-onset sepsis and NEC stage II or greater in preterm infants without adverse effects. Clarifications regarding optimum dosing regimens, type of lactoferrin (human or bovine), and long-term outcomes are still needed.

Probiotics

Probiotic bacteria are live microbial supplements which colonize the gastrointestinal tract and potentially provide health benefits the host. Probiotics protect high risk infants from developing NEC or sepsis, by different mechanisms including an increased barrier to bacterial migration across the mucosa, competitive exclusion of potential pathogens, modification of host response to microbial products, enhancement of IGA mucosal responses, enhancement of enteral nutrition inhibiting the growth of pathogenic bacteria, and up-regulation of host immune responses. The most frequently used probiotics are lactobacillus and bifidobacterium. As per Cochrane Database Syst Rev 2014, enteral supplementation of probiotics prevents severe NEC and all cause mortality in preterm infants and they strongly support a change in practice. However, the most effective preparations, timing, and length of therapy are yet to be assessed.

What are the differential diagnoses of neonatal sepsis?

The conditions which may mimic neonatal sepsis and should be excluded are hypoglycemia, hypothermia, perinatal asphyxia and associated hypoxic-ischemic encephalopathy, other causes of respiratory distress in a neonate like respiratory distress syndrome, transient tachypnea of newborn, meconium aspiration syndrome, polycythemia, congenital hypothyroidism and rarely, inborn errors of metabolism.

What are the complications of neonatal sepsis?

Sepsis can lead to many severe life-threatening complications during the NICU stay including acute lung injury, cardiac dysfunction, capillary leak syndrome, coma, critical care neuromyopathy, thrombosis, coagulopathy, hemorrhage, hepatic failure, renal failure, reactive hemophagocytic syndrome, hyperglycemia, multi-organ dysfunction syndrome (MODS), and death. Overall there is an increased risk of death in neonatal sepsis, mortality is inversely related to gestational age.

Survivors of neonatal sepsis are at a high risk of adverse outcomes especially in VLBW infants. VLBW infants with a history of EOS have a significantly higher risk of:

- Severe intraventricular hemorrhage or periventricular leukomalacia.
- Bronchopulmonary dysplasia.
- Impaired neurodevelopmental outcomes at 18–22 weeks corrected gestational age (low Bayley Scales of Infant Development II scores on the mental development index and psychomotor development index) and cerebral palsy.
- Vision impairments.
- A head circumference <10th percentile.
- Poor cognitive function, academic achievement, and behavior at school age.

What preventive measures of infection can you take in neonates?

The following controls should be taken to prevent infections in newborn:

- All mothers should be provided with regular antenatal check up and immunized against tetanus. All infections during pregnancy should be diagnosed early and treated appropriately.
- Babies should be fed early and exclusively with expressed breast milk (or breastfed) without any pre-lacteal feeds.
- Cord should be kept clean and dry.
- Approskin care is must in preterm neonates.
- Avoid overcrowding and maintain hygiene.
- **Hand washing:** This is the simplest and the most effective method for control of infection in the hospital. All persons taking care of the baby should strictly follow hand washing policies before touching any baby.
- All procedures should be done under strict aseptic precautions. Unnecessary interventions should be avoided.
- The use of prophylactic antibiotics for prevention of nosocomial infections is strongly discouraged.
- All units should have a written disinfection and housekeeping policy which should be strictly followed. Waste disposal policy should be practiced.

CONCLUSIONS

- Neonatal sepsis is a common cause of neonatal mortality and morbidity. Early anti-microbial administration and supportive care are the mainstays of treatment of neonatal sepsis. More reliable diagnostic criteria are required for rapid identification of sepsis or to exclude it, in order to prescribe antibiotics only to infected newborns and to stop empirical antibiotics early. The treatment of neonatal sepsis is inconsistent. Many controversies still exist in the management including the choice and optimum duration of antibiotic therapy.

TAKE HOME MESSAGES

- Neonatal sepsis is a major cause of morbidity and mortality. Prevention and early management can go a long way to decrease the mortality and long-term sequelae life.
- The signs and symptoms of neonatal sepsis are non-specific, which makes the diagnosis difficult. High index of clinical suspicion is, therefore, essential.
- The early diagnosis of neonatal sepsis continues to be a major clinical challenge as most of the routinely used laboratory tests are often not useful. Use of serial CRP measurement can be a simple tool to diagnose and guide antibiotic therapy.
- The current practice of starting empirical antibiotic therapy in all neonates results in adverse drug effects, nosocomial complications, and emergence of resistant strains.
- Proper antenatal care, maintenance of asepsis during delivery, promotion of breastfeeding, decreased interventions and health care hygiene are the best management strategies to reduce the incidence of neonatal sepsis and its sequelae.

FURTHER READING

1. Polin RA. Committee on Fetus and Newborn. Management of neonates with suspected or proven early-onset bacterial sepsis. *Pediatrics* 2012;129:1006–1015.
2. Ganatra HA, Stoll BJ, Zaidi AK. International perspective on early-onset neonatal sepsis. *Clin Perinatol* 2010; 37:501–523.
3. Stoll BJ, Hansen NI, Bell EF, *et al*. Neonatal outcomes of extremely preterm infants from the NICHD Neonatal Research Network. *Pediatrics* 2010;126:443–456.
4. Ng PC, Lam HS. Biomarkers for late-onset neonatal sepsis: Cytokines and beyond. *Clin Perinatol* 2010; 37:599–610.
5. Lever A, Mackenzie I. Sepsis: Definition, epidemiology and diagnosis. *BMJ* 2007;335(7625):879–883.
6. Benitz WE. Adjunct laboratory tests in the diagnosis of early-onset neonatal sepsis. *Clin Perinatol* 2010; 37:421–438.
7. Makkar M, Gupta C, Pathak R, Garg S, Mahajan NC. Performance evaluation of hematologic scoring system in early diagnosis of neonatal sepsis. *J Clin Neonatol* 2013;2:25–29.
8. Wynn JL, Neu J, Moldawer LL, Levy O. Potential of immunomodulatory agents for prevention and treatment of neonatal sepsis. *J Perinatol* 2009;29:79–88.
9. Dessì A, Corsello G, Stronati M, *et al*. New diagnostic possibilities in systemic neonatal infections: Metabolomics. *Early Hum Dev* 2014;90 (Suppl 1):S19–S21.

Chapter

14 Inborn Errors of Metabolism

Susanta Kumar Badatya, Anup Thakur

ABSTRACT

Inborn errors of metabolism are group of disease conditions which may present with varied clinical presentation in neonatal period including emergencies. Both diagnosis and management of inborn error of metabolism is challenging to physicians due to varied symptomatology and rarity of some conditions. Nevertheless, high index of suspicion is important to diagnose them as delay in diagnosis may lead to increased risk of mortality and significant neurological dysfunction. Moreover, recent advancement in molecular and biochemical genetics has been able to offer prenatal and postnatal diagnosis and treatment option to selected condition which should not be missed out.

This chapter discusses the case-based clinical features, investigations, treatment and a basic approach to the inborn disorders of metabolism.

Key Words: Encephalopathy, Hypoglycemia, Hyperammonemia, Inborn errors of metabolism (IEM), Postnatal diagnosis, Prenatal diagnosis.

INTRODUCTION

Inborn errors of metabolism (IEM) are disorders resulting from the absence or abnormality of an enzyme or its cofactor, leading to either accumulation or deficiency of a specific metabolite. There is a block at some point in the normal metabolic pathway caused by a genetic defect of a specific enzyme. They can present with non-specific findings, such as poor feeding, drowsiness, lethargy, hypotonia and failure to thrive. The clinical manifestations of inborn errors of metabolism (IEM) may include findings in virtually every system. The history should focus on previous episodes of metabolic decompensation, identification of potential triggering events, and family history of metabolic disease or members with similar presentations.

CASE SCENARIO

A neonate was delivered vaginally at 38 weeks of gestation to parents with second degree of consanguinity. Baby had uneventful postnatal course and Apgar scores were 9 at 1 minute and 10 at 5 minutes. Baby remained active, was started on breast feed and was discharged after 24 hours.

Contd...

Contd...

On day 4 of life, he presented with poor feeding, vomiting and lethargy. He had hepatomegaly, was grossly hypotonic and encephalopathic. A complete sepsis workup, including CBC, micro ESR, CRP, blood culture and lumbar puncture, was performed to rule out sepsis/meningitis and empirical antibiotics started.

Over the next 12 hours he deteriorated and required intubation for apneas.

CBC, blood sugar, serum electrolytes, and sepsis workup were normal. First line tests for IEM like ABG, serum lactate, ammonia and urine ketones were performed. Serum ammonia level was very high 1500 μmol/L. Tandem mass spectrometry and Urine gas chromatography and mass spectrometry revealed raised serum and urine citrulline.

This child was diagnosed to have a urea cycle defect, precisely "citrullinemia".

CRITICAL CASE ANALYSIS

This is a classical clinical profile of a case of inborn error of metabolism. The history is of a term baby with uneventful postnatal period becoming symptomatic after period of well-being. Symptoms of vomiting, lethargy being non-specific to point out any specific diagnosis and mostly mimicking sepsis. History of consanguinity here is a good pointer, however, may not be always present. Hypoglycemia, thrombocytopenia, hyperammonia, metabolic acidosis may be other important clues in such a patient. High index of suspicion in such cases often helps clinicians to clinch the diagnosis.

INTERACTIVE TOPIC REVIEW

Can inborn errors of metabolism manifest in a fetus antenatally?

Prenatal Onset: Fetuses in most condition escape the inborn errors of metabolism as either the substrate is not formed or placenta excretes the accumulated substrate. Similarly, most maternal inborn errors do not affect the developing fetus with exceptions as discussed below.

Maternal Diseases Affecting the Fetus: Maternal Phenylketonuria has increased risk for spontaneous abortion and increased risk of having a child with major birth anomalies, including intrauterine growth restriction, microcephaly, mental retardation, and a congenital heart defect. The risk of birth defects is proportional to the mother's serum phenylalanine concentration.

Fetal Diseases Affecting the Mother: As a rule, inborn errors of metabolism of the fetus do not affect the pregnant mother. However, reports began to appear in the 1990s describing mothers who had experienced acute fatty liver of pregnancy (AFLP) while carrying a fetus that subsequently manifested evidence of a fatty acid oxidation defect after birth.

How do inborn errors of metabolism present in neonates?

Inborn errors of metabolism often present as muti-system disorder. The presenting complaints can be categorised for simplifying approach to baby with IEMs and are mentioned in Table 14.1.

Table 14.1: Inborn errors of metabolism and predominant feature

Features	Disease conditions
Metabolic encephalopathy	Amino acid disorder, organic academia, respiratory chain defects, urea cycle defects
Metabolic seizures	Neurotransmitter disorders, pyridoxine dependency, pyridoxal phosphate dependency, folinic acid responsive seizures, glucose transporter 1 deficiency
Cardiomyopathy	Fatty acid oxidation defects, glycogen storage diseases, lysosomal storage diseases, respiratory chain defects
Hepatic dysfunction	Amino acid defects (Tyrosinemia), bile acid biosynthetic defects, carbohydrate defects, congenital disorders of glycosylation, fatty acid oxidation defects
Hepatomegaly/splenomegaly	Fatty acid oxidation defects, lysosomal storage disorders, organic acidemias
Sepsis	Galactosemia, defects of biotin metabolism
Cataracts	Peroxisomal disorders, carbohydrate defects, lysosomal storage disease
Hypoglycemia	Galactosemia, fatty acid oxidation defects, organic acidemias, glycogen storage disorders and disorders of gluconeogenesis
Dysmorphic features	Peroxisomal disorders, pyruvate dehydrogenase deficiency, congenital disorders of glycosylation (CDG), lysosomal storage diseases

What are the pointers to the presence of IEM?

IEMs should be suspected when there are following features:

- History of acute deterioration after a period of normalcy after birth and few days after feeding (refusal to feed, lethargy, vomiting, hypotonia, coma, seizures).
- History of consanguinity in the parents or of an unexplained death of siblings in the neonatal period may have possibilty of an inherited metabolic disease in the sick infant.
- Rapidly progressive encephalopathy and seizures of unexplained cause.
- Severe metabolic acidosis.
- Peculiar odor and dysmorphism.
- Jaundice, visceromegaly.

Is there any specific pattern in IEM?

Yes, **specific pattern** is noticed in most of inborn errors.

- Peculiar age of onset–usually presenting after a period of normalcy.
- Temporal profile, i.e., evolution of the disease with characteristic symptom and sign as the disease advances; affected sibs usually show a similar temporal profile.
- IEM has a characteristic inheritance pattern, e.g., ornithine transcarbamylase deficiency (OTC), Fabry's disease, Menkes disease and Hunter's disease are X–linked recessive and most others are autosomal recessive.

What are the investigations to be done in a suspected case of IEM?

Investigations should be based on index of suspicion. First line investigations may be done in all suspected cases. These include:

- Complete blood count–Neutropenia and thrombocytopenia seen in propionic and methylmalonic academia.
- Arterial blood gases and electrolytes – Metaboic acidosis/Respiratory alkalosis.
- Blood glucose–Hypoglycemia, e.g., organic acidemias.
- Plasma ammonia – Raised in Urea cycle defect.
- Arterial blood lactate – Increased lactate, e.g., Pyruvate carboxylase deficiecy.
- Liver function tests – Abnormal, e.g., Tyrisonemia.
- Urine ketones–Fatty acid oxidation defect, e.g., absent urine ketones in the setting of hypoglycemia.
- Urine reducing substances, e.g., Galactosemia.

Specialized Investigations

- Gas chromatography mass spectrometry (GCMS) of urine–for diagnosis of organic acidemias.
- Plasma amino acids and acyl carnitine profile by tandem mass spectrometry (TMS)–for diagnosis of organic acidemias, urea cycle defects, aminoacidopathies and fatty acid oxidation defects.
- High performance liquid chromatography (HPLC) for quantitative analysis of amino acids in blood and urine; required for diagnosis of organic acidemias and aminoacidopathies.
- Lactate/pyruvate ratio–in cases with elevated lactate.
- Serum uric acid (low in molybdenum cofactor deficiency).
- Urinary orotic acid–in cases with hyperammonemia for classification of urea cycle defect.
- Enzyme assay: biotinidase assay–in cases with suspected biotinidase deficiency and GALT (galactose 1- phosphate uridyl transferase) assay–in cases with suspected galactosemia.

What precaution should be taken while collecting sample for diagnosis?

Samples should be collected before starting specific treatment and withholding feed report may be falsely normal when feed is withheld. Samples for blood ammonia and lactate should be transported in ice and immediately tested. Lactate sample should be arterial and should be collected after 2 hours fasting in a preheparinized syringe. Ammonia sample is to be collected approximately after 2 hours of fasting in EDTA vacutainer while avoiding air mixing. Sample should arterial and be free flowing. Detailed history including drug details must be kept in mind while analyzing the report, for example, sodium valproate therapy may increase ammonia levels.

What are the principles of management of IEM?

The basic principles of management of inborn errors are:

- **Reduce formation of toxic metabolites** by decreasing substrate availability (by stopping feeds and preventing endogenous catabolism) and to enhance the excretion of toxic metabolites.
- **Co-factor therapy** for specific disease should be started even empirically if diagnosis not established.
- **Supportive care** treatment of seizures and maintaining euglycemia and normothermia, fluid, electrolyte and acid-base balance, treatment of infection, mechanical ventilation if required.
- **Definitive therapy** is available in few conditions with enzyme replacement or gene replacement along with long-term dietary modification. Once diagnosis is established then treatment is directed to specific disease process.

What is the acute management of neonate presenting with inborn errors?

When **hyperammonemia** is confirmed ruling out spurious result following measures are taken to curb hyperammonemia:

- Stop all feeds and adequate calories to be given to decrease endogenous catabolism by intravenous glucose and lipids. Maintain glucose infusion rate 8–10 mg/kg/min. Start intravenous lipid 0.5 gm/kg/day (up to 3 gm/kg/day). After stabilization gradually add protein 0.25 gm/kg till 1.5 gm/kg/day.
- Rapid removal of ammonia is only possible with dialysis and hemodialysis is more effective and faster than peritoneal dialysis.
- Excretion of nitrogen can be enhanced by use of Sodium benzoate (IV or oral) – loading dose 250 mg/kg then 250–400 mg/kg/day in 4 divided doses. Sodium phenylbutyrate – loading dose 250 mg/kg followed by 250–500 mg/kg/day. L-arginine (oral or IV) – 300 mg/kg/day. L-carnitine (oral or IV) – 200 mg/kg/day.

When **organic acidemia** is suspected, patient should be kept nil per orally and intravenous glucose to be started. Supportive care with hydration, treatment of sepsis, seizures, ventilation to be continued. Carnitine supplementation 100 mg/kg/day IV or oral and acidosis must be corrected. Biotin (10 mg/day orally),Vitamin B_{12} 1–2 mg/day I/M (useful in B_{12} responsive forms of methylmalonic acidemias) and Thiamine 300 mg/day (useful in thiamine-responsive variants of MSUD) can be considered in specific cases.

When **refractory metabolic seizures** are in question, trial of pyridoxine 100 mg intravenously can be considered. If intravenous preparation not available, oral pyridoxine can be given (15 mg/kg/day). If patient persists to have seizures despite pyridoxine, give trial of biotin 10 mg/day and folinic acid 5 mg twice daily (folinic acid responsive seizures). Trial of pyridoxal phosphate 10 mg/kg/dose × 2 doses is also recommended. CSF glucose transport defect should also be ruled out by performing paired CSF and blood glucose level.

What is the long-term treatment option for IEMs?

- **Dietary Treatment:** This is the mainstay of treatment in phenylketonuria (PKU), maple syrup urine disease (MSUD), homocystinuria, galactosemia and glycogen storage disease Type I and III. Special diets for PKU and MSUD are commercially available. These special diets are, however, very expensive. Some disorders like urea cycle disorders and organic acidurias require dietary modification (protein restriction) in addition to other modalities. The ketogenic diet is the treatment of choice for glucose transporter 1 defiency and pyruvate dehydrogenase deficiency.
- **Enzyme Replacement Therapy (ERT):** ERT is now commercially available for some lysosomal storage disorders. However, these disorders do not manifest in the newborn period, an exception being Pompe's disease (Glycogen storage disorder Type II) which may present in the newborn period and for which ERT is now available.
- **Cofactor Replacement Therapy:** The catalytic properties of many enzymes depend on the participation of non-protein prosthetic groups, such as vitamins and minerals, as obligatory cofactors. The following co-factors may be beneficial in certain IEM.
  1. *Thiamine:* Mitochondrial disorders, thiamine responsive variants of MSUD, PDH deficiency and complex I deficiency).
  2. *Riboflavin:* Glutaric aciduria Type I, Type II, complex I deficiency.

3. *Pyridoxine:* Fifty percent of cases of homocystinuria due to cystathionine β-synthetase deficiency, pyridoxine dependency with seizures, xanthurenic aciduria, primary hyperoxaluria type I, Hyperornithemia with gyrate atrophy.
4. *Cobalamin:* Methylmalonic academia (cblA, cblB), Homocystinuria and methylmalonic academia (cblC, cblD, cblF).
5. *Folinic acid:* Hereditary orotic aciduria, Methionine synthase deficiency, Cerebral folate transporter deficiency, hereditary folate malabsorption, Kearns-Sayre syndrome.
6. *Biotin:* Biotinidase deficiency, holocarboxylase synthetase deficiency.

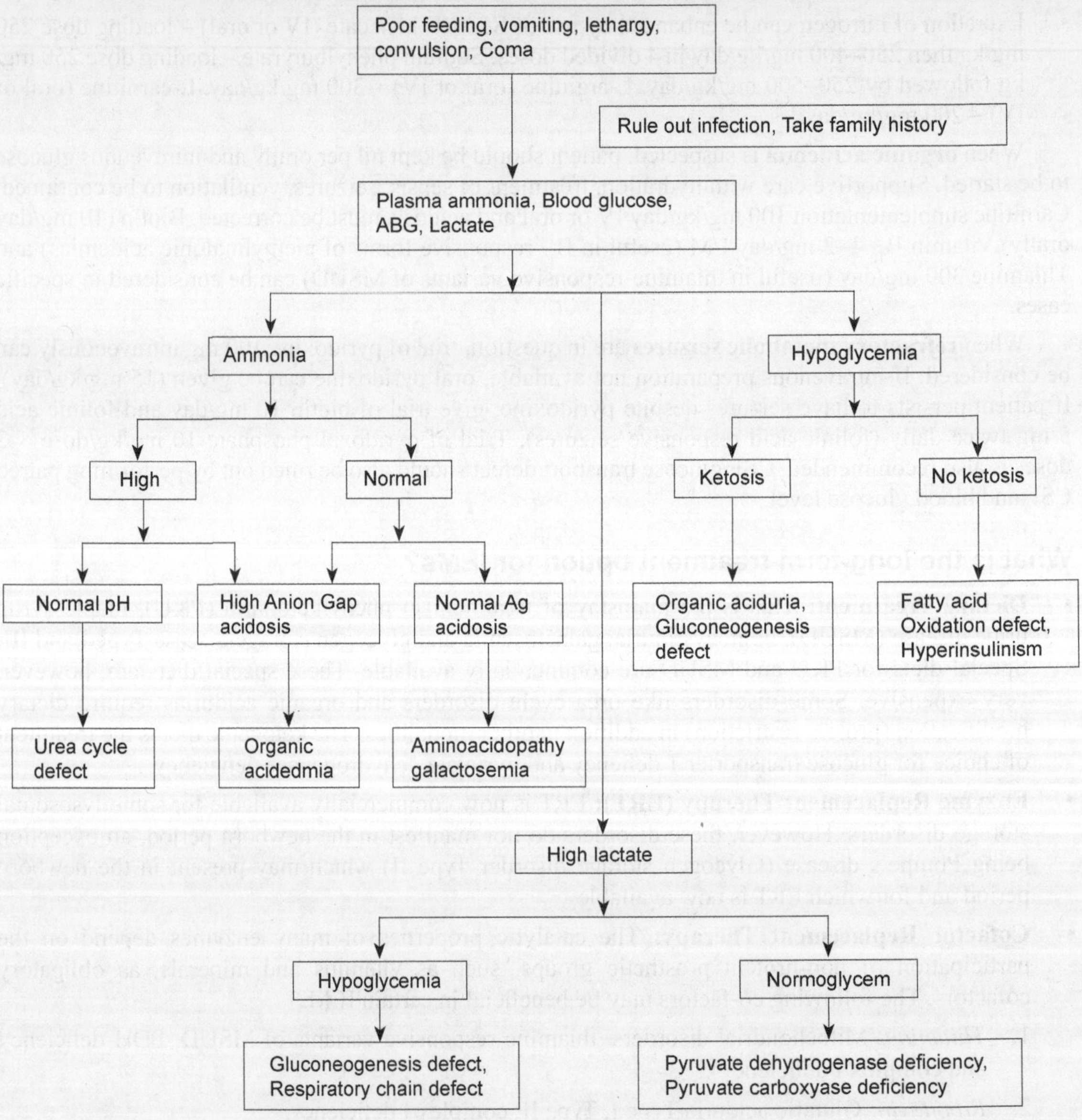

Flowchart: Approach to a neonate with suspected IEM

What can be offered to parents with affected infant for future pregnancy?

Antenatal Screening: As most of the IEM are inherited as single gene defects in an autosomal recessive manner, with a 25% recurrence risk. So when the diagnosis is confirmed in the index case, prenatal diagnosis can be offered, wherever available for the subsequent pregnancies. Chorionic villus tissue or amniotic fluid can be examined.

- *Substrate or metabolite detection:* Useful in phenylketonuria, peroxisomal defects.
- *Enzyme assay:* Useful in lysosomal storage disorders like Niemann-Pick disease, Gaucher disease.
- *DNA based (molecular) diagnosis:* Detection of mutation in proband/ carrier parents is a prerequisite.

Neonatal Screening: Tandem mass spectrometry is used in some countries for neonatal screening for IEM. Disorders which can be detected by TMS include aminoacidopathies (phenylketonuria, MSUD, Homocystinuria, Citrullinemia, Argininosuccinic aciduria, hepatorenal tyrosinemia), fatty acid oxidation defects, organic acidemias (glutaric aciduria, propionic acidemia, methylmalonic acidemia, isovaleric acidemia). The appropriate time for collection of samples is between 1 and 3 days of life. However, the results needs to be interpreted with caution and a metabolic expert should review all abnormal reports.

CONCLUSIONS

Inborn errors of metabolism are an important cause of morbidity and mortality in newborn infants. These disorders are probably under diagnosed because of their rarity, the non-specific way many of them are expressed, and the difficulty clinicians have with their diagnosis. This chapter reduces this difficulty by providing a practical approach to the diagnosis of these disorders based on sets of common clinical and laboratory findings.

TAKE HOME MESSAGES

- Inherited metabolic diseases are to be considered as cause of disease in the neonate who present after period of normalcy.
- The possibility of a genetic metabolic disease should be considered even if there is no family history of the disease as not always positive family history is available.
- Possibility of metabolic disorder should be kept in sick newborn infant especially if sepsis workup is negative repeatedly.
- Systemic approach to metabolic diseases as per symptom and basic laboratory parameter will lead to diagnosis and avoiding high cost investigations.
- Both antenatal and neonatal management option should be provided as new diagnostic and treatment modalities are available.
- Observe the precautions as explained while collecting and storing samples.

FURTHER READING

1. Zinn AB. Inborn errors of metabolism. In: Fanaroff and Martin's (eds): *Neonatal-Perinatal Medicine*, 10th edn. Philadelphia: Elsevier 2015:1553–1615.
2. Cederbaum S, Berry GT. Inborn errors of carbohydrate, ammonia, amino acid, and organic acid metabolism. In: Gleason, Christine A (eds): *Avery's Diseases of the Newborn,* 9th edn. Philadelphia: Elsevier 2012:869–889.
3. Sharma S, Kumar P, Agarwal R, *et al*. Approach to inborn errors of metabolism presenting in the neonate. *Indian J Pediatr* 2008;75:271–276.

Chapter

15 Infant of Diabetic Mother

Abhishek Chopra, Arun Soni

ABSTRACT

The term, *gestational diabetes mellitus*, denotes the glucose intolerance diagnosed for first time during pregnancy. Management includes lifestyle modification, insulin and drugs. Infants born to mother with gestational diabetes mellitus are at increased risk for complications during delivery such as brachial plexus injury, clavicular fractures and in postnatal period such as polycythemia, hypoglycemia, respiratory distress, hypertrophic cardiomyopathy.

Such a neonate should be appropriately monitored for the complications and managed accordingly.

Key Words: Gestational diabetes mellitus (GDM), Glucose tolerance test (GTT), Infant of diabetic mother (IDM), Oral glucose tolerance test (OGTT).

INTRODUCTION

Gestational diabetes mellitus (GDM) is defined as glucose intolerance beginning or diagnosed for first time during pregnancy. GDM complicates approximately 7% of all pregnancies in United States. Infants born to mothers with diabetes mellitus (IDM) are at high risk of complications and need close monitoring.

CASE SCENARIO

A baby weighing 4020 gm was born to the mother with gestational diabetes mellitus at 38 weeks by Cesarean section done for fetal distress. In view of mild respiratory distress, baby was shifted to nursery, started on tube feeds @ 60 ml/kg/day and blood sugar monitoring was done. At 4 hours of life, baby had blood sugar of 30 mg%. Baby was started on intravenous glucose infusion @ 6 mg/kg/min. Baby became euglycemic at glucose infusion of 8 mg/kg/min. Blood sugar monitoring was continued, glucose infusion was tapered and stopped over next 48 hours. As the respiratory distress settled, he was started on breast feeds and shifted with mother.

CRITICAL CASE ANALYSIS

This baby had weight more than 90th centile (LGA) which is common in infants of mothers with poorly-controlled diabetes. Respiratory distress could be due to transient tachypnea of newborn, respiratory distress syndrome or hypertrophic cardiomyopathy. As respiratory distress settled in a short-time, it appeared to be due to transient tachypnea of newborn (TTN). Babies born to diabetic mothers are at high risk for hypoglycemia. This baby required glucose infusion up to 8 mg/kg/min to control hypoglycemia.

IDM are at high risk for various complications such as birth injuries, congenital anomalies, polycythemia, hypertrophic cardiomyopathy for which they should be monitored.

INTERACTIVE TOPIC REVIEW

What should be the screening and diagnostic strategy for gestational diabetes mellitus?

In sequential two-step testing, a 50 gm glucose challenge test (GCT) is performed in pregnant women between 24 and 28 weeks gestation unless a high risk for developing GDM exists (glycosuria, diabetes in first degree relative, history of glucose intolerance, previous GDM, marked obesity and previous infant with macrosomia).

At risk women should be screened by 50 –g GCT at their first prenatal visit. Screening cut-off values is 130 mg/dl (90% sensitivity) or 140 mg% (80% sensitivity). Random or fasting glucose measurements are not recommended because of poor specificity.

In women who screen positive?

100 gm–3 hours Oral Glucose Tolerance test (OGTT) is used to diagnose gestational diabetes (GDM). GDM is diagnosed if two or more plasma glucose measurements are abnormal.

	Fasting	1 hour	2 hours	3 hours
Abnormal blood sugar	>95 mg%	>180 mg%	>155 mg%	>140 mg%

How should women with GDM be managed antenatally?

First line therapy for women with GDM is nutritional and life style modification (known as GDM A1). Pharmacotherapy is indicated when nutritional control is inadequate (Known as GDM A2), especially in patients with elevated fasting glucose levels because diet is largely ineffective to control these levels. The American College of Obstetrics and Gynecologists recommends insulin therapy for women if fasting glucose levels exceed 95 mg%, 1 hour post-prandial glucose is greater than 130–140 mg% and 2 hours level greater than 120 mg% despite nutritional modifications. Intermediate and short acting insulin are first line of therapies for GDM. Some clinicians use Glyburide as first line therapy in clinical practice, though its placental transfer is not known. Metformin may be another option but clearly crosses the placenta.

What is White's classification of maternal diabetes?

White's classification of maternal diabetes is as per Table 15.1.

Table 15.1: White's classification of maternal diabetes

Gestational diabetes	Diabetes not known to be present before pregnancy
	Abnormal glucose test in pregnancy
GD diet	Euglycemia maintained by diet alone
	Diet alone insufficient; insulin required
Class A	Chemical diabetes; glucose intolerance before pregnancy; treated by diet alone; rarely seen
	Prediabetes; history of large babies >4 kg or unexplained still births after 28 weeks
Class B	Insulin dependent; onset after 20 years of age; duration <10 years
Class C	C_1: Onset at 10–19 years of age
	C_2: Duration 10–19 years
Class D	D_1: Onset before 10 years of age
	D_2: Duration 20 years
	D_3: Calcifications of vessels of the leg (macrovascular disease)
	D_4: Benign retinopathy (microvascular disease)
	D_5: Hypertension (not preeclampsia)
Class F	Nephropathy with >500 mg/day of proteinuria
Class R	Proliferative retinopathy or vitreous hemorrhage
Class RF	Criteria for both classes R and F coexist
Class G	Many reproductive failures
Class H	Clinical evidence of arteriosclerotic changes
Class T	Prior renal transplantation

What are the fetal effects of maternal hyperglycemia?

Congenital Anomalies: In normoglycemic pregnancy, the risk of major birth defect is 1 to 2% and the risk increasing 4 to 8-fold in women with pregestational diabetes. Time frame for risk of anomalies is during organogenesis. Jensen compared risks of serious adverse pregnancy outcome at different glycosylated hemoglobin level (HbA_1C). The risk of anomalies was significantly increased when periconceptional HbA_1C was more than 6.9% and risk was 16% when HbA_1C exceeded 10.4%. Major malformations include:

- Cardiovascular (Transposition of great arteries, Truncus arteriosus, Ventricular septal defects, Septal hypertrophy).
- Neurological (Caudal regression syndrome, anencephaly).
- Renal (Hydronephrosis, renal agenesis); and
- Gastrointestinal (Duodenal atresia, Imperforate anus).

Macrosomia: If is defined as birthweight above 90th percentile for age and occurs in 15 to 45% of diabetic pregnancies. During first two trimesters, there is undetectable difference between fetuses born to diabetic and non-diabetic mothers. After 24 weeks, in IDM fetus' abdominal circumference begins to rise above normal. Greater growth of abdominal circumference is caused by deposition of fat in abdominal and interscapular area. Fetal hyperinsulinemia in response to fetal hyperglycemia which reflects maternal hyperglycemia acts as growth factor. Macrosomic babies are at high risk of birth injuries, shoulder dystocia. Strict glycemic control in second and third trimester may reduce risk of fetal macrosomia.

Birth Injury: This includes brachial plexus injury and shoulder dystocia with macrosomic infants being at greater risk. Shoulder dystocia is defined as difficulty in delivering fetal body after expulsion of head and occurs in 0.3–0.5% of vaginal deliveries among pregnant women. Incidence is 2 to 4-folds higher in women with diabetes.

Polycythemia: It defined as hematocrit >65% is not uncommon in IDM and is related to glycemic control. Insulin raises metabolic rate, increases oxygen demand leading to mild chronic hypoxemia which stimulates erythropoietin production.

Hypoglycemia: Approximately 15–20% IDMs develop hypoglycemia during immediate newborn period. This complication is less in pregnancies where glycemic control was good during pregnancy and labor.

Hyperbilirubinemia: Prematurity and polycythemia are chief contributing factors with most babies usually managed by phototherapy.

Respiratory Distress: Hyperinsulinemia retards production and secretion of pulmonary surfactant both phospholipids and surfactant associated proteins and thus increases the risk of respiratory distress syndrome. Other causes of respiratory distress are cardiac or pulmonary anomalies (4%), hypertrophic cardiomyopathy, transient tachypnea of newborn and polycythemia. Elective cesarean section without labor leads to increased risk of Transient Tachypnea of newborn.

Hypertrophic Cardiomyopathy: Late exposure to hyperinsulinemia contributes to cardiac manifestations. Echocardiographic findings include hypercontractile thickened myocardium, often with septal hypertrophy disproportionate to ventricular free walls. This condition often resolves within few months after birth. Beta blockers are the treatment of choice whereas cardiotonic agents might worsen the condition.

What is the pathophysiology of hypoglycemia?

Pathophysiology is explained by Pederson's maternal hyperglycemia-fetal hyperinsulinism hypothesis. Maternal hyperglycemia stimulates insulin secretion and thus causing hypoglycemia. Strong relationship exists between poor maternal glycemic controls (HbA_1C), neonatal hypoglycemia and macrosomia.

What is optimal fetal monitoring?

Monitoring is based on degree of metabolic control, therapy (diet/drugs/insulin) used and presence of any other complications such as hypertension. Non-stress test and Biophysical profile (Table 15.2) should be done biweekly beginning in early third trimester.

Table 15.2: Biophysical profile

Parameter	Normal (2 points)	Abnormal (0 points)
Non-stress test/Reactive fetal heart rate	At least two accelerations in 20 minutes	Less than two accelerations to satisfy the test in 20 minutes
Fetal breathing movements	At least one episode of rhythmic breathing for 30 seconds or more within 30 minutes	Does not meet the criteria
	Baby moves his or her body or limbs three times or more within 30 minutes	Does not meet the criteria
Fetal muscle tone	At least one episode of active bending and straightening of the limb or trunk	No movements or movements slow and incomplete
Qualitative amniotic fluid index	At least one vertical pocket > 2 cm or more in the vertical axis	Largest vertical pocket </=2 cm

When and how should baby be delivered?

Macrosomia is a strong risk factor for birth injuries, shoulder dystocia occurs in 50–86% of these fetuses. Hence, Cesarean section is generally performed for macrosomic babies.

Are mothers with GDM at risk of developing diabetes later in life?

Most women with GDM do not require insulin post-partum but these women have 50% risk to develop type 2 diabetes in next 5 years and also at risk for GDM in subsequent pregnancies. Oral Glucose tolerance test at 3 year intervals is a costeffective management strategy.

CONCLUSIONS

Gestational diabetes mellitus should be diagnosed by glucose challenge test and oral glucose tolerance test. Fetal monitoring should be done and baby must be monitored for various complications postnatally and managed accordingly.

TAKE HOME MESSAGES

- GDM can be easily diagnosed with Glucose challenge test and Oral Glucose Tolerance Test.
- IDM are at higher risk of congenital anomalies.
- Babies born to mothers with GDM are at high risk for various complications like hypoglycemia, hyperbilirubinemia, polycythemia, respiratory distress etc.
- Adequate fetal well-being monitoring is essential.

FURTHER READING

1. HAPO Study Cooperative Research Group. Hyperglycemia and adverse pregnancy outcome (HAPO) Study: Associations with neonatal anthropometrics. *Diabetes* 2009;58:453–459.
2. Jensen DM, Korsholm L, Ovesen P, *et al*. Peri-conceptional A1C and risk of serious adverse pregnancy outcome in 933 women with type 1 diabetes. *Diabetes Care* 2009; 32:1046–1048.
3. Metzger BE, Lowe LP, Dyer AR, *et al*. (For HAPO Study Cooperative Research Group). Hyperglycemia and adverse pregnancy outcomes. *N Engl J Med* 2008;8;358(19):1991–2002.

Chapter

16 Neonatal Hypoglycemia

Susanta Kumar Badatya, Manoj Modi

ABSTRACT

Hypoglycemia in neonatal period is defined as blood sugar value below 40 mg/dL. Presence of untreated hypoglycemia is shown to be associated with poor neurodevelopmental outcome and neurological sequelae. Neonatal conditions like prematurity, intrauterine growth restriction, and maternal diabetes, asphyxia, sepsis predispose to hypoglycemia. Asymptomatic hypoglycemia may be treated with supervising feeding and monitoring whereas symptomatic hypoglycemia must be managed with a continuous infusion of intravenous glucose. Persistent and refractory hypoglycemia should be investigated furthermore for a definite cause of hypoglycemia.

Key Words: Asphyxia, Asymptomatic hypoglycemia, Glucose infusion rate (GIR), Hypoglycemia, Intrauterine growth restriction (IUGR), Maternal diabetes, Neurodevelopmental outcome, Persistent hypoglycemia, Prematurity, Refractory hypoglycemia, Sepsis.

INTRODUCTION

Transition from intrauterine to extra uterine life accompanies shift of continuous transplacental glucose supply to intermittent enteral supply. Hypoglycemia, especially in the early neonatal period is further accentuated by developmental immaturity of normal adaptive mechanisms like gluconeogenesis, hepatic glycogenolysis and ketogenesis. Although level at which hypoglycemia is detrimental is debatable, the effect of neonatal hypoglycemia on the developing brain, with the potential for long-term damage is of great concern.

CASE SCENARIO

A male infant weighing 1800 gm was born at 36 weeks of gestation to a 28-year-old primigravida woman, who had history of pre-eclampsia. Baby was small for gestational age with birthweight less than 3rd centile. There was no requirement of resuscitation and baby was shifted to nursery in view of severe growth restriction and prematurity. He appeared slightly jittery at that time and lethargic. A blood glucose concentration of 26 mg/dL was obtained using a glucometer. Baby was given intravenous

Contd...

Contd...

glucose bolus followed by continuous dextrose infusion. Clinically, baby improved over next 1 hour. Baby was started on feeds and intravenous glucose infusion was tapered after next 24 hours. Blood sugars were monitored for next 48 hours, which were normal. Breastfeeding was started and baby was discharged on day 4 of life.

CRITICAL CASE ANALYSIS

This is a clinical profile of a case of hypoglycemia presenting in neonatal period. Hypoglycemia is although defined by lab parameter; suspicion for a baby being hypoglycemia should be high when baby is premature or sick or small for gestational age. Prompt management of hypoglycemia is needed when baby is symptomatic as in this case with intravenous glucose bolus followed by supplementation. Once blood sugars are maintained, intravenous fluids can be gradually tapered and stopped while blood sugar monitoring is to be continued.

INTERACTIVE TOPIC DISCUSSION

What is definition of hypoglycemia in neonatal period?

Diagnosis of clinically significant hypoglycemia is dependent on the clinical setting and cannot solely be based on a specific blood glucose level. Ideally, neonatal hypoglycemia would be defined as the blood glucose concentration at which intervention should be initiated to avoid significant morbidity, especially neurologic sequelae. In 2011, a report from the American Academy of Pediatrics (AAP) proposed an operational threshold of 45 mg/dL (2.5 mmol/L) as a target glucose level prior to routine feeds. WHO defines hypoglycemia as blood glucose level of less than 45 mg/dL.

Which neonates should be screened for hypoglycemia and what should be the screening schedule?

Around 97 to 98% of hypoglycemic episodes occur within the first 24 hours of birth in asymptomatic neonates at risk. Hypoglycemia usually occurs in LGA infants and IDMs within 12 hours of birth, and screening beyond this period is not required provided blood glucose is maintained at > 45 mg/dL and feeding has been established. Preterm and SGA infants may be vulnerable up to 36 hours of age.

All asymptomatic, at-risk neonates should be screened at 2 hours after birth and surveillance is continued 4–6 hourly thereafter, until feedings are well-established and glucose values have normalized which is generally till 48 hours of life. Monitoring before 2 hours may be required if mother has been starving or vomiting. The maximum risk for hypoglycemia is in first 24 hours but usually persists till 72 hours.

At-risk infants who should be screened are:

- Preterm infants (< 35 weeks)
- Low birthweight infants (<2000 grams)
- Small for gestational age infants (SGA): birthweight < 10th percentile
- Infant of diabetic mothers (IDM)

- Large for gestational age (LGA) infants: birthweight >90th percentile
- Infants with Rh-hemolytic disease
- Infants born to mothers receiving therapy with terbutaline/propranolol/lebatolol/oral hypoglycemic.

What should be the schedule to monitor at-risk infants?

The schedule recommended by the American Academy of Pediatrics to monitor blood sugars in "at-risk infants" is given in Table 16.1.

Table 16.1: Schedule for monitoring the "at-risk infants"

Condition	Risk period for hypoglycemia	Schedule
Prematurity, intrauterine growth retardation	First 72 hours	2, 6, 12, 24, 48 and 72 hours
Asphyxia, hypothermia	First 72 hours	6–8 hours
Sepsis	Transient	6–8 hours
Infant of diabetic mother	First 72 hours	1, 2, 3, 6, 12, 24, 36 and 48 hours
Inborn errors of metabolism	Prolonged	To be individualized
Familial hyperinsulinism	Prolonged	To be individualized

How should blood glucose be tested in neonates and when should a sample be sent to the laboratory for confirmation?

Whenever possibility of hypoglycemia is in question; the plasma or blood glucose concentration must be done immediately by using laboratory enzymatic methods like glucose oxidase or hexokinase method. Plasma blood glucose reading is usually approximately 10 to 18% higher than whole-blood values because of the higher water content of plasma. Capillary blood glucose measurement is usually done in almost all nurseries perform as it is rapid and easy. But there is concern of large variations in values compared to laboratory methods, especially at low glucose concentrations and questionable reliability to document hypoglycemia in newborns. Any glucose value in intervention zone as determined by a glucose meter or infant with signs consistent with hypoglycemia should be confirmed by laboratory measurement laboratory confirmation of the plasma glucose concentration should be performed in any infant with hypoglycemic record. However, treatment should be started immediately after the blood sample is obtained and before confirmatory results are available.

What should be approach to management of a hypoglycemic neonate? What should be criteria for parenteral glucose administration for hypoglycemia?

Approach to baby with hypoglycemia is determined with initial blood glucose level of baby and presence of symptoms of baby as depicted in the flowchart (Fig. 16.1).

A. **Asymptomatic Hypoglycemia:** In asymptomatic hypoglycemic infants, Spoon feed with measured amount of breast or formula milk to be given initially. Factors like hypothermia and sepsis should be identified and treated. Blood glucose level should be checked after 30–60 minutes to ensure euglycemia. If repeat blood glucose is above 40 mg/dL, 2–3 hourly feed is ensured with 4–6 hourly monitoring for glucose up to 48 hours.

Flowchart showing approach to Hypoglycemia

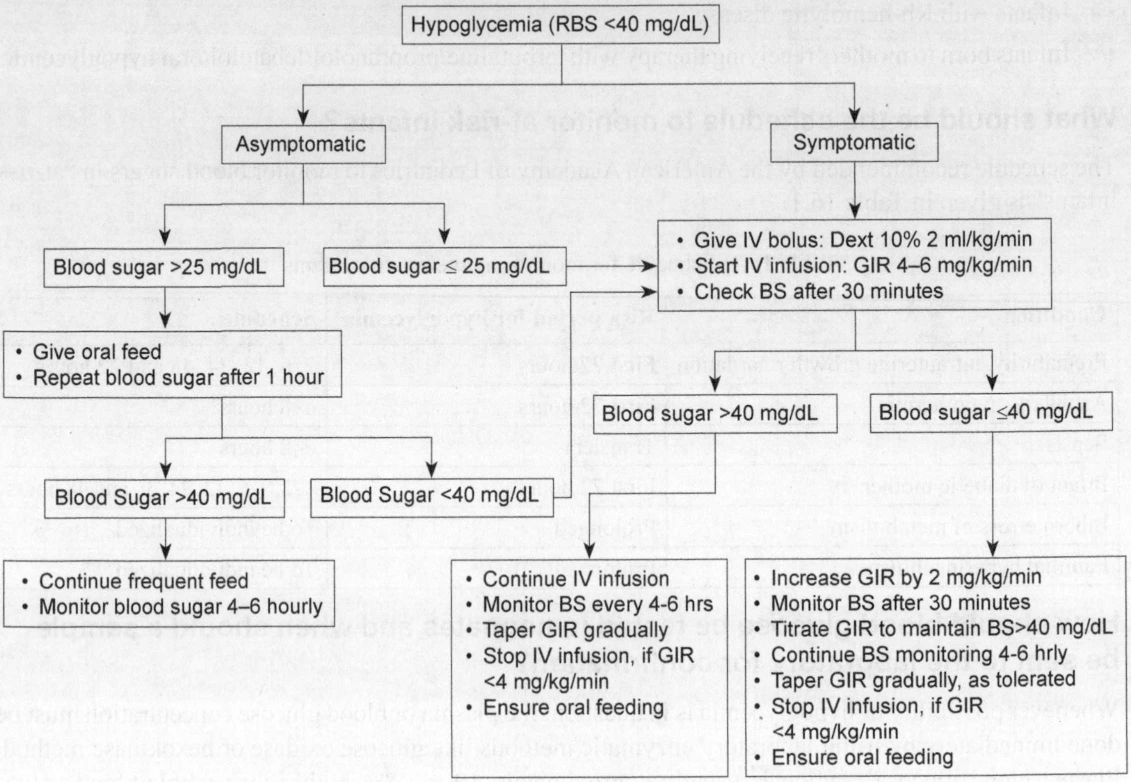

Fig. 16.1: Algorithmic approach to neonatal hypoglycemia

Following conditions where intravenous glucose administration will be warranted are:

1. Blood glucose is < 25 mg/dL.
2. Blood glucose remains below 40 mg/dL despite one attempt of feeding breast milk.
3. Enteral feeding is contraindicated as in case of shock, surgical abdomen, NEC.

B. Symptomatic Hypoglycemia: Any baby with blood glucose value less than 45 mg/dL and associated symptoms should be managed on emergency basis as there is high incidence of neurological injury.

1. A bolus of 200 mg/kg of glucose (2 ml/kg of 10% dextrose) is given intravenously immediately (after sending a sample to the laboratory for confirmation of the diagnosis).
2. After a bolus, an intravenous infusion of glucose with glucose infusion rate (GIR) of 6 mg/kg/min should be started. This GIR is to keep balance between the requirement of glucose and the risk of iatrogenic hyperglycemia which in turn may cause rebound hypoglycemia.
3. Blood glucose is monitored after 15–30 minutes. If it remains above 45 mg/dL, GIR of 6 mg/kg/min is continued. The frequency of checking can be gradually decreased from every hour to 4–6 hourly.

4. If the blood glucose remains < 45 mg/dL, the GIR is increased in steps of 2 mg/kg/min. Every 15–30 minutes with repeat checks on blood glucose till the values is > 45 mg/dL.
5. Tapering of glucose infusion is started when blood glucose values remain stabilized above 45 mg/dL for about 24 hours. Rate of tapering the infusion must be 2 mg/kg/min every 6 hours. Once a GIR of 4 mg/kg/min is reached, the infusion can be stopped if the neonate is euglycemic. In neonates who cannot be fed orally, the GIR is gradually brought down to the minimum at which euglycemia is maintained.
6. When there is requirement of GIR of > 12 mg/kg/min, a diagnosis of resistant hypoglycemia should be done and investigations and management should be modified accordingly. An infant requiring IV glucose for > 7 days should be investigated for persistent hypoglycemia.

What is the role of hydrocortisone in resistant hypoglycemia?

Glucocorticoids physiologically reduce insulin secretion and increase insulin resistance and promote both gluconeogenesis and glycogenolysis. These effects lead to increase in serum glucose concentrations. Dexamethasone and hydrocortisone are the two agents of interest. But due to side effect profile of these steroids like growth suppression, feed intolerance, and hypertension, spontaneous perforation of the gastrointestinal tract, hyperetension, these are rarely used in presence of agents like diazoxide and glucagon. When used, hydrocortisone is used in dose of 5 mg/kg in 2 divided doses. Serum cortsiol level should be documented prior to hydrocortisone use.

What is the role of glucagon in hypoglycemia?

Hypoglycemia induces the secretion of glucagon to raise serum glucose levels. Glucagon is less effective in infants with hyperinsulinemia condition like persistent hyperinsulinism of infancy and familial hyperinsulinism. But it is quite effective in elevating serum glucose concentrations in preterm and term neonates not exhibiting hyperinsulinemia. Occurrence of severe hyponatremia with the use of glucagon is reported. Dose is 0.025–0.2 mg/kg (max 1.0 mg) intramuscular, intravenous or subcutaneously. It is only a temporary measure to mobilize glucose.

What are the causes of resistant or persistent hypoglycemia?

Following causes are known for refractoriness of hypoglycemia:

- **Hyperinsulinism:** Congenital Hyperinsulinisms, Infant of Diabetic mother.
- **Endocrine Disorders:** Congenital hypopitutarism, Adrenal insufficiency, Congenital glucagon deficiency, epinephrine deficiency.
- **Inborn Error of Metabolism:** Galactosemia, Glycogen storage disorders, Maple syrup urine disease, Mitochondrial disorders, propionic academia, methylmalonic academia, Fatty acid oxidation defect.

What are the first and second line investigations in cases resistant or persistent hypoglycemia?

When we are confronted with persistent hypoglycemia.

First set of investigation must include a critical laboratory sample. This is done to rule out hyperinsulinemia in relation to present blood glucose level. An arterial blood gas, serum ammonia, lactate and urine ketone are done as a screening test to rule out hyperinsulism and inborn errors of metabolism. Critical sample includes–Glucose, Serum Insulin, C-Peptide, Serum cortisol, free fatty acids and plasma ketones.

Second tier of investigations advised if insulin levels are found to be normal for the given glucose level. Investigations required as per the likely etiology are listed in Table 16.2.

Table 16.2: Tests needed according to the anticipated causative condition

Condition anticipated	Test
Congenital hypopitutarism	Growth hormone, TSH levels
Adrenal insufficiency	Serum cortisol levels, S ACTH level
Inborn error of metabolism	Plasma amino acid–Tandem Mass sphectrometry Urine ketone, pH Urine reducing substances Urine aminoacids Urine organic acids–Urine GCMS

If congenital hyperinsulism is suspected, then genetic test for Kir 6.2 and SUR1 mutation to be considered. PET Scan, ^{18}F DOPA Positron emission Tomography imaging is of use to localize the lesion in pancrease in this mutation positive condition.

What is the role of neuroimaging in hypoglycemia? What are the common MRI findings?

Neuroimaging in form of MRI brain may demonstrate some common findings in neonates suffering from symptomatic hypoglycemia. White matter changes in parieto occipital cortex and subcortical area in occipital lobe are reported in most of symptomatic babies acutely. Both computed tomography and MRI scans show extensive cortical loss predominantly in the occipital regions.

How should one follow-up infants who had hypoglycemia in neonatal period?

All confirmed and persistent hypoglycemia cases during NICU stay should be planned for follow-up as there are concerns of neuro-developmental delay in these babies. All domains should be paid attention. Serial assessment for neurodevelopment, vision and hearing loss at 3, 6, 9, 12 and 18.

CONCLUSIONS

Hypoglycemia is a potential problem in preterms and IUGR babies. Prompt recognition of symptoms is key to diagnosis and baby should be managed depending upon clinical status. Causes of refractory hypoglycemia should be kept in mind when treating difficult to control hypoglycemia case.

TAKE HOME MESSAGES

- Establishing a single numerical blood glucose level which predicts significant neonatal hypoglycemia at which intervention should be initiated to prevent morbidity is debatable.
- The American Academy of Pediatrics uses an operational level of 45 mg/dL in asymptomatic neonates.
- Blood glucose should be measured in infants who are symptomatic or at risk for hypoglycemia.

Contd...

Contd...

- Most nurseries do capillary blood glucose measurements with a glucometer as a rapid screening method. A low screening glucose value should always be confirmed by laboratory measurement.
- Treatment is initiated after the blood sample is obtained, while awaiting confirmatory laboratory results.
- Oral feedings of breast milk or formula in asymptomatic infants is recommended.
- Parenteral glucose infusion of at least 6 mg/kg per minute in infants who are symptomatic, have severe hypoglycemia or non-responding to oral supplement.
- Infants who require glucose infusions of greater than 8 mg/kg per minute to maintain plasma glucose concentrations greater than 50 mg/dL for more than 1 week should be evaluated by a pediatric endocrinologist for unusual causes of hypoglycemia.

FURTHER READING

1. Clinical Report. Postnatal glucose homeostasis in late-preterm and term infants. *Pediatrics* 2011;127:3: 575–579.
2. Jain A, Aggarwal R, Jeeva Sankar M, Agarwal R, Deorari AK, Paul VK. Hypoglycemia in the newborn. *Indian J Pediatr* 2010;77:1137–1142.
3. Wilker RE. Hypoglycemia and hyperglycemia. In: Cloherty JP, Eichenwald EC, Hansen AR, Stark AR (eds): *Manual of Neonatal Care*, 7th edn. Philadelphia: Lippincott Williams and Wilkins 2012:284–296.
4. Devasker SU, Garg M. Disorders of carbohydrate metabolism in neonate. In: Martin RJ, Fanaroff AA, Walsh MC (eds): *Fanaroff and Martin's Neonatal Perinatal Medicine,* 10th edn. Philadelphia, Elsevier 2015; 1434–1459.

Chapter

17 Electrolyte Imbalance in the Newborn

Ajit Kumar, Anup Thakur

ABSTRACT

Fluid and electrolyte imbalance are common in neonatal intensive care settings. For maintaining such homeostasis in neonate, a thorough concept of its physiology is required. Some of them pose as true emergencies in critical care and needs to be managed expediently for preventing neonatal morbidity and mortality.

Key Words: Electrolyte imbalance, Hyponatremia, Hypernatremia, Hypokalemia, Hyperkalemia.

INTRODUCTION

Physiological adaptation following birth affects water and electrolyte homeostasis in newborn infants. After parturition, there is a sudden efflux of fluid from the intracellular fluid (ICF) to the extracellular fluid (ECF) compartment followed by diuresis at 48–72 hours later. Fluid and electrolyte therapy must account for these factors in determining maintenance requirements and correction of any abnormalities. Electrolyte imbalance is often encountered in a critically sick neonate and includes hyponatremia, hypernatremia, hypokalemia and hyperkalemia.

CASE SCENARIO 1

A term infant was born following a difficult vaginal delivery with shoulder dystocia. The baby required extensive resuscitation at birth, with Apgar scores of 0 at 1 minutes and 4 at 5 minutes. He started to make irregular breathing efforts at 10 minutes and was extubated 2 hours after delivery. He was initially started on IV 10% dextrose at 60 ml/kg/day and switched to electrolyte free parenteral nutrition to prevent catabolic state. Baby was monitored for his urine output, weight, serum sodium, potassium, and BUN and creatinine (Table 17.1). Baby had persistent oliguria with rising serum BUN and creatinine and gained excessive weight. We restricted IV fluid (40 ml/kg/day) for 2 days and cautiously increased his fluid on 3rd day of life to adjust these changes. The baby remained stable after this point, with a gradual return to normalization of electrolytes and a stable urine output.

Contd...

Contd...

Table 17.1: Progressive renal function

Hours of life	Sodium (mEq/L)	Potassium (mEq/L)	BUN/Creatinine (mg/dL)	Weight (g)	Urine output (mL/kg/h)
12	145	4.8	18.8 [1.6]	3990	0.06
24	128	6.5	40.4 [2.4]	4040	0.6
36	132	5.8	50.2 [4.6]	4018	0.8
48	142	5.2	32.6 [3.9]	3995	0.9
60	148	4.8	23.4 [1.1]	3890	1.2
72	144	4.6	16.8 [0.8]	3860	2.2

CRITICAL CASE ANALYSIS

In babies in whom one can anticipate renal problems, the fluid volume should be restricted early on. In this case, acute kidney injury was due to perinatal asphyxia which led to hyponatremia secondary to relative fluid overload. In such a scenario, fluid restriction is the correct approach rather than adding sodium to correct hyponatremia.

INTERACTIVE TOPIC DISCUSSION

What is hyponatremia?

Serum sodium less than 130 mEq/L. Serum sodium < 125 mEq/L are more likely to produce symptoms and are of clinical concern. Hyponatremia may be associated with Normal/Increased/Decreased total body sodium.

How to differentiate pseudo vs true hyponatremia?

Most laboratories measure sodium using a so-called indirect ion-selective electrode (ISE). The formula used to calculate plasma sodium concentration from the activity of sodium ions in the sample assumes that water comprises 93% of plasma volume, but this assumption fails in plasma samples with abnormal protein or lipid content, the so-called ion-exclusion effect. This process leads to the well-recognized phenomenon of pseudohyponatremia in lipemic samples or those with excess protein content.

What are the common causes of hyponatremia in NICU?

1. *Positive free water balance*:
   (a) Increased maternal free water intake during labor.
   (b) Excess free water administration in the postnatal period.
   (c) Perinatal nonosmotic release of vasopressin (SIADH):
      (i) Perinatal asphyxia, respiratory distress, bilateral pneumothoraces and intraventricular hemorrhage.
      (ii) Medications: Morphine, Barbiturates, or Carbamazepine.

2. *Negative sodium balance*:
   (a) Inadequate sodium intake or
   (b) Excessive renal losses:
      (i) High fractional excretion of sodium (FENa) in extremely premature neonates.
      (ii) Rare causes: Bartter syndrome, congenital adrenal hyperplasia, pseudo-hypoaldosteronism.

How to evaluate a case of hyponatremia?

Assess the hydration status of the newborn, whether it is excess fluid intake, poor diuresis or net salt loss. In this case, weight and blood pressure are either stable or increased and there is normal skin turgor and peripheral perfusion. Once the assessment of water excess versus salt loss has been made, biochemical evaluation of the urine can help delineate the etiology.

One important point to remember is that kidney maintains euvolemia by regulating sodium re-absorption. Therefore, with excess water the kidneys will excrete more sodium to restore euvolemia. Weight and blood pressure can be stable and not increased with water excess. Thus, an elevated urine sodium level does not necessarily indicate primary renal salt loss, but may be the appropriate physiologic response to water overload. Biochemical and clinical data needs to be integrated to generate a reasonable diagnosis (Box 17.1).

Box 17.1: Clinical parameters for the assessment of dysnatremias

- Weight
- Urine output
- Type and volume of administered fluids
- Blood pressure
- Peripheral perfusion
- Insensible water losses
- Skin turgor
- Renal ultrasonography

How to manage a case of hyponatremia?

- *Symptomatic infant or serum sodium <120 mEq/L*: IV bolus of 3% NS at 1–2 mL/kg will correct the symptoms. This should be followed by a gradual sodium correction [weight × 0.75 × (130-observed Na)].
- *Asymptomatic child with excess water (wt gain, euvolemic/Hypervolemic)*: The simplest treatment is to restrict fluid intake. The excess volume can be calculated: weight (kg) × Total body water (TBW) × (130-observed Na)/130. Thus, a euvolemic 3 kg neonate with a sodium level of 120 mEq/L would be estimated to have 3 × 0.75 × (130–120)/130 = 0.173 l excess water. Reduction of water administration by this amount over the next 24–48 hours would be expected to normalize plasma sodium to 130 mEq/L over the same time period, assuming that other factors, such as insensible water losses and urine output, remain unchanged.
- *Asymptomatic infant with true sodium deficit (wt loss, hypovolemic)*: Sodium supplementation is the correct treatment, and the sodium deficit can be calculated in similar fashion to water excess:

weight (kg) × TBW × (130 – observed Na). In an asymptomatic child, slow correction of the plasma sodium concentration is generally advised (up to 10 mEq/L per day) because of concerns of osmotic demyelination syndrome, especially in chronic hyponatremia.

HYPERNATREMIA

CASE SCENARIO 2

A term neonate born to a primigravida mother through elective LSCS and was discharged home on 3rd day of life on formula milk. Baby was readmitted on 21st day of life with history of poor feeding and lethargy for 2 days along with failure to thrive. Examination revealed a markedly wasted, lethargic neonate with signs of moderate dehydration and sclerema. His birthweight was 3.0 kg and current weight is 2.5 kg. An intravenous line was started shortly thereafter, and blood was drawn for complete blood count, culture, electrolytes, urea (blood urea nitrogen) and creatinine. Investigation revealed serum Na 170 mEq/L, serum K 3.8 mEq/L, BUN = 48 mg/dL and Cr: 1.2 mg/dL. Baby was rehydrated slowly with N/3 and gradually his serum Na normalized to 148 mEq/L over 2 days. Once adequate urine output was established, K was added to provide maintenance requirements or replace urinary losses. Baby was started on breast feeds and lactational counseling as well as support for the mother was ensured. Baby was neurologically normal at discharge and parents counseled about need for close follow-up.

CRITICAL CASE ANALYSIS

This is a classical case of hyponatremia presenting in NICU. Neonates with hypernatremic dehydration are often more dehydrated than is apparent by physical examination, because the increased osmolality helps maintain the extracellular fluid space. Dehydration was corrected slowly with the hypotonic saline (N/3) over 3 days to avoid a rapid fall in serum osmolality, which would cause rapid movement of water into cells and potentially lead to cerebral edema. Body weight, serum electrolytes, urine volume and specific gravity was monitored regularly so that fluid therapy can be adjusted appropriately.

INTERACTIVE TOPIC DISCUSSION

What is hypernatremia?

Hypernatremia is defined as serum sodium level ≥150 mEq/L.

What are the common causes of hypernatremia?

- Free water loss: increased insensible or urinary water losses (Diabetes Insipidus).
- Water loss > Na loss (Diarrhea, Lactational failure, Osmotic diuresis).
- Absolute Na gain: Excess oral/IV Na intake, excess sodium bicarbonate use.

What is the pathophysiology of hypernatremia?

Hypernatremia results in movement of organic acid and free H^+ ion into the extracellular fluid (ECF) leading to acidosis. Hyperglycemia may occur due to inappropriately low level of insulin. Hyperosmolality of the ECF causes a shift of water from the cells, which in case of brain, leads to distension of cerebral vessels. These may rupture causing intracerebral, subdural or subarachnoid hemorrhage. Idiogenic osmoles are generated in the cells in patients with sustained and severe hypernatremia. This is a protective phenomenon, which reduces the efflux of intracellular fluid (ICF) to ECF, thereby preventing from cell shrinkage.

What are the impacts of hypernatremia?

- *Acute Hypernatremia:* Hypertonic ECF leads to Cell shrinkage-Intracranial bleed or thrombosis.
- *Chronic Hypernatremia:* Cells generate osmoprotective idiogenic osmoles–no cell shrinkage and baby may be asymptomatic.

What are the clinical features and morbidities of hypernatremia?

- Usually present at around 10 days (3–21 days) of life.
- Very variable presentation.
- May be asymptomatic, alert and hungry to irritable or lethargy to moribund and comatose.
- Fever, irritability, drowsiness alternating with irritability.
- Excessive or high pitched crying, lethargy, restlessness, hyperreflexia, spasticity, seizures and coma.
- Doughy skin (> loss of 10% of weight).
- Hyperpnea, apnea, bradycardia, hypertension.
- May not look dehydrated (ECF loss is compensated by ICF efflux).
- May appear sicker than expected for the clinical signs of dehydration.
- Shock is rare and late as intravascular volume is preserved.
- Cerebral edema, intracranial hemorrhage, hemorrhagic infarcts and cerebral sinovenous thrombosis, seizures, focal neurological deficits.
- Arteriovenous thrombosis (renal vein thrombosis, cerebral sinus venosus thrombosis), intracranial hemorrhage or infarct.

How to evaluate a case of hypernatremia?

After establishing that the hypernatremia is true and not a measurement artefact, the most important step is to determine whether the cause is a deficiency of water or an excess of salt. Once this distinction is made, urinary indices can help delineate the etiology (Fig.17.1).

How to manage a neonate with hypernatremic dehydration?

- No fluid boluses should be given unless the infant is in shock.
- If in shock, IV NS bolus (better to give fluid with Na concentration equal to current serum Na level).
- Calculate free fluid and Na deficit, the desired IV fluid and correct it over 48–72 hours.
- Follow serum Na, and adjust fluid composition and rate based on clinical response.
- Initial boluses (RL or NS) should be accounted to minimize excessive dropping of serum sodium.
- Sodium level >200 mEq/L: Peritoneal/hemodialysis, especially when no urine output.

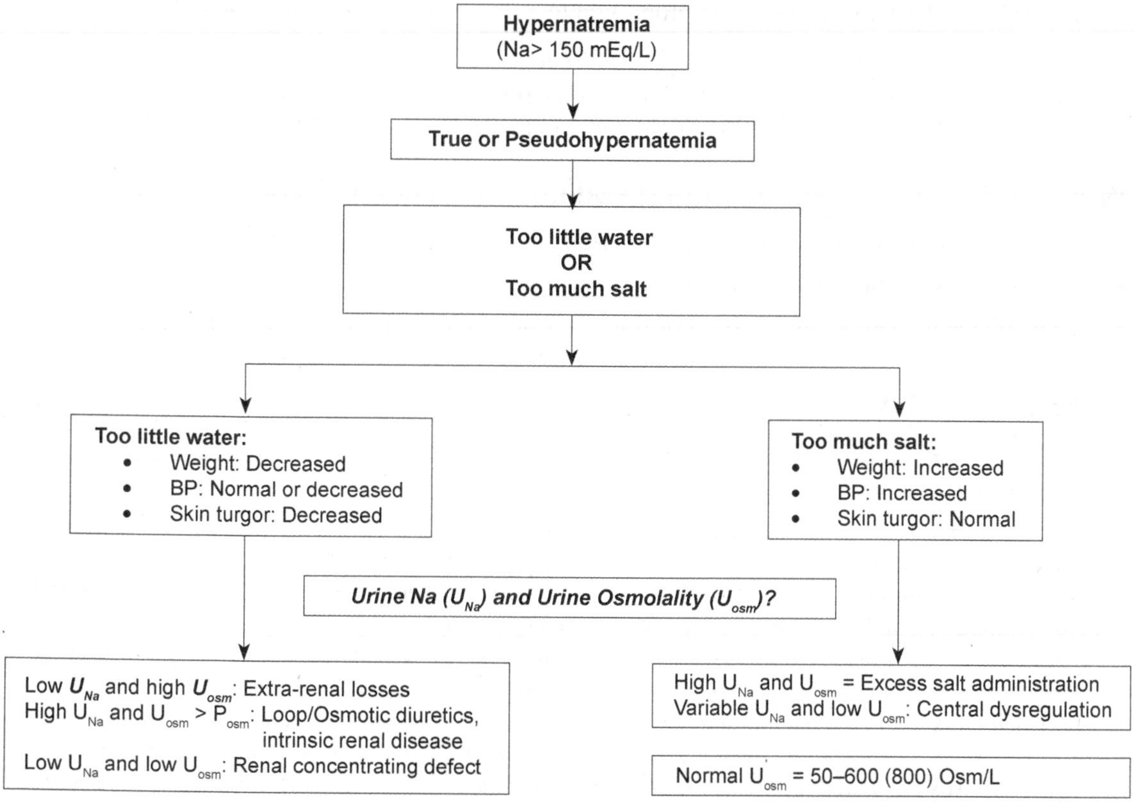

Fig. 17.1: Flowchart for the evaluation of hypernatremia

Calculations:

- *Total Fluid Deficit* (TFD): Pre-illness weight – Current weight (3.0 2.5) = 0.5 L.
- *Free Fluid Deficit* (FFD): The amount of additional water needed to correct serum Na to the desired level.

$$\text{Free Fluid Deficit} = \left(\frac{Na_{obs} - Na_{target}}{Na_{target}}\right) \times 0.75 \times \text{Birthweight} \ \{*Na_{target} = 150\}$$

$$= (Na_{obs} - 150) \times 5 \text{ mL/kg}$$

$$= (170 - 150) \times 5 \times 3 = 300 \text{ mL} = 0.3\text{L}$$

- *Solute Fluid Deficit* (SFD): The amount of additional fluid volume loss beyond free water loss (Isonatremic dehydration) in a patient with hypernatremic dehydration. The SFD is subsequently used to calculate Na and K^+ deficits in these patients. [SFD = TFD – FFD]. In this case, SFD would be 0.5 – 0.3 = 0.2 L.
- Na deficit (mEq/L) = SFD (L) × fluid proportion lost from ECF × Na concentration in ECF

  = 0.2 × 0.75 × 145 = **22 mEq.**

  Maximum Na correction allowed: 12 mEq/day (0.5 mEq/L/hr)

- K+ deficit (mEq/L) = SFD × fluid proportion lost from ICF × K concentration in ICF
  = 0.2 × 0.4 × 150 = **12 mEq.**

In the above case, the desired fall in serum Na – 20 mEq/L and the maximum Na correction allowed: 12 mEq/L/24 hours. Therefore, free fluid defict in this case should be corrected over 48 hours.

What are the complications during sodium correction in hypernatremia?

- Rapid correction of chronic hypernatremia leads to extrapontine myelinolysis.
- Increased CSF protein due to leakage from damaged blood vessel.
- Hyperglycemia: Do not give insulin (insulin may precipitous lowered serum osmolality).

HYPERKALEMIA

CASE SCENARIO 3

A 38 weeks neonate born to a G2P1L1 mother through vacuum assisted vaginal delivery and was born limp and cyanosed. Baby was resuscitated with positive pressure ventilation for 5 minutes and was shifted to NICU for post-resuscitative care. Baby was continued on CPAP for respiratory distress and was monitored for urine output. Baby had decreased urine output on day 2 of life with abnormal gain in weight. Investigations showed rise in creatinine with Serum potassium value of 7.9 mEq/L. Baby was started on restricted renal regime. ECG showed presence of tall t waves with sinus rhythm. Baby was continued on potassium free fluid and was given intravenous calcium gluconate. Potassium lowering resin was started per rectally. Repeat potassium done after 12 hours showed declining trend. ECG monitoring was continued. Urine output increased over next 3 days with normalisation of creatinine levels. Resins were stopped as potassium normalized.

CRITICAL CASE ANALYSIS

This case scenario describes the presentation of acute kidney injury secondary to an asphyxial event. Complications like hyperkalemia should be screened in settings of acute renal failure. Other causes of hyperkalemia should be ruled out including spurious lab value and medication error. On diagnosing hyperkalemia, ECG should be done to look for rhythm disturbance. All sources of potassium intake should be stopped and membrane stabilising drug like calcium gluconate was given immediately. Potassium lowering agents should be started as soon as possible.

What is hyperkalemia?

Serum $K^+ > 6.5$ mEq/L.

What are the common causes of hyperkalemia in a neonate?

- Acidosis: PH 0.1 unit ≈ K 0.6 mEq/L.
- Increase K release:
  - Hemolysed blood sample (most common innocuous cause).
  - Hemolysis, Intracranial hemmorrhage, cephalhematoma.
  - Tissue destruction, hypothermia, perinatal asphyxia.

- Decreased K Clearance:
  - ARF, oliguria, hyponatremia, congenital adrenal hyperplasia.
- Misc: Exchange transfusion, dehydration.
- Non-oliguric Hyperkalemia of VLBW infants: It is due mainly to a shift of potassium from the intracellular to the extracellular space associated with a decrease in the erythrocyte Na, K^+ - ATPase activity.

What are the clinical manifestations and progressive ECG changes in hyperkalemia?

- Skeletal muscle weakness, parentheses and ECG changes.
- Typical ECG changes of hyperkalemia progress with increasing serum K^+ values:
  - Peaked T waves, prolongation of PR interval.
  - Loss of P waves, widened QRS complex.
  - ST-segment depression.
  - Progressive widening of QRS complex.
  - Sine wave pattern.
  - Torsade de pointes, Ventricular fibrillation, Asystole, AV block.

Characteristic ECG changes in hyperkalemia are depicted in Figure 17.2.

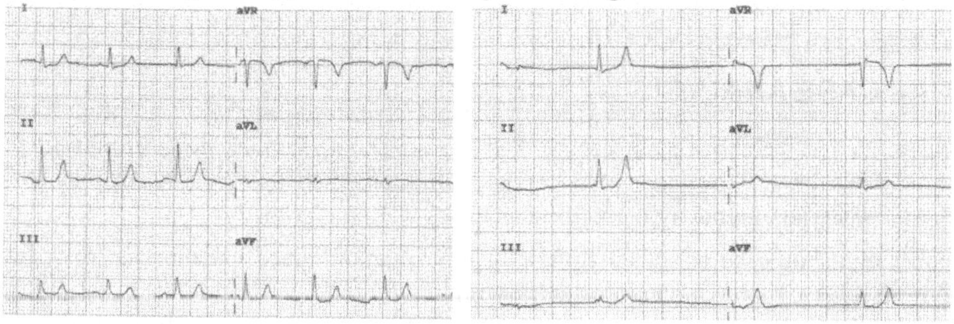

Fig. 17.2: ECG change in hyperkalemia: Peaked T, loss of P wave and effect of IV calcium gluconate

How to manage a case of hyperkalemia?

- Reconfirm K^+ level and rule out Pseudohyperkalemia.
- Urgent ECG.
- Discontinued all source of K^+.
- Established the cause and managed accordingly:
  - ECG changes: IV Calcium gluconate (10%) 2 ml/kg under cardiac monitor to **stabilize the myocardium,** may repeat in 10 minutes. It does not lower the serum potassium concentration.
  - Sodium bicarbonate 1–2 mEq/kg IV over 5–10 minutes may be used in cases of metabolic acidosis. Sodium bicarbonate is not compatible with IV Calcium gluconate, therefore, flush line between infusions; and/or

- Regular insulin: Bolus 0.1 u + 4 ml 10% D/kg over 30 minutes, repeat dose or begin infusion @ 0.05–0.1 units/kg/hr + 2–4 ml/kg/hr of D10 and monitor hourly blood glucose – **Most effective.**
- B-2 agonist-nebulized Salbutamol 2.5 mg inhalation every 1–2 hr, less effective in preterm infants.

Negative K balance:

- K-bind (Kayexalate) 1 gm/kg q4–6 hourly: Rectal route.
- Furosemide 1 mg/kg/dose if good renal function-very rarely used in neonate.
- Peritoneal or hemodialysis in case of oliguria/anuria or refractory to above measures.

HYPOKALEMIA

CASE SCENARIO 4

A 40 weeks neonate born to a primigravida mother presented on day 5 of life with persistent bilious vomiting. Baby was investigated and found to have mal-rotation with volvulus. Investigation showed presence of serum K of 2.8 mEq/L. ECG was normal. Baby was started on potassium supplementation and fluid replacement. Baby was operated on day 6 of life and kept nil per orally with continuous nasogastric tube decompression. Volume by volume replacement of aspirates was done. Electrolytes were monitored every 12 hourly. Repeat potassium normalized over next 48 hours. Feeds were started on day 14. Baby was discharged on day 17 of life.

CRITICAL CASE ANALYSIS

Neonate described in the above case scenario had hypokalemia secondary to gastrointestinal losses in form of bilious vomiting. Baby was started on potassium supplement as well as replacement of on-going losses. Serum potassium gradually normalized as losses were replaced.

Hypokalemia should be corrected slowly. In this situation, since patient was NPO, intravenous correction was done. The maximum infusion rate of potassium via peripheral line is 0.3–0.5 mEq/kg/hr and via central line is 1mEq/kg/hr (up to 20 mEq/hr). Potassium should never be pushed intravenously or given IM as bolus. Electrolyte monitoring should be done at least 12 hourly to notice trend of serum potassium and avoiding iatrogenic hyperkalemia.

What is hypokalemia?

Serum K<3.5 mEq/L.

Mild: 3–3.5 mEq/L, Moderate: 2.5–3.0 mEq/L and severe <2.5 mEq/L.

What are the causes of hypokalemia?

1. Normal Store: Hyperinsulinism, Catecholamine, Xanthenes, Hypothermia and Alkalosis (↑0.1 U pH ≈↓K^+ 0.3–1.3 mEq/L).
2. Decreased Sore:
   (a) Hypertensive: Renovascular disease, excess rennin/mineralcorticoid/steroids use.

(b) Normotensive:

(i) Renal loss: Diuretics, Antibiotics, Ampho-B, RTA, Fanconi syndrome, Bartter syndrome.

(ii) Extra-renal loss: Skin losses, GI losses, enema.

How to evaluate a case of hypokalemia?

The most important step is to determine the cause whether it is redistribution or net loss of K store either renal or extra-renal losses (Table 17.2).

Table 17.2: Evaluation of hyperkalemia in a neonate

Urinary indices	Renal losses	Extra-renal losses (GI losses)
K: Cr ratio	> 1.5	<1.5
Cl (mEq/L)	>20	<20
Anion Gap (Na + K–Cl)	<10	>10

What are the impacts of hypokalemia?

Generalized muscle weakness, paralytic ileus, and cardiac arrhythmias (AT, AV dissociation, VT/VF).

Severe untreated hypokalemia: Rhabdomyolysis, myoglobinuria, and acute renal failure.

What are the progressive ECG changes in hypokalemia?

- ST segment depression
- T wave flattening or inversion
- U wave
- Prolong QT interval.

Figure 17.3 shows typical ECG changes in hypokalemia.

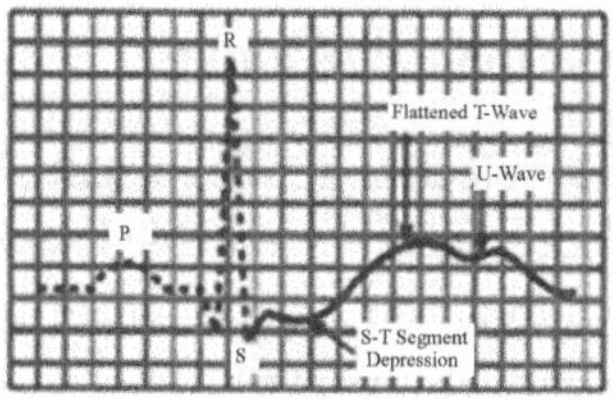

Fig. 17.3: Shows typical ECG changes in hypokalemia

How to manage a case of hypokalemia?

The most important steps in the management of hypokalemia is to address the cause, such as improving the K^+ supplementation, treating losses or stopping offending medications.

- **Oral KCl solution supplementation:** Mild to moderate hypokalemia

  Increasing dietary potassium intake is not completely effective in replacing the potassium loss associated with chloride depletion (e.g., diuretic therapy, vomiting, or nasogastric drainage) because dietary potassium is almost entirely coupled with phosphate, rather than with chloride. Oral Potassium chloride solution USP 20% is a sugar-free, clear colorless solution. Each 15 ml (table spoonful) contains potassium chloride 3.0 gm (supplying 40 mEq of potassium and chloride) =20 mEq K^+/15 ml.

- **Intravenous KCl (0.5 mEq/kg/dose):** Cardiac arrhythmias, extreme muscle weakness, respiratory distress, NPO or K <2.5 mEq/L
  - IV KCl must be prescribed in meq of potassium and must specify the **dose**, **route**, **dilution**, **volume and rate (mEq/hr).**

- **Never IM or IV push (bolus).**
- The maximum infusion rate via peripheral line is 0.3–0.5 mEq/kg/hr and via Central line @ 1 mEq/kg/hr (up to 20 mEq/hr).

KCl supplementation:

Serum K 3–3.5 mEq/L — 30 mEq/L

Serum K 2.5–3 mEq/L — 40 mEq/L

Serum K 2–2.5 mEq/L — 60 mEq/L

Serum K <2 mEq/L — 0.5–1 mEq/kg IV over 1 hour ↓ECG

IV $MgSO_4$: Refractory hypokalemia: 50 mg/kg/dose

DON'T treat concomitant Hypocalcemia and Acidosis till K level improve.

TAKE HOME MESSAGES

- Electrolyte homoeostasis is maintained by the kidneys.
- During management of dyelectrolytemia, rule out factious causes and address the critical situations.
- Sodium handling by the kidneys is determined by volume homeostasis rather than plasma sodium.
- Low glomerular filtration rate and tubular immaturity contribute to an increased frequency of electrolyte abnormalities in the neonatal period.

CONCLUSIONS

Dyselectrolytemia (usually hyponatremia, hypernatremia, hypokalemia and hyperkalemia), a common occurrence in the NICU, should be addressed on urgent basis to prevent the short and long-term morbidities. Since, electrolyte homoeostasis is maintained by the kidneys, during management of dyselectrolytemia, factitious causes should be ruled out. Critical situations should be addressed on priority.

FURTHER READING

1. Bell EF, Oh W. Fluid and electrolyte management. In: Avery GB, Fletcher MA, MacDonald MG (eds): *Neonatology: Pathophysiology of the Newborn*, 5th edn. Philadelphia: Lippincott Williams and Wilkins 1999;345–361.
2. Bockenhauer D, Zieg J. Electrolyte disorders. *Clin Perinatol* 2014;41:575–590.
3. Lorenz JM. Assessing fluid and electrolyte status in the newborn. *Clin Chem* 1997;43:205–210.

Chapter

18 Neonatal Hyperthyroidism

Jay Kishore, Satish Saluja

ABSTRACT

Neonatal thyrotoxicosis is rare and is mainly caused by placental transfer of thyroid stimulating antibodies to the fetus from a mother with Graves' disease or Hashimoto's thyroiditis. Other rarer causes of neonatal thyrotoxicosis may occur in conditions leading to overactivation of the TSH receptor and in Mc-Cune Albright syndrome. Neonatal Graves' disease occurs in 1 to 5% of pregnant mothers with Graves' disease. Neonatal hyperthyroidism manifests as irritability, flushing, diarrhea, vomiting, tachycardia, hypertension, poor weight gain, thyroid enlargement, and exophthalmos. Thrombocytopenia, hepatosplenomegaly, jaundice, and hyperviscosity syndrome also have been observed.

Neonatal hypothyroidism is managed with antithyroid medication propylthiouracil or carbimazole. Propranolol is also used for symptomatic management.

Key Words: Carbimazole, Exophthalmos, Graves' disease, Neonatal hypothyroidism, Propylthiouracil, Propranolol, Thyrotoxicosis.

INTRODUCTION

Autoimmune or transient neonatal hyperthyroidism (Neonatal Graves' disease) is more common form of neonatal hyperthyroidism (incidence-1:25,000–50,000) and occurs in 1 to 5% of the offspring of mothers with active or inactive Graves' disease. Non-autoimmune or permanent congenital hyperthyroidism, a form of neonatal thyrotoxicosis, is a very rare, but potentially serious disease. It can be non-familial or familial (autosomal–dominant inheritance). The non-familial variation may be either a de novo germline or somatic thyrotropin receptor-activating mutation.

CASE SCENARIO

A baby of gestational age 35 weeks presented at 2 weeks with poor weight gain, irritability and neck swelling. On examination, baby had heart rate–220/min, blood pressure was more than 99th centile for that gestational age. Baby had mid-line swelling of neck with hepatosplenomegaly. Skull examination

Contd...

Contd...

revealed craniosynostosis. Detailed antenatal history revealed that mother was a case of Graves' disease and was on propyl thiouracil treatment.

Lab investigation revealed high total and free T4 level and low TSH. TSH receptor antibody was also present.

CRITICAL CASE ANALYSIS

This baby was diagnosed as suffering from neonatal thyrotoxicosis as a result of placental transfer of TSH receptor antibody. If a mother is on antithyroid medication, baby usually manifests after 1 week (after depletion of transferred antithyroid drug). Clinical symptomatology in above mentioned case revealed goitre, tachycardia, hypertension, craniosynostosis and hepatosplenomegaly suggestive of neonatal thyrotoxicosis. Maternal history of Graves' disease is another clue to neonatal thyrotoxicosis.

INTERACTIVE TOPIC DISCUSSION

What are the common types of neonatal hyperthyroidism?

There are two types:

(a) Autoimmune or transient neonatal hyperthyroidism: more common form

(b) Non-autoimmune or permanent congenital hyperthyroidism: very rare, but serious disease

1. Non-familial
2. Familial (autosomal-dominant inheritance)

What is the pathogenesis of transient neonatal hyperthyroidism?

The transplacental passage of maternal TRSAb is important in the pathogenesis of this disease. The elevated TRSAb level leads to hyperthyroidism in utero from the second trimester as the fetal thyrotropin receptors respond to fetal thyrotropin or maternal TRSAB.

After how much time does the transient neonatal hyperthyroidism recover?

After 2–5 months of anti-thyroid drug treatment, transient neonatal hyperthyroidism recovers.

Does breastfeeding transmit TRSAb to baby?

Breastfeeding transmits TRSAb to the baby. Thus, transient neonatal hyperthyroidism can result in a breastfed baby of a mother having Graves' disease.

What is the clinical symptomatology of neonatal hyperthyroidism?

Infants may be born prematurely from such a mother. Sweating, increased appetite, weight loss or lack of weight gain, irritability, excessive movement, tremor, flushing of the cheeks, supraventricular tachycardia, goiter, and exophthalmos are found in the newborn. A distinctive feature in neonate with severe Graves' disease is generalized enlargement of the reticuloendothelial system, causing generalized lymphadenopathy, hepatosplenomegaly, *thrombocytopenia and hypoprothrombinemia.*

What are the side effects to the fetus if mother is taking beta blocker during pregnancy?

Use of beta blockers will lead to retarded fetal growth or postnatal bradycardia and hypoglycemia of the newborn.

What are the medical modalities for the management of neonatal hyperthyroidism?

The common medical modalities are:

1. Antithyroid drug: methimazole or propylthiouracil
2. High dose iodine treatment
3. Intravenous immunoglobulin

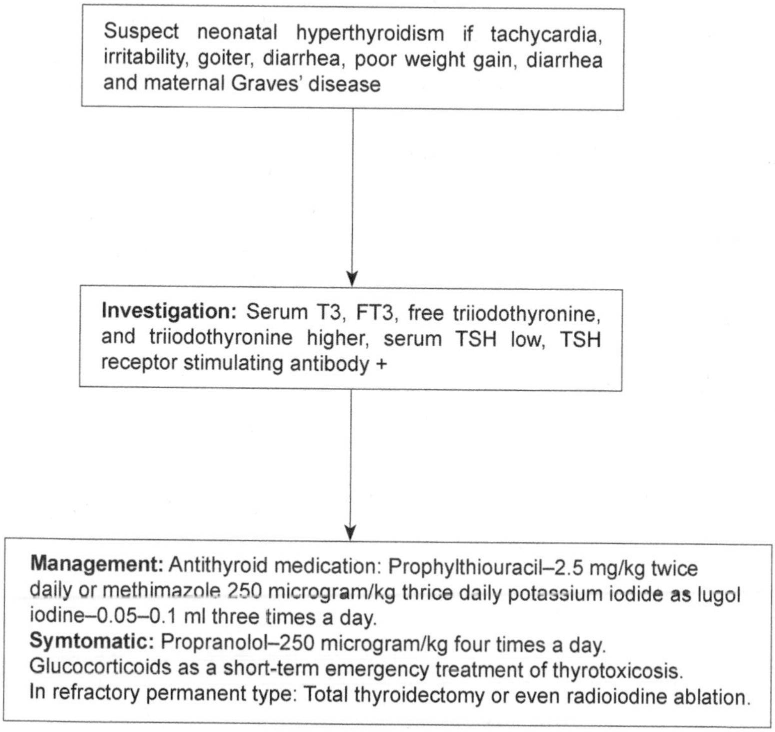

Fig: 18.1: Neonatal hyperthyroidism

CONCLUSIONS

Neonatal hyperthyroidism is a rare clinical condition. There are two forms: autoimmune and non-autoimmune. Non-autoimmune are of two types: Familial and non-familial. More common form is autoimmune or transient neonatal hyperthyroidism. Autoimmune type is seen in 1–5% offspring of mothers having Graves' disease. Neonatal hyperthyroidism is managed with antithyroid drug, high dose iodine treatment and IVIG. In permanent non-autoimmune form, thyroidectomy or radioactive iodine ablation is required in refractory cases.

TAKE HOME MESSAGES

- He prognosis of the autoimmune neonatal hyperthyroidism depends upon the severity of the fetal hyperthyroidism.
- TRSAb level at birth, and also its clearance rate in the newborn.
- In most cases, the antibodies clear by the end of the first year of life.
- If thyrotoxicosis persists beyond this time, it is likely that the infant has an activating mutation of the TSH receptor or endogenous thyroid stimulating antibody production.

FURTHER READING

1. Bollepalli S, Rose SR. Disorders of thyroid gland. In: Gleason, Christine A (eds). *Avery's Diseases of the Newborn,* 9th edn. Philadelphia: Elsevier 2012:1307–1319.
2. Chuang J, Gutmark-Little I, Rose SR. Thyroid disoders in the neonate. In: Martin, Richard J (eds): *Fanaroff and Martins' Neonatal-Perinatal Medicine* 10th edn. Philadelphia: Elsevier 2015:1490–1515.
3. CJ Peters, Hindmarsh PC Management of neonatal endocrinopathies—Best practice guidelines. *Early Human Develop* 2007;83:553–561.

Chapter

19 Congenital Adrenal Hyperplasia

Jay Kishore, Satish Saluja

ABSTRACT

Congenital adrenal hyperplasia is an autosomal disorder of cortisol synthesis. Most common enzyme deficiency is 21-hydroxylase deficiency. About 70% manifest as salt wasting crisis with virilization of genitalia in females. Males may show increased pigmentation of genitalia. A small proportion manifest as hypertension.

Salt wasting type is managed with hydrocortisone, fludrocortisones and sodium chloride while non-salt wasting variant is managed by hydrocortisone only.

Prenatal diagnosis and treatment is available.

Key Words: Congenital adrenal hyperplasia, 21-hydroxylase deficiency, Fludrocortisones, Hydrocortisone, Hypertension, Salt-wasting type, Salt-wasting crisis, Sodium chloride, Virilization.

INTRODUCTION

Congenital adrenal hyperplasia (CAH) is a lifelong endocrine disorder that presents acutely in the neonatal period. It comprises a group of autosomal recessive disorders of adrenal steroidogenesis. This condition is caused by an enzyme defect in the adrenal steroid synthesis pathway. The most common form is due to 21-hydroxylase deficiency which blocks the pathways for the synthesis of cortisol and aldosterone. It leads to an accumulation of 17-hydroxyprogesterone (17-OHP) and drives the steroid precursors into the pathway synthesising androgens and testosterone. Therefore, the neonate may present as a virilised female with high levels of 17-OHP on blood testing. The lack of glucocorticoid and mineralocorticoid place the baby at risk of an adrenal crisis with hyponatremia, hyperkalemia, hypoglycemia and hypotension. Plasma electrolytes must, therefore, be monitored closely if this condition is suspected.

The five enzymes or enzymatic steps involved in the synthesis of cortisol from cholesterol are cholesterol side chain cleavage enzyme complex (P450scc), 3β-hydroxysteroid dehydrogenase

(3βHSD), 17-α-hydroxylase, 21-hydroxylase, and 11β-hydroxylase. All except 3βHSD are members of the cytochrome P450 group of oxygenases. Except for 17α-hydroxylase, these enzymes are also necessary for mineralocorticoid (aldosterone) biosynthesis. The first three enzymes are present in gonadal tissue, where they are necessary for synthesis of the sex steroids. A deficiency in males results in inadequate testosterone formation and incomplete male sex differentiation; in females, it results in deficient estrogen synthesis, which is clinically significant at puberty.

CASE SCENARIO

A 15-day-old term newborn, initially diagnosed as a male, was referred to NICU because of vomiting, dehydration and jaundice and poor weight gain. Physical examination showed hyperpigmentated ambiguous external genitalia, IV stage of virilization following Prader classification (phallus sized almost as a normal penis and an empty scrotum).

Adrenal insufficiency was diagnosed according to the severe electrolyte abnormalities, hyponatremia of 110 mmol/l, hyperkalemia of 7 mmol/l, mild hypoglycemia and metabolic acidosis during an acute infection—osteomyelitis of the left lower limb. The karyotype in combination with the extremely increased 17-hydroxyprogesterone (17-OHP) confirmed the diagnosis of a 46,XX female sex with androgen excess caused by congenital adrenal hyperplasia due to 21-hydroxylase deficiency. Treatment with hydrocortisone and fludrocortisone resulted with electrolyte normalization. Female sex was reassigned and further reconstructive surgery advised to the parents.

CRITICAL CASE ANALYSIS

This neonate, aged 15 days, appeared to have penis and had, hence, been initially diagnosed as male. However, detailed examination showed that the scrotum was empty. There was also pigmentation. In fact, grade IV virilization was present according to the Prader classification. The problem related to misdiagnosis was because initially scrotum had not been palpated for testes.

Invariably (95%), CAH is due to 21 hydroxylase deficiency.

Two forms are seen in neonates: A simple virilizing form, in which the enzyme deficiency is partial, and a salt-losing form, in which the enzyme deficiency is more complete. A third form, late-onset or non-classic 21-hydroxylase deficiency represents a mild enzyme deficiency that does not have clinical manifestations in the fetus, neonate, or infant.

The symptoms or signs of adrenal insufficiency are not present at birth and rarely occur before 3 to 4 days of age. About half of the untreated patients with salt-losing CAH have onset of adrenal crisis between 6 and 14 days of age; by 1 month of age, more than three-fourths have developed adrenal crisis. In this case, the baby was 16 days old.

Diagnosis of 21-hydroxylase deficiency in a neonate or infant should be considered in females with any masculinization of the external genitalia, in presumed males with impalpable gonads (including males with hypospadias), in females or males who develop symptoms or signs of adrenal insufficiency or crisis (females should be recognized by their genital abnormalities), and in those who have a family history of CAH or an unexplained death in infancy.

INTERACTIVE TOPIC DISCUSSION

What is the pathway of cortisol synthesis?

Figure 19.1 gives pathway of cortisol synthesis.

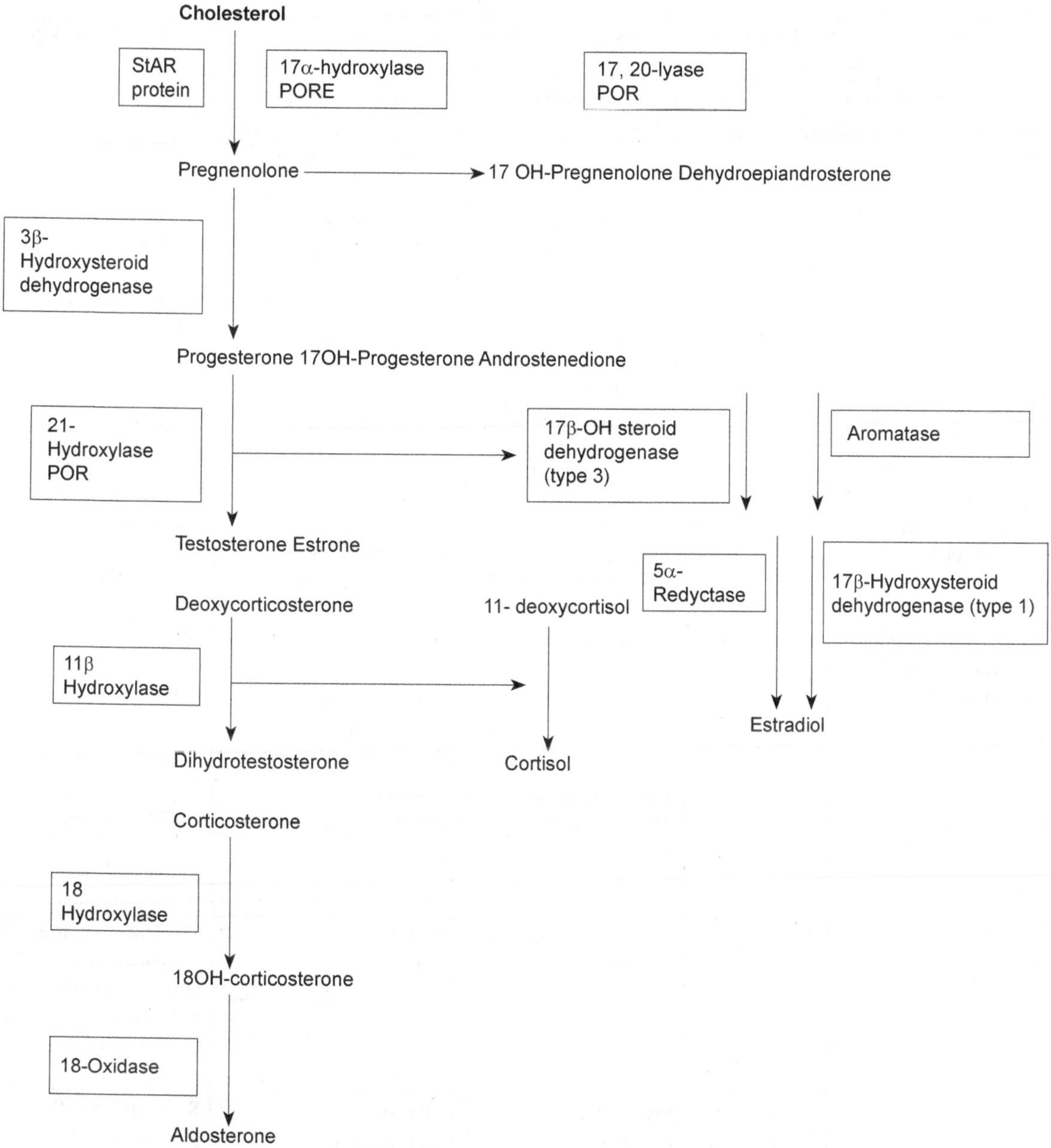

Fig. 19.1: Algorithm highlighting the pathway of cortisol synthesis

What are the different types of CAH? Summarise the salient features, clinical parameters and management of different types?

Different types of CAH and their salient features are listed in Table 19.1.

Table 19.1: Salient features of different types of CAH

Disorder	Affected gene and chromosome	Signs and symptom	Lab finding	Therapeutic measure
21 Hydroxylase deficiency classic form	CYP21 6p21.3	Glucocorticoid deficiency	↓ Cortisol, ↑ACTH ↑↑ Baseline and ACTH-stimulated 17-hydroxy-progesterone	Glucocorticoid (hydrocortisone) replacement
		Mineralocorticoid deficiency (salt-wasting crisis)	Hyponatremia, hyperkalemia ↑ Plasma renin	Mineralocorticoid (fludrocortisone) replacement; sodium chloride supplementation
		Ambiguous genitalia in females	↑ Serum androgens	Vaginoplasty and clitoral recession
		Postnatal virilization in males and females	↑ Serum androgens	Suppression with glucocorticoids
21-Hydroxylase deficiency, non-classic form	CYP21 6p21.3	May be asymptomatic; precocious adrenarche, hirsutism, acne, infertility	↑ Baseline and ACTH-stimulated 17-hydroxyprogesterone ↑ Serum androgens	Suppression with glucocorticoids
3 β-Hydroxysteroid dehydrogenase deficiency, classical form	*HSD3B2* 1p13.1	Glucocorticoid deficiency	↓ Cortisol, ↑ ACTH ↑ ↑ Baseline and ACTH-stimulated Δ5 steroids (pregnenolone, 17-hydroxy pregnenolone)	Glucocorticoid (hydrocortisone) replacement
		Mineralocorticoid deficiency (salt-wasting crisis)	Hyponatremia, Hyperkalemia, ↑ Plasma renin	Mineralocorticoid (fludrocortisone) replacement; sodium chloride supplementation
		Ambiguous genitalia in females and males	↑DHEA, ↓androstenedione, testosterone, and estradiol	Surgical correction of genitals and sex hormone replacement as necessary, consonant with sex of rearing
		Precocious adrenarche, disordered puberty	↑ DHEA, ↓ androstenedione, testosterone, and estradiol	Suppression with glucocorticoids

Contd...

Contd...

1 11β-Hydroxylase deficiency	*CYP11B1* 8q24.3	Glucocorticoid deficiency	↓ Cortisol, ↑ ACTH	Glucocorticoid (hydrocortisone) replacement
			↑ ↑ Baseline and ACTH-stimulated 11-deoxycortisol and deoxycorticosterone	
		Ambiguous genitalia in females	↑ Serum androgens	Vaginoplasty and clitoral recession
		Postnatal virilization in males and females	↑Serum androgens	Suppression with glucocorticoid
		Hypertension	↓ Plasma renin, hypokalemia	Glucocorticoid
17α-Hydroxylase/17, 20-lyase deficiency	*CYP17* 10q24.3	Cortisol deficiency	↓ Cortisol, ↑ ACTH ↑ DOC, corticosterone	Glucocorticoid
		Ambiguous genitalia in males	↓ Serum androgens; poor response to hCG	Orchidopexy or removal of intra-abdominal testes; sex hormone replacement consonant with sex of rearing
		Sexual infantilism	↓ Serum androgens or estrogens	Sex hormone replacement consonant with sex of rearing
		Hypertension	↓ Plasma renin; hypokalemia	Suppression with glucorticoid
Congenital lipoid adrenal hyperplasia	*STAR* 8p11.2	Glucocorticoid deficiency	↑ ACTH Low levels of all steroid hormones, with decreased or absent response to ACTH	Glucocorticoid (hydrocortisone) replacement
		Mineralocorticoid deficiency (salt-wasting crisis)	Hyponatremia, hyperkalemia ↓ Aldosterone, ↑ plasma rennin	Mineralocorticoid (fludrocortisone) replacement; sodium chloride supplementation
		Ambiguous genitalia in males	Decreased or absent response to hCG in males	Orchidopexy or removal of intra-abdominal testes; sex hormone replacement consonant with sex of rearing
		Poor pubertal development or premature ovarian failure in females	↑ FSH, ↑ LH, ↓ estradiol (after puberty)	Estrogen replacement

Contd...

Contd...

P-450 oxidoreductase deficiency	*POR* 7q11.3	Glucocorticoid deficiency	↓↓ Cortisol, ↑ ACTH ↑ Pregnenolone, ↑ progesterone	Glucocorticoid (hydrocortisone) replacement
		Ambiguous genitalia in males and females	↑ Serum androgens prenatally, ↓ androgens and estrogens at puberty	Surgical correction of genitals and sex hormone replacement as necessary, consonant with sex of rearing
		Maternal virilization	Decreased ratio of estrogens to androgens	

Which type is the most common type of CAH?

21-hydroxylase enzyme deficiency is the most common cause of CAH, accounting for 95% of all cases.

What are the different forms of 21-hydroxylase enzyme deficiency?

Two forms are seen in neonates:

1. Simple virilizing form: Enzyme deficiency is partial.
2. Salt-losing form: Enzyme deficiency is more complete. A third form.

Late-onset or nonclassic 21-hydroxylase deficiency: A mild enzyme deficiency that does not have clinical manifestations in the fetus, neonate, or infant.

What is the incidence of classic forms of 21-hydroxylase enzyme deficiency?

The incidence of classic forms of 21-Hydroxylase enzyme deficiency is 1 in 15,000 live births, and the carrier frequency of classic CAH is about 1 in 60 individuals. Seventy percent of all reported cases of CAH are salt wasting, and 30% are not salt wasting.

How does the simple virilizing form clinically manifest?

Spectrum of masculinization in females ranges from mild clitoromegaly, usually with some posterior labial fusion, to perineal or penile hypospadias to occasionally complete male differentiation, with the urethra opening at the tip of a male-sized phallus; the latter phenotype may have a normal male appearance except that the gonads are impalpable. In males, external genitalia are usually normal at birth; some enlargement of the penis may occur, but it is rarely recognizable as such. Female and male neonates may have increased pigmentation of the genitalia or areolae. Usually, there are no symptoms of adrenal insufficiency unless they are exposed to major stress or significant salt depletion.

How does the salt-wasting type manifest?

Symptoms rarely occur before 3 to 4 days of age. About half of the untreated patients with salt-losing CAH have onset of adrenal crisis between 6 and 14 days of age; by 1 month of age, more than three-fourths have developed adrenal crisis.

A. Marked impairment of cortisol and aldosterone synthesis, increased levels of ACTH and angiotensin.
B. In females, complete virilization of the external genitalia and some are incorrectly identified as males at birth. Males generally receive medical attention when they develop a salt-losing crisis caused by adrenal insufficiency.

C. Early symptoms and signs of adrenal crisis are non-specific and include lethargy, a poor appetite, and regurgitation of feedings, failure to thrive, and weight loss. Hyperkalemia, hypoglycemia, hyponatremia, and metabolic acidosis may be seen early. The regurgitation of feedings may progress to projectile vomiting. Severe symptoms and signs may occur within 1 to 2 days, including dehydration (with azotemia), hypotension, muscle weakness, altered sensorium, a gray or cyanotic appearance, cold and clammy skin, hyperkalemic cardiac conduction abnormalities, and hyponatremic or hypoglycemic seizures.

How can one make the diagnosis of 21-hydroxylase enzyme deficiency?

1. In females with any virilization of the external genitalia, in presumed males with impalpable gonads (including males with hypospadias), in females or males who develop symptoms or signs of adrenal insufficiency or crisis and in those who have a family history of CAH or an unexplained death in infancy.
2. Most important diagnostic test: Increased level of serum 17-OHP (>80 times higher than normal in a full-term infant). Elevated androstenedione, testosterone, DHEA, renin, ACTH and decreased level of aldosterone and cortisol.

How to manage a case of 21-hydroxylase enzyme deficiency?

- **Salt wasting type:**
  - Glucocorticoids: hydrocortisone - Maintenance: 12–20 mg/sq m per day PO divided in 3 doses. Stress dosing: Acute illness with stable hemodynamics: 40 mg/sq m per day PO/IV/IM divided q 6-8 h.

    Severe stress, such as major surgery or sepsis, or if hemodynamically unstable 100 mg/sq m (or 25 mg) IV/IM STAT once, then 25 mg/sq m/dose q 6 h for 24–48 hours. Assess the need for ongoing stress dosing as per clinical status. General anesthesia (either for surgery or procedure): 50 mg/sq m IV/IM once 30–60 minutes before anesthesia induction.
  - Mineralocorticoids: Fludrocortisone: 0.05–0.3 mg/day PO once or twice daily.
  - Sodium chloride: 0.5–5 mmol/kg per day divided in 4–6 doses as tolerated. Measurements of blood pressure and the level of plasma renin activity are used to adjust the mineralocorticoid dosage and sodium supplementation. The dose of Fludrocortisone does not change with increases in body size or during stress. In acute salt-losing adrenal crisis, fluid replacement (beginning with 20 ml/kg of bodyweight of 0.9% saline), sodium replacement, continuous glucose infusion, glucocorticoid therapy at 50 to 100 mg/sq m (initially given intravenously as the phosphate or succinate ester of hydrocortisone), and mineralocorticoid replacement (Florinef Acetate, 0.1–0.2 mg orally every 12–24 hours) are needed.
  - Correction of acidosis, hypoglycemia, and hyperkalemia.

Won't just cortisol replacement cause normalization of ACTH in the simple virilizing form?

Yes, in **simple virilizing** form of 21-hydroxylase deficiency, normalization of ACTH requires only cortisol replacement. The adequacy of cortisol replacement is monitored by the measurement of serum 17-OHP and androstenedione with the aim to keep them normal for age reference values.

How should gender be assigned to a baby with CAH?

Female gender assignment is usually recommended in 46, XX CAH individuals regardless of the extent of virilization of their genitalia. These patients have normal ovaries and mullerian structures and have the potential to lead normal, fertile lives as females. Typically, they have a female gender identity.

How about surgical correction of virilized clitoris?

Surgical correction and its timing in females with virilized external genitalia are controversial. If done, it is usually performed when a reasonable body size has been achieved, commonly in the first 2 to 6 months.

Can 21- hydroxylase deficiency CAH be diagnosed prenatally?

Yes, gene-specific diagnosis in utero can be made on fetal cells obtained by chorionic villus sampling or amniotic fluid analysis.

Is there any prenatal treatment of 21 hydroxylase deficiency CAH?

Yes, prenatal dexamethasone is effective with success rate 80 to 85% in preventing or minimizing the virilization of the classical 21-hydroxylase CAH affected female infants. Dexamethasone dose is 20 μg/kg prepregnancy maternal weight daily in 2–3 divided doses and started by 6 weeks gestation. As the genetic diagnosis cannot be made until 10 to 12 weeks, all pregnancies at risk for CAH are treated empirically with dexamethasone as soon as pregnancy is confirmed and preferably before 9 weeks of gestation. Treatment is discontinued once the genetic results confirm either a male fetus karyotype and or unaffected female fetus.

Do we have possibility of newer diagnostic modality which will stop undesirable antenatal dexamethasone treatment to male fetuses?

Recent genetic advances may soon permit the determination of fetal sex by quantitative polymerase chain reaction of fetal Y-chromosomal DNA obtained directly from maternal blood. Such an approach can improve the probability of treating affected female fetuses from 1 in 8 to 1 in 4 by eliminating the unnecessary treatment of male fetuses. Currently, this test is not routinely available.

Is there any side effect to babies and mothers treated with antenatal dexamethasone?

Children exposed to this therapy have slightly lower birth weights. Effects on personality or cognition, such as increased shyness, have been suggested but not consistently observed. At present there is insufficient information to determine whether there are any long-term risks, particularly in the males and unaffected females who derive no direct benefit from the treatment. Maternal side effects of prenatal treatment have included edema, excessive weight gain, hypertension, glucose intolerance, cushingoid facial features and severe striae.

Is there any screening test for 21 hydroxylase deficiency CAH? What precaution should be taken in interpretation of screening test?

The method of detection is based on finding an increased level of 17-OHP in blood collected on filter paper at 2–5 days of age (>50 ng/ml: abnormal). False-positive results are usually associated with prematurity (due to decreased metabolic clearance of 17-OHP) or low birthweight and, less often, with serious illness (probably caused by increased 17-OHP production associated with stress), age less than 24 hours (fetoplacental contribution of 17-OHP), or technical problems.

How do we counsel the family for next pregnancy?

Since most of these disorders are autosomal recessive, the risk of having a baby with CAH in each subsequent pregnancy is 25%.

Will a child with CAH attain a normal adult height?

Theoretically, with meticulous treatment it should be possible for children with CAH to achieve a normal adult height. However, in practice, even with the very best treatment it is not always possible to achieve perfect control and some children with CAH do not reach their potential adult height. If a child is not treated until a later age, he or she may become short-statured.

Is steroid therapy harmful for the CAH baby?

In appropriate dose, there should be no side effects as the treatment is replacing natural deficient hormone. However, if too much hydrocortisone is given over a long period of time it can result in slowing of growth and weight gain.

Higher dose of fludrocortisone can cause high blood pressure, but this is usually temporary and responds to dose reduction.

At what time of the day should treatment be given?

Opinions vary on the best time to give hydrocortisone. It should usually be given three times throughout the day. The child's paediatric endocrinologist will advise the exact dose and times of treatment that suits the child.

How is the dosage of steroid determined?

The dose varies between individuals. In general, non-salt-losers will require lower doses than salt-losers. As the child grows, the dose will be increased and may rise significantly at puberty. Each child should be monitored closely by the paediatric endocrinologist and doses adjusted to their individual needs. The child's growth rate is one of the most reliable markers for determining hydrocortisone dose although blood tests are also useful. Blood pressure monitoring and blood tests are also usually done to monitor the levels of adrenal hormones including 17 Hydroxyprogesterone (17-OHP) and a test is done to assess the adequacy of salt replacement.

How often should a CAH child be medically monitored?

Regular medical assessment and monitoring of treatment is the essential for the successful management of CAH. Regular assessment of growth, bone maturation, blood pressure and blood tests help the pediatric endocrinologist decide on the best treatment plan. Generally, a visit to the paediatric endocrinologist four times a year will be necessary. It is also important to have a local doctor who is easily accessible and familiar with the child's condition.

Can a CAH child live a normal life?

Yes. Although not curable, CAH is a very treatable condition. With careful management, children with CAH can lead normal lives and should have a normal life expectancy. Although there are many issues that a person with CAH may face, there are people who can help. Pediatric and adult endocrinologists, gynecologists, fertility specialists, psychologists, counsellors and family support groups can all play vital roles in helping children and adults with CAH live healthy lives and assist with any issues that may arise.

What should be the algorithmic approach in CAH?

The flowchart for such an approach is presented in Figure 19.2.

Female baby with virilized genitalia/male baby with hyperpigmented genitalia presenting with vomiting, dehydration and failure to thrive hypotension, hypothermia and shock.

↓

- Glucose/dextrose stick at bedside
- RFT with electrolyte and liver function test
- Arterial blood gas/serum pH
- Cortisol
- ACTH
- 17-OHP
- Pelvic ultrasonography
- Karyotype

↓

Suspect CAH if hypoglycemia, hyponatremia, hyperkalemia, metabolic acidosis, ↓ cortisol, ↑ ACTH, ↑ 17-OHP

↓

Management of acute adrenal crisis

- Fluid resuscitation with a 20 ml/kg bolus of 0.9% normal saline. Repeated boluses may be needed.
- Replacement of fluid loss with isotonic crystalloid solutions containing dextrose (typically 5% dextrose with normal saline) at a rate of 1.5 to 2 times maintenance.
- Stress doses of hydrocortisone (100 mg/sqm per day).
- Central venous access and vasopressors, along with higher glucose concentrations, may be required in profoundly ill patients.
- Management with hyperkalemia with potassium-lowering resin, IV calcium, insulin and bicarbonate.

↓

Contd...

Contd...

Long-term Management:
- Maintenance dose: Oral hydrocortisone, in three divided doses of 10–20 mg/sq m per day.
- Monitoring by ACTH, 17-OHP, DHEA and androstenedione level.
- Target 17-OHP range of 500–1,000 ng/dL.
- Annual bone age radiograph and careful monitoring of linear growth.
- During times of mild-to-moderate stress, such as fever: doubling or tripling the usual maintenance dose of oral hydrocortisone.
- For severe stress and major surgery, administration of hydrocortisone (100 mg/sq m per day), divided in three to four IV doses, for at least 24 hours peri- and postoperatively before tapering over several days to a maintenance dose.
- Replacement with fludrocortisones: Usually 0.1 to 0.2 mg, but occasionally patients require up to 0.4 mg/day.
- Supplementation with 1 to 2 g of sodium chloride often is required (each gram of sodium chloride contains 17 mEq of sodium).
- Surgical reconstruction, with reduction clitoroplasty and construction of a vaginal opening.

↓

Management: Antithyroid medication: Prophylthiouracil – 2.5 mg/kg twice daily or methimazole 250 mcg/kg thrice daily Potassium iodide as Lugol iodine – 0.05–0.1 ml three times a day.
Symtomatic: Propranolol–250 mcg/kg four times a day.
Glucocorticoids as a short-term emergency treatment of thyrotoxicosis.
In refractory permanent type: Total thyroidectomy or even radioiodine ablation.

↓

Investigation: Serum T3, FT3, free triiodothyronine, and triiodothyronine higher, serum TSH low, TSH receptor stimulating antibody +

Fig. 19.2: Congenital adrenal hyperplasia

CONCLUSIONS

CAH connotes a family of disorders of the cortisol synthesis pathway in which more than 90% of cases are caused by 21OHD. The hallmark of 21OHD is excessive androgen production that varies in degree among its different subtypes. The severe classic form of CAH is the most common cause of ambiguous genitalia in a genetically female fetus.

Antenatal treatment of mothers with dexamethasone in early gestation results in significantly less virilization in female fetuses affected with classic CAH. Newborn screening has had an important impact on identifying the salt-wasting subtype in male infants and preventing adrenal crisis. Lifelong treatment with steroids is required for most patients. The consequences of the disease and complications of the treatment remain a challenge and require the involvement of multiple subspecialties.

TAKE HOME MESSAGES

- In an unexplained hyponatremia with hyperkalemia during 2nd week of life, diagnosis of CAH should always be considered.
- High index of suspicion in a doubtful male baby is helpful.
- Universal newborn screening should be done to pick up cases early and prevent mortality.
- Long-term comprehensive follow-up and parental education is essential part of management of CAH.
- Offer genetic counseling and antenatal diagnosis and treatment in subsequent pregnancy.

FURTHER READING

1. Antal Z, Zhou P. Congenital adrenal hyperplasia: Diagnosis, evaluation and management. *Pediatr Rev* 2009; 30;e49–e57.
2. Lin-Su K, New MI. Ambiguous genitalia in the newborn. In: Gleason, Christine A (eds). *Avery's Diseases of the Newborn,* 9th edn. Philadelphia: Elsevier 2012:1286–1306.
3. Remeithi SA, Wherrett DK. Disorders of Sex Development. In: Martin, Richard J (eds): *Fanaroff and Martin's Neonatal-Perinatal Medicine,* 10th edn. Philadelphia: Elsevier 2015:1516–1552.
4. White PC. Congenital adrenal hyperplasia and related disorders. In: Kliegman RM, Stanton BF, St Geme JW, Schor NF, (eds): *Nelson Textbook of Paediatrics,* 19th edn. Philadelphia: Elsevier 2016.

Chapter

20 Neonatal Shock

Anup Thakur, Anita Singh

ABSTRACT

Shock is a state of inadequate perfusion resulting from an inability of heart to satiate tissue oxygen demand. In neonates, it may complicate several clinical conditions, causing hemodynamic compromise which, if left untreated, invariably proves fatal. The clinical parameters for its diagnosis have insufficient sensitivity and specificity. Management is further complicated in premature and low birthweight neonates because of the Immature myocardium, presence of fetal channels, increased pulmonary pressure, pressure passive cerebral circulation and relative adrenal insufficiency.

Treatment involves fluid infusion, inotropes and sometimes steroids.

Key Words: Functional echocardiography, Hypotension, Inotropes, Low birthweight, Neonatal shock, Prematurity, Systemic blood flow.

INTRODUCTION

Shock is a state of inadequate perfusion resulting from an inability of heart to satiate tissue oxygen demand. In neonatal intensive care unit, it results in hemodynamic compromise of sick neonates. Several parameters are used for diagnosis and monitoring of shock but for simplification, low blood pressure has been traditionally used as main criterion. However shock can present with normal blood pressure and furthermore blood pressure may remain low with normal systemic blood flow and organ perfusion. Immature myocardium, presence of fetal channels, increased pulmonary pressure, pressure passive cerebral circulation and relative adrenal insufficiency further complicate the management of the condition especially in preterm infants.

CASE SCENARIO

A 3.2 kg male baby, appropriate for gestational age, was delivered at 38 weeks gestation to second gravida mother through meconium stained liquor. Baby was born limp and required resuscitation. APGAR scores were 4, 7 and 9.

Contd...

Contd...

He was shifted to neonatal intensive care unit for post-resuscitation care.

At 1 hour of life baby was ventilated for worsening respiratory distress (PIP/PEEP–26/5, FiO_2 = 80%). Capillary filling time was 4 seconds, mean arterial pressure 32 mm of Hg and a faint systolic murmur was heard on auscultation. Pre- and post-ductal saturations were 86 and 74% respectively. Chest X-ray revealed heterogeneous infiltrates. Echocardiography revealed elevated pulmonary pressures with normal cardiac contractility, under-filled inferior vena cava, low systemic blood flow and bi-directional shunting through ductus arteriosus. Baby was managed on high frequency ventilator (Mean airway pressure = 16 and FiO_2 = 60%). A normal saline fluid infusion was given by 20 ml/kg over 1 hour followed by dopamine and epinephrine infusion to increase systemic pressure. After 6 hours, mean arterial pressure increased to 55 mm of Hg. Oxygen requirement decreased to 40% at 24 hours. Baby was shifted to conventional ventilation after 48 hours and non-invasive ventilation after another 72 hours. Baby was weaned off respiratory support at day 10 of life and was discharged on day 14 of life. Parents were advised for regular follow-up in high-risk clinic and neurodevelopmental follow-up.

CRITICAL CASE ANALYSIS

This is a case of shock in a term infant whose clinical course is complicated by perinatal asphyxia along with meconium aspiration syndrome and persistent pulmonary hypertension. Circulatory failure and cardiovascular compromise is an important organ dysfunction in case of babies who have perinatal depression. Asphyxia and meconium aspiration both are risk factor for elevated pulmonary pressure. Increased pulmonary pressure contributes to shock and complicates its management. Treatment involves volume expanders to support preload, inotropes to increase systemic pressures, pulmonary vasodilators to reduce pulmonary pressure and supportive management. This baby responded to inotropes, fluid infusion and ventilation.

INTERACTIVE TOPIC DISCUSSION

What is shock?

Shock is a pathological state of circulatory compromise in which tissue oxygen delivery is inadequate to meet the demand.

What is normal blood pressure range for the neonates and how hypotension should be defined?

Blood pressure in neonates has direct relationship with gestational age and birthweight. There are a lot of controversies regarding normal blood pressure range according to available literature. Many investigators have tried to generate normative data for blood pressure for neonate but the values may be influenced by management protocol within given institution. More appropriate would be data which relates the blood pressure value with systemic blood flow and cardiac output. Nomograms given by Zubrow, *et al.* from Philadelphia Neonatal Blood Pressure Study Group are widely used in neonatal intensive care. Le Flore, *et al.* have given blood pressure range for very low birthweight babies during initial 72 hours of life when there is maximum risk of hypotension leading to loss of auto regulation and intraventricular hemorrhage.

Hypotension can be statistically defined as value less than – 2SD for each postmenstrual and gestational age. An operational definition would be valuable, i.e., a threshold pressure below which intervention will improve outcome. Early hypotension has been defined as mean blood pressure less than 30 mm of Hg in any gestation age infant in the first postnatal days. This cut-off is based on association of cerebral injury in the form of intraventricular hemorrhage and white matter injury in babies with mean blood pressure less than 30 mm of Hg. There is also suggestion from near infrared spectroscopy studies that cerebral blood flow decreases below threshold of around 30 mm of Hg. Another simplified cut-off which is supported by Joint Working Group of the British Association of Perinatal Medicine, is mean arterial pressure value below gestational age in weeks mainly in first 24–48 hours of life.

What is permissive hypotension?

It has been found by several investigators that many hypotensive neonates have normal systemic blood flow, good perfusion and tend to have good short-term and long-term outcome even without intervention. If these babies are treated only on the basis of low blood pressure cut-off, as much as 98% of extremely preterm babies will require intervention in intensive care units. On the other hand, if intervention for these babies is withheld and treatment is instituted for only those babies who have evidence of poor perfusion with hypotension, then only 16% of extremely low birthweight babies will require treatment. Permissive hypotension is the concept of withholding intervention for hypotension in babies with normal perfusion.

What are the peculiarities of neonatal cardiovascular system which are important for assessment of shock?

Assessment of shock in neonates is complicated by following peculiarities in preterm and term infants:

- *Immature myocardium*: Myocardium in neonates lacks sarcoplasmic reticulum and has poorly formed t-tubule system. Myocardium contains much of non-contractile fibrous tissue and has reduced sympathetic innervations. They have limited capacity to increase cardiac output but enhanced sensitivity to increase afterload which can ultimately results in decreased cardiac output.
- *Increased pulmonary pressure*: After birth pulmonary pressure fall over days to weeks during transitional circulation. Failure of pulmonary pressure to decrease can complicate the conditions as respiratory distress syndrome, perinatal asphyxia and meconium aspiration syndrome. Persistence of elevated pulmonary pressure can result in decreased cardiac output.
- *Presence of fetal channels*: Ductus arteriosus and foramen ovale are fetal channels which close after birth over few days. Patency of ductus arteriosus is inversely proportional to gestational age and birthweight. Ductus arteriosus if remains patent can result in overloading of left heart failure and lead to cardiac failure.
- *Relative adrenal insufficiency*: Adrenal gland plays important role in maintenance of cardiovascular homeostasis. Mineralocorticoid exerts their effect on intravascular volume while glucocorticoids promote developmental increase in blood pressure by enhancing expression of angiotensin II receptors. Very low birthweight babies and preterm infants are only capable of producing corticosteroids to meet their metabolic demand when they are not stressed. When critically sick they may not be able to mount an adequate stress response which is termed as relative adrenal insufficiency.

- *Hypovolemia*: Extremely preterm neonates especially who have not been exposed to antenatal steroids may have increased transepidermal loss during first few days of life resulting in significant hypovolemia and shock.

What are the causes of shock in neonates?

Etiologies of shock in neonates are following:

- **Hypovolemic Shock:**
    - o Antenatal hemorrhage-placenta previa, placental abruption, feto-maternal transfusion, twin-to twin transfusion.
    - o Perinatal-birth injuries (subgaleal hemorrhage), slipped ligature, rupture of umbilical vessels, spleen or liver.
    - o Postnatal-iatrogenic or secondary to disseminated intravascular coagulation or vitamin K deficiency, massive pulmonary hemorrhage.
    - o Fluid and electrolyte loss in newborns secondary to gastrointestinal abnormalities, vomiting, diarrhea or heat stress.
    - o Increased trans epidermal loss in extremely preterm babies.
- **Cardiogenic Shock:**
    - o Severe intrapartum asphyxia resulting in myocardial depression.
    - o Structural heart disease like coarctation of aorta, hypoplastic left heart, pulmonary atresia or tricuspid atresia.
    - o Myocardial failure due to neonatal tachy or bradyarrythmia or cardiomyopathy.
    - o Disturbance of cardiovascular function due to conditions related to transitional circulation like persistent pulmonary hypertension of newborn and patent ductus arteriosus.
- **Distributive Shock:**
    - o Septic shock.
- **Obstructive Shock:**
    - o Tension pneumothorax.
    - o Cardiac tamponade.
    - o Diaphragmatic hernia.
- **Dissociative Shock:**
    - o Anemia.
    - o Methemoglobinemia.

Conditions like sepsis and perinatal asphyxias have simultaneous presence of multiple etiologies.

What are the phases of shock?

There are three phases of shock:

1. *Compensated shock:* In this stage, perfusion of vital organs is maintained and there is minimal alteration of vital signs like blood pressure and heart rate.

2. *Uncompensated shock:* In this stage compensatory mechanism have failed and hypotension and decreased perfusion to vital organs starts ultimately leading to metabolic acidosis. From this phase, baby may either recover or progress to final irreversible stage.
3. *Irreversible shock:* In this stage, irreparable damage to end organ result manifesting as acute tubular necrosis, gastrointestinal bleeding and uncorrectable acidosis.

   Mortality is significantly improved if shock is diagnosed and anticipated in early stages.

What are parameters for assessment of shock in neonates?

Shock in neonates can be assessed by following methods:

- **Clinical:**
  - Increased heart rate.
  - Prolonged capillary filling time.
  - Low blood pressure.
  - Poor peripheral pulses.
  - Cool peripheries.
  - Increased core and peripheral temperature difference.
  - Mottling of skin.
  - Altered sensorium or lethargy.
  - Decreased urine output.
- **Laboratory:**
  - Progressive increased anion gap acidosis.
  - Increased lactate.
  - Increased Troponin T, I and CK-MB reflecting myocardial injury.
- **Echocardiographic:**
  - Preload assessment.
  - Myocardial contractility.
  - Systemic blood flow.
- **Tissue perfusion:**
  - Near infrared spectroscopy to measure oxygen extraction.
- **Continuous cardiac output monitoring by electrical impedance cardiometry.**

What investigations are done in cases of shock in neonates?

- Neonatal shock is a medical emergency and infants should be stabilized first. Investigations in case of shock in neonates are mainly addressed to determine type of shock, cause of shock, status of end organ damage and to monitor shock. The following investigations may be required:
  - Complete blood count, hematocrit and peripheral smear–for assessment of anemia and evidence of sepsis in form of leucopenia/neutropenia and presence of band cells and toxic granules.

- o Blood culture for identification of organism in case of neonatal sepsis.
- o Blood glucose, calcium (total/ionized), electrolytes for supportive care.
- o Arterial blood gas and serum lactate for monitoring of shock.
- o Blood urea nitrogen, serum creatinine and hepatic function test.
- o Platelet count and coagulation profile in case of bleeding.
- o Chest X-ray helps in identifying cardiomegaly and pulmonary parenchymal status.
- o Functional echocardiography.
- o Cranial ultrasound to detect complication like intraventricular hemorrhage.

What is the role of functional echocardiography in shock in neonates?

In case of shock to monitor hemodynamic status, functional ECHO can used to evaluate myocardial contractility, ventricular output, superior vena cava flow, preload assessment, presence of ductus arteriosus and pulmonary hypertension.

- **Myocardial contractility:** It can be assessed by shortening fraction. Normal value is 25–41% in healthy term and 23–40% in preterm neonates.
- **Cardiac output:** Left ventricular output is a direct measure of blood pumped out of left ventricular output. In the absence of ductus, it is surrogate marker of perfusion of the body. The normal value is 150–325 ml/kg/min. In the presence of ductus, left ventricular output is not a reliable marker of systemic perfusion, as part of this output is diverted to pulmonary circulation. In this case right ventricular output is a better marker. Normal range in neonate is same as left ventricular output i.e., 150–325 ml/kg/min. However in case of patent foramen ovale and atrial septal defect, right ventricular output may be falsely increased and is not a reliable marker of systemic perfusion. Superior vena cava flow has advantage of reflecting global flow to upper body and brain and also avoiding the transitional shunts that confound the early measurement of ventricular output. Normal range is 40–120 ml/kg/min.
- **Preload assessment:** A relatively small right atrium and ventricle size is a marker of decreased preload. Inferior vena cava (IVC) diameter and variation in inferior vena cava size can give some indirect idea of intravascular volume. Though nomogram of normal inferior vena cava diameter is not available for neonate, a visibly collapsed IVC suggest hypovolemia and visibly distended IVC suggest euvolemia/hypervolemia.
- **Assessment for patent ductus arteriosus and persistent pulmonary hypertension of newborn:** Ductus arteriosus is an important cause of hemodynamic compromise in extremely preterm babies. Functional echocardiography helps in identification and assessment of hemodynamically significant ductus and its response to treatment. Elevated pulmonary pressure is another common associated morbidity in some disorders presenting with shock, i.e., perinatal asphyxia, sepsis, meconium aspiration syndrome. Functional echocardiography is important for diagnosis and monitoring of pulmonary pressure in sick neonates.

Discuss the management of neonatal shock.

Management of shock involves initial stabilization, supportive treatment and management of hypotension. A simplified management algorithm is illustrated in Figure 20.1.

- Identification on the basis of clinical parameters.
- Initial stabilization-maintain temperature, position airway, start oxygen, consider elective ventilation.
- Obtain vascular access.
- Give antibiotic dose in suspected sepsis, send requisition for packed cell in suspected blood loss.
- Start intravenous fluid with glucose infusion rate adequate to maintain euglycemia.

Consider volume expansion by normal saline (0.9%) by 10 ml/kg over 30–60 minutes in babies suspected to have hypovolemic (one more infusion can be repeated in case of non-response)

→ Non-response

Start dopamine @ 10 mcg/kg/minute, increase in increment of 2.5 mcg/kg/min up to 15–20 mcg/kg/min

→ Non-response

Dobutamine @ 10 mcg/kg/min, increase in increment of 2.5 mcg/kg/min up to 15–20 mcg/kg/min

→ Non-response

Epinephrine in dose of 0.05–0.3 mcg/kg/min

→ Non-response

Hydrocortisone 2 mg/kg/dose stat, then 1 mg/kg/dose 6–8 hourly for 24–48 hours

→ Non-response

Consider Functional Echo. May consider trial of vasopressin/norepinephrine/milrinone.*Evaluate for pneumothorax and pneumopericardium, inhaled nitric oxide for PPHN and closure of hemodynamically significant ductus

Fig. 20.1: A simplified algorithm for management of shock in neonates

1. **Initial Stabilization:**
   - *Temperature:* Babies in shock frequently have hypothermia. Neonate should be nursed under radiant warmer. Incubator may be required in extremely preterm babies to take care of transepidermal losses.
   - *Airway:* Airway should be maintained by positioning and suctioning.
   - *Breathing:* Babies with shock may need to be electively ventilated to decrease the energy required for work of breathing because as much of 40% of neonatal cardiac output may be consumed on work of breathing. Pre- and post-ductal SpO_2 monitoring is preferable for neonates.
   - *Circulation:* Peripheral intravenous access can be difficult in babies with shock, so a central venous access is preferable. Central venous access is also needed for infusion of inotropes in higher doses. Volume expanders and vasopressors help to support circulation. Arterial line is ideal for accurate monitoring of blood pressure. Continuous ECG monitoring should be started. Input/output charting, blood gas analysis and serum lactate will help in further monitoring.
2. **Supportive treatment:**
   - Prompt antibiotic treatment should be started in case of suspected septic shock.
   - Maintain hematocrit-Packed red cell can be transfused in neonates with hemoglobin <12 g/dL.
   - Maintain glucose and calcium level within normal range.
3. **Management of Hypotension:**

   Volume expanders and inotropes are mainstay of treatment for hypotension. Inotropes are contraindicated in infants of diabetic mother with hypertrophied interventricular septum in which case propranolol is indicated for treatment for cardiovascular insufficiency.
4. **Treatment of the Cause:**
   - Nitric oxide therapy is required for associated persistent pulmonary hypertension.
   - Pneumothorax requires chest tube drainage. Babies with pnemopericardium and pericardial effusion resulting in tamponade will improve with drainage.
   - Prostaglandin infusion should be started for suspected duct dependent cardiac lesion.
   - Medical/surgical closure of hemodynamically significant ductus arteriosus may be required in extremely preterm babies.
   - Triiodothyronine (T3) is effective in newborns with thyroid insufficiency.
   - Adenosine or cardioversion is required in cases presenting with supraventricular tachycardia.

What is the role of volume expanders in management of shock in neonates?

Hypovolemia an important cause of shock in pediatric population, is not frequently encountered in neonates. In most hypotensive infants circulating blood volume is normal. Routine use of volume infusion is not recommended and should be preferably avoided in immediate postnatal period, unless there is strong suspicion of low blood volume. It has been found in studies that neonates who received rapid volume infusion were at increased risk of cerebral injury. Multiple fluid boluses have been associated with increased risk of mortality and bronchopulmonary dysplasia in preterm neonates.

Beyond first postnatal days and in term neonates maximum of two infusions of 10 ml/kg of crystalloid or colloid over 20–30 minutes can be given. There have been no differences in clinical outcomes in studies comparing crystalloid vs. colloid for volume expansion.

Discuss the role of inotropes and vasopressors in neonatal shock.

Inotropes and vasopressors are pharmacological agents which increase myocardial contractility and heart rate, and reduce or increase peripheral vascular resistance. The effects of these medications are dose dependent and depend on receptors which are stimulated. The commonly used inotropes and vasopressors in neonates are:

- **Dopamine**–It is most frequently used inotrope in neonates with hypotension. It stimulates dopaminergic, β and α-receptors in dose dependent manner. It has no β_2 activity and its β_1 activity is less potent than epinephrine. It primarily has α_1, some α_2 and dopaminergic effects. Established dose range is 5–20 mcg/kg/min. At low doses up to 5 mcg/kg/min, it primarily stimulates vascular dopaminergic receptors in mesenteric and renal circulation. At moderate doses of 5-10 mcg/kg/min it stimulates myocardial contractility and increases the heart rate by stimulation of β_1 receptors. At high dose >10 mcg/kg/min, vasoconstriction occurs due to stimulation of vascular α_1 receptors, which results in increased systemic and pulmonary vascular resistance. Cochrane meta-analysis has shown that dopamine produces greater increase in blood pressure in hypotensive infants than dobutamine. Dopamine is an important neurotransmitter and may decrease release of prolactin and thyroid stimulating hormone in neonates resulting in decrease in thyroxine and triiodothyronine.
- **Dobutamine**–It has α adrenergic effect that leads to increase in myocardial contractility and heart rate, and β adrenergic effect resulting in vasodilation. Thus, it is helpful in situation where there is myocardial dysfunction with increased peripheral vascular resistance. The cardiovascular effects are dose dependent and recommended dose range is 5–20 mcg/kg/min. In preterm infants with low systemic blood flow, there is some evidence that dobutamine is better than dopamine at increasing and maintaining systemic blood flow. Side effects include arrhythmia and hypertension.
- **Epinephrine**–It stimulates both α (α_1, α_2) and β (β_1, β_2) receptors. At low dose, it increases cardiac output and blood pressure while at higher doses, increase in systemic vascular resistance become significant. At higher doses it also increases pulmonary vascular resistance. Dose range is 0.05–0.3 mcg/kg/min. It has been found to be effective in cases of shock refractory to other inotropes. It can result in increase in lactate levels due to increase in lactate production and decrease in lactate metabolism. At higher doses, there may be impairment of mesenteric circulation.
- **Nor-epinephrine**–It is not much used in neonates. It has decreased β_2 activity in comparison to epinephrine, so it results in more pronounced vasoconstriction. Since warm phase of septic shock is not frequently encountered in neonates, its use is limited only to cases refractory to other inotropes. Recommended dose range is 0.05–0.5 mcg/kg/min.
- **Milrinone**–It is a selective class III phosphodiesterase inhibitor and its cardiovascular property include increase in myocardial contractility, improvement in myocardial relaxation and reduction of both systemic and pulmonary vascular resistance. It may have beneficial effects in cases of PPHN unresponsive to nitric oxide therapy. The recommended dose is 0.75 mcg/kg/min, followed by 0.2 mcg/kg/min.
- **Vasopressin**–Its main physiologic role in the body is to maintain extravascular osmolarity. Vascular effects occur by V_{1a} and V_2 receptors resulting in vasoconstriction and vasodilation respectively. When used as infusion, its vasoconstrictor action dominates. Its use in neonates is restricted to case reports in few preterm neonates unresponsive to conventional inotropes.

- **Isoprenaline**–Its acts exclusively on β receptors. It causes greater increase in the heart rate than cardiac output. In neonates, it is used in neonates with congenital heart block.
- **Levosimenden**–It is a new cardiovascular medication which exerts its inotropic effects by enhancing the binding of calcium to troponin C. It also has some vasodilator effects. It is a promising agent as inotrope in neonatal cardiac patients.

What is the role of corticosteroids in management of shock in neonates?

Relative adrenal insufficiency and down regulation of adrenergic receptors are important underlying pathophysiology in vasopressor resistant shock. Corticosteroids can help by improving the vascular sensitivity to inotropes, inhibiting nitric oxide synthase enzyme activity, suppressing immune responses or ameliorating relative adrenal insufficiency. Use of corticosteroids in neonates with shock have resulted in improved systemic blood pressure and reduced need for inotropes in several randomized controlled trial, however, there was no difference in clinical outcomes.

Its use should be restricted to shock refractory to epinephrine or in suspected cases of relative or absolute adrenal deficiency. It can be used in 1–2 mg/kg every 6–8 hourly for 24–48 hours.

What are therapeutic end points in management of shock?

- Capillary filling time < 2 seconds
- Normal blood pressure for age
- Good pulse volume
- Warm extremities
- Urine output > 1 ml/kg/hour
- SpO_2 = 90–95%
- <5% difference in pre- and post-ductal saturation
- Normal anion gap and lactate
- SVC flow > 40 ml/kg/min.

How should babies with shock followed?

Babies with shock should be followed in high risk clinic for assessment of neurodevelopmental outcome and early intervention and rehabilitation of associated morbidities.

CONCLUSIONS

Shock in neonates has complex pathophysiology involving cardiogenic, hypovolemic and distributive causes. If not identified early, it can progress to irreversible stage resulting in mortality. Integrated management with clinical and echocardiographic parameters can result in better understanding of hemodynamics and management of shock. Vigilant use of volume expanders and inotropes results in better outcome in terms of reduced cerebral injury especially in preterm and very low birthweight babies with shock.

TAKE HOME MESSAGES

- Neonates both preterm and term have peculiar cardiovascular physiological differences from pediatric and adult patients which needs to be understood for proper management.
- Neonates who may be categorized as hypotensive by statistical definition may have normal perfusion.
- Clinical markers of hemodynamic assessment are less reliable.
- Identification of shock in early phase improves the outcome.
- Functional echocardiography is an important adjunct in management of shock.
- Neonates in shock require individualized assessment according to pathophysiology and etiology.

FURTHER READING

1. Caresta E, Papoff P, Benedetti Valentini S, Mancuso M, Cicchetti R, *et al*. What's new in the treatment of neonatal shock. *J Matern Fetal Neonatal Med* 2011;24 (Suppl 1):17–19.
2. Kleinman CS, Seri I. *Hemodynamics and Cardiology Neonatology Questions and Controversies,* 2nd edn. Philadelphia: Saunders/Elsevier 2012.
3. LeFlore JL, Engle WD, Rosenfeld CR. Determinants of blood pressure in very low birth weight neonates: Lack of effect of antenatal steroids. *Early Hum Dev* 2000;59:37–50.
4. Noori S, Friedlich P, Seri I. Pathophysiology of Neonatal shock. In: Polin RA, Fox WW, Abman S (eds): *Fetal and Neonatal Physiology,* 3rd edn. Philadelphia: Saunders 2003;772–782.
5. Noori S, Seri I. Neonatal blood pressure support: The use of inotropes, lusitropes, and other vasopressor agents. *Clin Perinatol* 2012;39:221–238.
6. Subhedar NV, Shaw NJ. Dopamine versus dobutamine for hypotensive preterm infants. *Cochrane Database Syst Rev* 2003;CD001242.
7. Turner MA, Baines P. Which inotrope and when in neonatal and pediatric intensive care? *Arch Dis Child Educ Pract Ed* 2011;96:216–222.
8. Zubrow AB, Hulman S, Kushner H, Falkner B. Determinants of blood pressure in infants admitted to neonatal intensive care units: A prospective multicenter study. *J Perinatol* 1995;15:470–479.

Chapter

21 Acyanotic Heart Disease with Heart Failure

Neeraj Aggarwal, Mridul Aggarwal, Raja Joshi

ABSTRACT

Neonates are susceptible to heart failure due to various factors. Congenital heart diseases are first possibility in the differential diagnosis of congestive heart failure (CHF) in any neonate. We aim to discuss the various presentations of neonatal CHF with emphasis on etiopathogenesis, clinical features and management of acyanotic congenital heart disease (ACHD). Also discussed are various clinical clues which give an insight into the diagnosis of congenital heart diseases in neonates.

Key Words: Congenital heart disease (CHD), Congestive heart failure (CHF), Left to right shunts, Left ventricle (LV), Left atrium (LA), Neonatal shock.

INTRODUCTION

The incidence of moderate to severe structural congenital heart diseases in live born infants is 6–8 per 1000 live births. The secondary effects of unoperated lesions can occur on the heart, lung and brain. These effects may be quite severe and may include chronic congestive heart failure, failure to thrive, frequent infections, irreversible pulmonary vascular changes, delayed cognitive development or focal neurological defect. In critical lesions, the prognosis depends on timely and accurate assessment of structural anomaly. It is, therefore, crucial that pediatricians and neonatologists should be rapidly able to evaluate and participate in initial management of congenital heart disease.

CASE SCENARIO 1

A normal full-term baby delivered vaginally is discharged on day 2 of life on breast feeds. On day 5 of life the neonate presented to emergency department with history of interrupted feeding, fast breathing, sweating with feeding and not passing urine since morning. On examination, the neonate is afebrile, there is respiratory distress with subcostal indrawing and pulses are feeble in lower limbs along with hypotension. There is discrepancy in the BP in upper and lower limbs (upper limb BP being 60/40 and lower limb BP being 40/20 mm of Hg. Saturation in all 4 limbs is between 95–97%.

Contd...

Contd...

Sepsis screen, serum creatinine, BUN, electrolytes, Chest X-ray and ABG were done. Echo performed showed coarctation of aorta (Fig. 21.1) with left ventricular dysfunction (left ventricular ejection fraction 35%). Prostaglandin infusion was started and corrective surgery was performed next day. Postoperative course was uneventful and the child was discharged on day 10 of life.

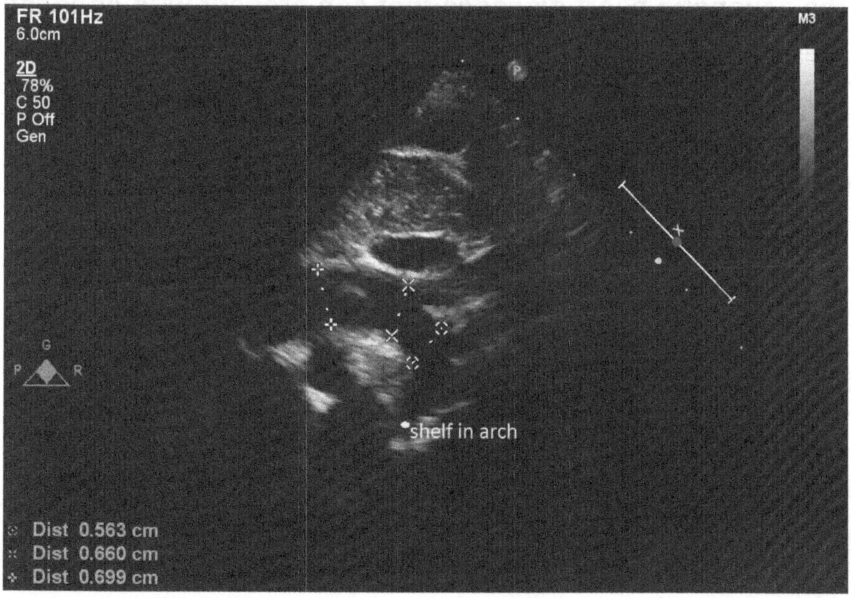

Fig. 21.1: 2D Echo in suprasternal view demonstrating coarctation of aorta. Shelf in the arch is seen indicative of coarctation of aorta. Proximal arch measurements are normal ruling out hypoplasia of arch

CRITICAL CASE ANALYSIS

The neonate who was well at discharge, presented in emergency with sudden onset of respiratory distress and shock. In such cases, the possibilities of septicemia, metabolic and cardiac causes should be kept in the differential diagnosis. A good clinical examination including peripheral pulses of upper and lower limbs, saturations in all four limbs and blood pressure almost established the diagnosis in this case. This child was in shock and and the BP discrepancy indicated a possibility of coarctation of aorta. If systolic BP difference between upper and lower limbs is more than 20 mm Hg, coarctation should be kept in diagnosis unless proved otherwise. Oliguria in this child may suggest reduced renal blood flow secondary to coarctation of aorta.

Coarctation of aorta is an obstructive lesion in the left ventricular outflow tract and so blood flow to descending aorta beyond coarctation of aorta will be diminished. When a child is born with coarctation, PDA maintains flow to the descending aorta and as PDA closes in 48–72 hours of life, the duct dependent lesion start manifesting. Other duct dependent acyanotic obstructive lesions presenting in 1st week of life are aortic stenosis (AS), interrupted aortic arch (IAA) and hypoplastic left heart syndrome (HLHS).

Any newborn presenting with uneventful perinatal period, suddenly presenting with shock in first few weeks of life, should be looked for duct-dependent systemic circulation. Feeble lower limb pulses strongly favor diagnosis of coarctation of aorta. Immediate intervention in such cases proves life-saving.

INTERACTIVE TOPIC DISCUSSION

What are the acyanotic heart diseases that can present with congestive heart failure in the fetal and neonatal period?

Table 21.1 provides the list of acyanotic lesions presenting with CHF in fetal and neonatal period.

Table 21.1: Causes of CHF in fetus and neonate

• **CHF in the Fetus** 1. Supraventricular tachycardia (SVT). 2. Severe bradycardia due to complete heart block (e.g., Maternal systemic Lupus Erythematosus). 3. Fetal anemia. 4. Valvular regurgitation–Severe tricuspid regurgitation (TR) due to Ebstein's anomaly of the Tricuspid valve, Mitral regurgitation (MR) from Atrioventricular canal defect. 5. Fetal myocarditis. 6. Systemic AV malformations. 7. Antenatal ductal closure leading to RV dysfunction (e.g., maternal intake of NSAID).
• **CHF on first day of life** 1. Myocardial dysfunction secondary to asphyxia, hypoglycaemia, hypocalcemia or sepsis. 2. Fetal SVT. 3. Severe valvular regurgitation like Severe MR, TR, Aortic regurgitation (AR) or Pulmonary Regurgitation (PR). 4. Critical obstructive lesions like Aortic stenosis (AS), Coarctation or HLHS may present with early PDA closure. • **CHF in first week of life** 1. Obstructive lesions like AS, coarctation. 2. Severe valvular regurgitation. 3. Premature infants have a poor myocardial reserve and a significant patent ductus arteriosus (PDA). 4. Non–cardiac causes like Adrenal insufficiency, neonatal thyrotoxicosis, severe anemia, systemic AV malformations, Arrhythmia. • **CHF beyond second week of life** 1. Post-tricuspid left to right shunts like VSD, PDA, Aorto-pulmonary window. 2. Origin of one of the branch PA from aorta (Hemi-Truncus). 3. Anomalous origin of left coronary artery from Pulmonary artery (ALCAPA). 4. Left-sided obstructive lesions and cardiomyopathy.
Note: Left to right shunts does not lead to CHF in the first 2 weeks of life unless associated lesions are present like coarctation of aorta, arrhythmias etc.

What are important presentations of CHD in neonate?

Three important presentation of congenital heart disease in a neonate are:

1. **Cyanosis:** Cyanosis should be confirmed by pulse oximetry in all newborns. Cyanosis is caused by either cyanotic congenital heart disease, primary pulmonary hypertension of the newborn, lung disease or hematological disorders.
2. **Decreased Systemic Perfusion:** This particular group is characterised by features of low cardiac output. Signs of decreased systemic perfusion including the temperature and color of the skin, blood pressure (including differential BP), peripheral pulses, and capillary refill in each extremity should be assessed. This group includes obstructive heart disease and myocardial dysfunction (resulting from sepsis, Persistent pulmonary hypertension of newborn (PPHN), anemia, hypertension, polycythemia, cardiomyopathy and metabolic disorders (such as hypocalcemia, hypoglycemia, metabolic acidosis). Newborns with obstructive heart disease mostly have an uneventful perinatal history, are stable during the first hours of life and develop signs over next few days with either obstruction getting severe or PDA getting closed. Subtle findings of irritability, pallor, poor feeding, cold feet or sweating may reflect inadequate systemic perfusion.
3. **Tachypnea:** This group of congenital heart diseases have the symptoms of increased pulmonary blood flow as the main pathophysiologic process.

Suppose a child presents with tachypnea and signs of low peripheral perfusion with obstructive cardiac lesion. What is the pathophysiology of tachypnea in such a case?

If there is obstructive lesion in LV inflow (e.g., Mitral stenosis) or outflow (e.g., Aortic stenosis/ coarctation), there is back pressure from LV or LA, leading to rise in pulmonary venous pressure with resultant pulmonary edema and respiratory distress. Also metabolic acidosis due to low perfusion will lead to tachypnea in such cases.

In critical aortic stenosis, PDA shunts right to left. Severe forms of PPHN also have PDA shunting right to left. What is the possibility of differential cyanosis in both of these cases?

In critical AS, as LV outflow is obstructed, systemic perfusion is compromised and PDA shunts from right to left will provide flow to descending aorta. Due to Aortic stenosis, LV is hypertrophied and LVEDP is raised leading to increased pressure in LA and more left to right shunt across PFO. Consequently blood in right-sided heart is more saturated and thus PDA shunt from right to left is also more saturated. Thus, the blood delivered to lower limbs is less desaturated than in PPHN. In cases of PPHN, if there is significant pulmonary hypertension, PDA shunting right to left gives a significant differential cyanosis.

To diagnose coarctation of aorta, which specific pulses and BP should be measured?

Lower extremity pulses are more easily palpated in the feet rather than in the inguinal area. If the infant has a normal dorsalis pedis or posterior tibial pulse, then pulsatile blood flow to the lower extremity is not impaired. Blood pressure should be measured in the upper and lower extremities; normally the lower extremity blood pressure is slightly greater than that in the upper extremity.

The left subclavian artery arises from the aortic isthmus and may be involved in a coarctation and in this situation, left arm BP and lower limb BP will be same and reduced in both. Thus, the systolic pressures in the right arm and either leg should be measured simultaneously. Rarely right sub-clavian artery may arise aberrantly from descending aorta distal to coarctation and right arm pressure may also be lower in such cases. Here both carotids should be palpated to see the differential pulses. Figure 21.2 shows a peak gradient of 83 mm Hg along with diastolic tailing in coarctation of aorta.

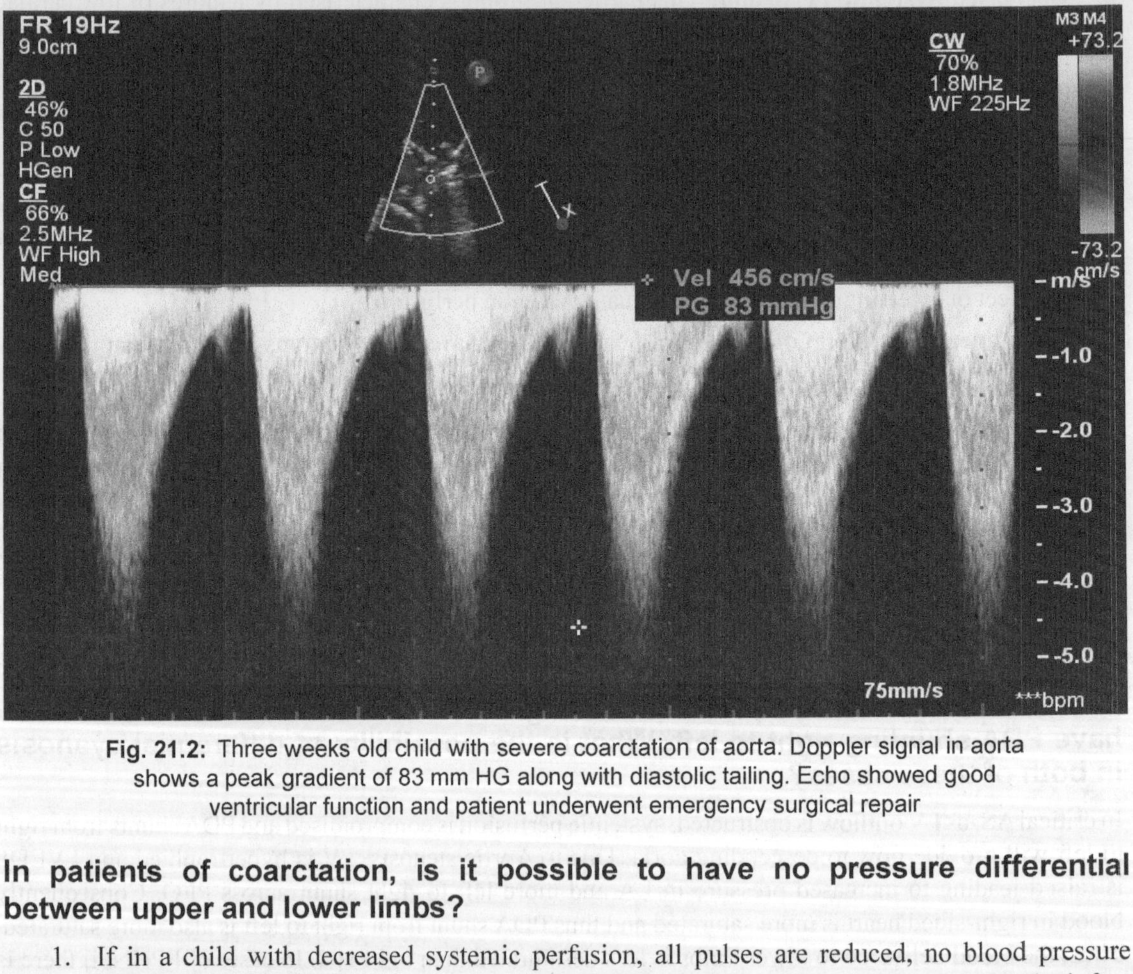

Fig. 21.2: Three weeks old child with severe coarctation of aorta. Doppler signal in aorta shows a peak gradient of 83 mm HG along with diastolic tailing. Echo showed good ventricular function and patient underwent emergency surgical repair

In patients of coarctation, is it possible to have no pressure differential between upper and lower limbs?

1. If in a child with decreased systemic perfusion, all pulses are reduced, no blood pressure differential is detected, the carotid arteries should be palpated. If they are increased, the infant may have a coarctation with right subclavian artery arising anomalously from the descending aorta (Fig. 21.3).
2. If these patients present late and continue to have low perfusion for long, then ventricular dysfunction may become so significant that all central pulses are lost and so the differential will not be significant.

In coarctation of aorta, mostly left ventricular dysfunction is seen but in neonates, RV dilatation and dysfunction is well-known. How can this be explained?

In neonates with severe coarctation of aorta, PDA is patent at birth and supports systemic circulation. In this setting of open PDA with coarctation, right ventricle support the systemic circulation and when the ductus closes, RV dilatation and dysfunction set in.

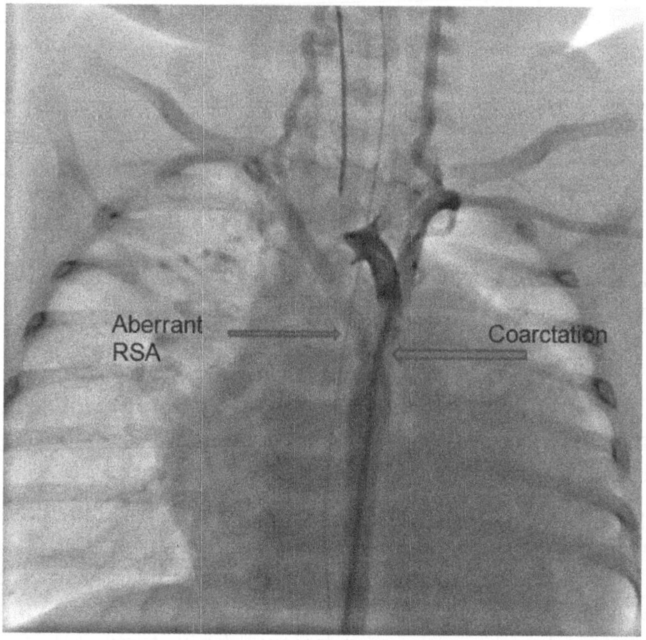

Fig. 21.3: One week old child came in emergency with severe LV dysfunction (LVEF 10). Both upper limb and both lower limb pulses were significantly weak but carotids were strongly palpable. Echo showed coarctation of aorta but Doppler gradient was not severe enough as gradient was not being generated due to significant ventricular dysfunction. Patient underwent immediate angiography and aberrant origin of right subclavian artery (RSA) was noted from descending aorta beyond the site of coarctation. Left subclavian origin was also noted to be at the site of coarctation of aorta. This explained the poor pulses in both upper limbs along with both lower limbs (all 4 limb pulses were beyond site of coarctation of aorta and so were weak). Patient underwent successful balloon dilatation of coarctation

What is the preferred choice of therapy in aortic stenosis or coarctation of aorta?

In valvar aortic stenosis, the aortic valve is frequently bicuspid or unicuspid and the leaflets are usually dysplastic and thickened. Balloon valvuloplasty for critical aortic valve stenosis can provide rapid hemodynamic relief. Results of balloon valvuloplasty are comparable to surgical valvotomy.

Surgical repair of coarctation of the aorta or aortic arch hypoplasia is the preferred treatment for native coarctation of the aorta in the newborn period. Balloon dilatation of coarctation as palliation is the treatment of choice for those cases where severe LV dysfunction has already set in and surgical risk becomes high.

CASE SCENARIO 2

A full-term neonate was discharged from hospital on breast feeds without a significant perinatal history. After 3 weeks, child was brought with poor feeding and excessive sweating. There is no history of fever and cough. On examination, child was found to have tachypnea, tachycardia, hepatomegaly and a systolic murmur in left second intercostal space. There was no cyanosis, saturation 98% and all 4 limbs had good peripheral pulses. There was no radio-femoral delay and no difference in BP was noted in upper and lower limbs. What are the pointers towards heart disease in this case? Critically review this case.

CRITICAL CASE ANALYSIS

This neonate had signs and symptoms consistent with congestive cardiac failure. Tachypnea (respiratory rate >60 breaths/min) without distress is an important sign of heart disease and is even more significant if associated with difficulty in feeding. Tachypnea with suck rest suck cycle is often a feature of shunt lesions, but develops over days or weeks, as pulmonary vascular resistance and hemoglobin concentration falls over 2–3 weeks. Before making a diagnosis of shunt, always ensure that child has good perfusion and normal saturations because obstructive lesions also present with tachypnea. On the other hand, tachypnea immediately after birth, in the absence of cyanosis or low cardiac output, usually points to pulmonary disease rather than heart disease. Another important clue is poor feeding with associated failure to thrive and diaphoresis (remember murmurs may be absent).

Shunt lesions typically present in neonates beyond 2 weeks, coinciding with fall in neonatal pulmonary vascular resistance (PVR). So, the lesions depending on PVR fall will typically present around 2–3 weeks of age and those independent of PVR may present earlier. Shunt lesions typically depend on PVR fall, where as obstructive lesions, regurgitant lesions or arrhythmias will not need PVR fall to manifest. Also remember the uncommon lesions like systemic AV malformations which also don't depend on PVR.

This baby was asymptomatic for first 3 weeks and when PVR fell, shunt started manifesting. Presence of good lower limb pulses and pulse oximetry confirmation of saturations is must in all cases suspected of CHD and so we came to a diagnosis of left to right shunt lesion in this baby. Remember there are few cyanotic lesions with high pulmonary blood flow (e.g., Truncus arteriosus, Total anomalous pulmonary venous connection, Transposition of great arteries with large VSD) where saturations are near 90% and these lesions will not be picked up as cyanotic lesions on examination unless pulse oximetry is done.

INTERACTIVE TOPIC DISCUSSION

Describe the pathophysiology of signs and symptoms seen in acyanotic newborns with CHF.

This group of congenital heart diseases have the symptoms of increased pulmonary blood flow as the main pathophysiologic process. These infants have heart failure with high cardiac output, which is very different than the low output failure that occurs in adults with acquired heart disease and in neonates with decreased systemic perfusion. The primary features of high pulmonary blood flow are tachypnea, tachycardia, mildly increased work of breathing, failure to thrive, sweating with feeds and cardiomegaly.

The heart is hyper-contractile and venous filling pressures are usually normal on both sides of the heart. Peripheral edema does not occur because venous pressures are not increased. Hepatomegaly is a common feature because the liver and hepatic veins are very compliant and enlarge to accommodate the increased circulating blood volume.

- *Pathophysiology of diaphoresis:* It is mainly due to increased adrenergic drive mediated by neural and hormonal drive. The increase in adrenergic drive is necessary to maintain the increased combined ventricular output.
- *Pathophysiology of failure to thrive:*
  1. Increased caloric requirements associated with increased oxygen consumption (Secondary to increased cardiac output).
  2. Infants feed poorly because of their increased respiratory effort. They also vomit frequently because of gastro-esophageal reflux in the presence of increased intra-abdominal pressure (caused by increased respiratory effort).
- *Pathophysiology of tachypnea:*
  1. The increased amount of fluid in the thorax caused by increased pulmonary blood flow, particularly distributed in the pulmonary veins, may make it more difficult for the infant to breathe by increasing the weight of the lungs.
  2. More likely, the increased production of interstitial fluid with the attendant increase in lymphatic flow is the primary cause of tachypnea in these infants. As blood flows normally through the lungs, interstitial fluid is produced. This fluid is drained from the interstitial spaces by the lymphatic vessels. As blood flow increases, lymphatic flow increases proportionately. The fluid is predominantly peribronchial, which may impair bronchial function. Airway size may decrease and airway resistance may increase, further increasing the work of breathing.
  3. In addition, the infant may be more likely to develop wheezing, as only a small further decrease in airway lumen would impair air exchange. This scenario explains not only the tachypnea universally seen in infants with a symptomatic increase in pulmonary blood flow, but also the radiographic findings of increased vascular markings, the presence of peribronchial edema, and other manifestations of interstitial, but not of alveolar fluid.

What is the logical explanation for delayed onset of symptoms in shunt lesions?

Infants do not develop tachypnea and failure to thrive until pulmonary blood flow is very high, usually exceeding two and one-half times the normal flow. The onset of symptoms tends to track with the time course over which pulmonary blood flow increases after birth. In the normal infant, systemic blood flow peaks at around 6–10 weeks of age, at the time of the nadir of hemoglobin concentration. Pulmonary vascular resistance also decreases during this time period. Thus, pulmonary blood flow increases greatly during this time in the infant with a heart defect associated with increased pulmonary blood flow because of the increase in systemic blood flow associated with physiologic anemia and an increase in the relative proportion of blood flow to the lungs (an increased pulmonary-to-systemic blood flow ratio) related to the decreased pulmonary vascular resistance.

In contrast, infants with intrinsic pulmonary disease (along with high pulmonary blood flow) may develop tachypnea and heart failure at a level of pulmonary blood flow only modestly higher than normal. A common situation is an infant born prematurely who develops bronchopulmonary dysplasia.

What is the common age of presentation of ASD and why it is different from VSD or PDA?

Type and magnitude of shunt across an atrial septal defect depends on the relative compliance of right and left ventricle. Right ventricle in a newborn has more thickness and stiffness compared to left ventricle so that the left-to-right shunt in the neonates is not significant and does not cause symptoms of high pulmonary blood flow. Although pulmonary vascular resistance (PVR) begins to fall immediately at birth and reduces to almost normal levels in next 2–3 weeks of life, Right ventricle takes months to remodel and accept a significantly greater amount of blood than the left ventricle. So, even a large atrial septal defect does not cause symptoms in newborns and young infants. The common age of presentation of ASD with symptoms is around 2 years with failure to thrive and only 10% present in first year of life with CHF.

In case of VSD, the magnitude of the left-to right shunt depends on the relative resistances of the pulmonary and systemic vascular beds. Also large VSD are associated with severe PAH due to direct transmission of systemic pressures and that also contributes to the symptomatology. Mostly in cases of VSD, murmur appears around 2–3 weeks of age when neonatal PVR has fallen and significant left to right shunting starts. PVR falls significantly at birth and further gradual fall in PVR happens over the next 2–3 weeks of life. This occurs simultaneously with physiologic anemia of infancy. Together, these processes produce symptoms around 3–6 weeks of life.

In case of patent ductus arteriosus, the shunt occurs during both systole and diastole and blood continues to flow from the resistance vessels of the lungs during diastole. Thus, PDA is more likely to cause symptoms of heart failure at an earlier age than VSD.

What are the reasons of a left to right shunt presenting early in neonatal life (in first or second week of life)?

As we have discussed earlier, left to right shunt lesions do not manifest in first 2–3 weeks of life. But if a neonate with left to right shunt presents early with CHF, we must look for additional causes of CHF.

In cases of atrio-ventricular septal defect, we must look for LV to RA jet or severe mitral insufficiency. Both of these conditions lead to a large atrial left-to-right shunt; the shunt is obligatory, in that atrial pressure is always much lower than left ventricular pressure during ventricular systole and in such cases a large shunt may cause early symptoms of heart failure. So, presence of an additional valvular regurgitation lesion in a shunt can precipitate early CHF.

In a newborn diagnosed with VSD or PDA presenting with CHF in first 2 weeks of life, possibility of associated coarctation should always be ruled out beyond doubt. Also equally important is to rule out associated non cardiac lesions like lung disease, anemia and systemic AV malformations which can precipitate heart failure.

Premature infants are at significantly high risk of CHF with a shunt lesion and PDA is a common accompaniment in these cases.

Congenital arteriovenous malformations are obligatory shunts because arteriolar pressure far exceeds venous pressure and thus the magnitude of the shunt is directly related to the size of the malformation and does not depend on pulmonary vascular resistance (so does not depend on age of child).

What are the cardiac lesions that present with bounding pulses and CHF – in the neonatal period?

PDA, aortopulmonary window (APW) and hemi-truncus (origin of pulmonary artery from aorta) – These lesions may manifest with signs of heart failure in the first few weeks of life with bounding pulses. These lesions share the feature of diastolic flow being diverted to pulmonary circulation from systemic circulation leading to wide pulse pressure.

What are the differences in mechanisms of closure of ductus arteriosus in premature vs. term neonate and why premature have high incidence of PDA?

In the term infant, normal postnatal closure of the ductus arteriosus occurs in two stages. Immediately after birth, contraction of the medial smooth muscle causes functional closure, usually within 12–24 hours. The second stage usually takes place in next 2–3 weeks. This is produced by infolding of the endothelium, disruption and fragmentation of the internal elastic lamina, proliferation of the subintimal layers, and hemorrhage and necrosis in the subintimal region. There is connective tissue formation and replacement of muscle fibers with fibrosis leading to permanent closure and converting the ductus to a ligamentum arteriosus.

The initial closure of the ductus arteriosus and its failure to close in premature infants has been the subject of debate. Closure of the ductus arteriosus is mediated by the high oxygen concentrations in post-natal period and the levels of prostaglandins E2 and I2. Other factors, such as the release of vasoactive substances (e.g., acetylcholine, bradykinin, or endogenous catecholamines), may also contribute to postnatal closure of the ductus arteriosus under physiologic conditions. Inhibitors of prostaglandin synthesis such as NSAID produce constriction of ductus arteriosus in fetal and premature infants signifying a prominent role of prostaglandins in PDA physiology.

The effects of prostaglandins, as well as of inhibitors of prostaglandin synthesis, vary at different gestational ages. Indomethacin constricts rings of ductus arteriosus from immature fetal lambs more than it does rings from close to term lambs. Both PGE_2 and PGI_2 relax the ductus arteriosus from immature lambs more than that from mature animals, reflecting the significantly greater sensitivity to PGE_2 and PGI_2 of the immature ductus arteriosus. This change in sensitivity is influenced by the increase in endogenous cortical toward term.The immature ductus is very sensitive to the dilating effects of prostaglandins and much less sensitive to the vasoconstricting effects of oxygen. As the ductus matures in the later stages of gestation, it becomes much more sensitive to oxygen and much less so to prostaglandins. Thus, the large increase in oxygen concentration likely induces complete closure of the ductus arteriosus in the term infant, but this is not the case in the preterm infant. Moreover, prostaglandin levels decrease to a greater extent in the term infant, further promoting ductal closure.

Why are premature infants more susceptible to PDA effects than term infants?

Because the pulmonary vascular musculature is less well-developed in preterm infants, pulmonary vascular resistance is particularly low and shunts of a large magnitude can develop rapidly. Furthermore, the immature alveoli may be more sensitive to the presence of increased fluid. Because of these factors, a moderate left-to-right shunt through a ductus arteriosus has a far greater effect on the lung function in a preterm infant than in a term infant.

The effects of a patent ductus arteriosus on the systemic circulation are also much more prominent and deleterious in the preterm infant. In a term infant with a PDA, the left ventricle is capable of greatly increasing output, systemic blood flow usually is maintained and organ ischemia does not occur. In contrast, the left ventricle of the preterm infant is less capable of increasing its output. The ventricle is less compliant because of higher water content and less organized myocyte architecture. Therefore, end-diastolic volume cannot increase as much in response to an increase in pulmonary venous return, limiting the increase in stroke volume. End-diastolic pressure increases to a greater extent, contributing to alveolar edema. Additionally, resting heart rate is greater and near the level at which a further increase causes a decrease in stroke volume. Premature infants often have lower than normal serum Ca_2+ concentrations, and this too may affect myocardial performance. Probably for one or all of these reasons, premature infants with left-to-right shunts through a PDA develop left ventricular failure earlier than their full-term counterparts and, in addition, with a smaller volume load.

For all of these reasons, systemic blood flow frequently falls in the premature infant with a large PDA which may lead to renal insufficiency, necrotizing enterocolitis, and intraventricular hemorrhage. Even the myocardium is susceptible to ischemia due to low diastolic pressures as coronary perfusion mainly happens in diastolic period.

What are the clinical manifestations of PDA in preterm infants?

Improvement of lung function with surfactant therapy has led to the clinical emergence of PDA earlier and more frequently in preterm infants (by decreasing PVR).

Clinical features depend on the magnitude of left-to-right shunt through the PDA (depends on PVR) and the ability of the infant to initiate compensatory mechanisms to handle the extra volume load (depends on gestational age). Because many premature infants have respiratory distress syndrome, the stage of development of this disease and the use of surfactant replacement therapy will determine the pulmonary vascular resistance and therefore, the shunt.

In premature with PDA without lung disease, a systolic murmur is first heard 24–72 hours after birth, and as the left-to-right shunt increases, this murmur becomes louder and more prolonged, extending into early diastole but it is not a classical continuous murmur. The murmur commonly is heard best at the left sternal border in the second and third intercostal spaces. A mid-diastolic flow rumble owing to increased diastolic flow across the normal mitral valve may be heard at the apex. The precordium becomes increasingly more hyperactive and pulse pressure widens with bounding pulses as the left-to-right shunt increases. If shunt is large, there may be tachycardia, tachypnea, and fine crepts on auscultation of the lung fields. Episodes of apnea and hepatomegaly may be seen in later stages. The chest X-ray may show enlargement of both the left atrium and left ventricle, if there is a moderately large shunt with increased pulmonary vascular markings.

Echocardiographic evaluation has become essential in the clinical management of PDA and in assessing the magnitude of the shunt (Figs. 21.4–21.6). The ratio of the left atrial (LA) diameter to the aortic root (Ao) diameter can be used to determine LA enlargement. The normal LA: Ao ratio in infants is between 0.8 and 1. A ratio >1.2 suggests left atrial enlargement indicating a significant left-to-right shunt.

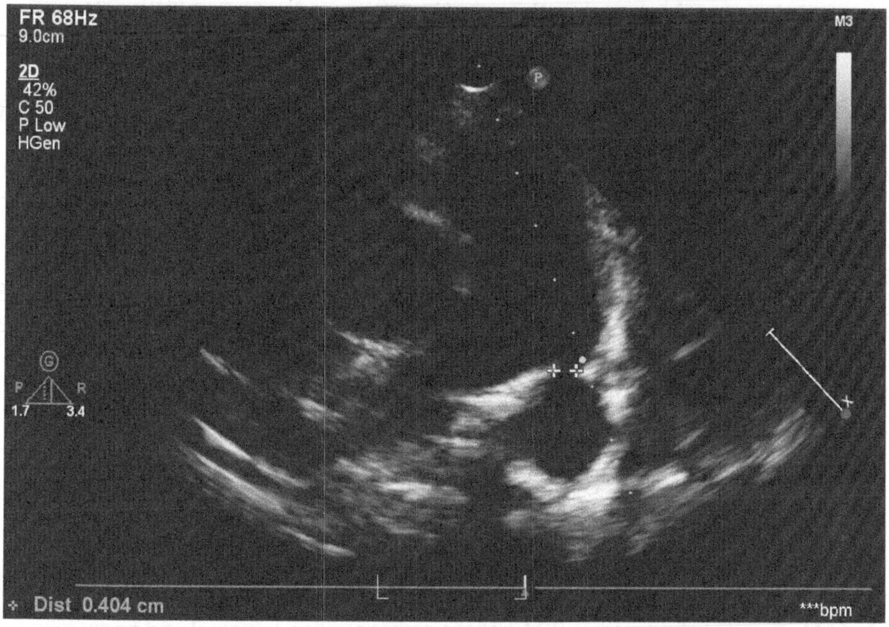

Fig. 21.4: Ductal view demonstrating a 4 mm large PDA in 2D Echo image

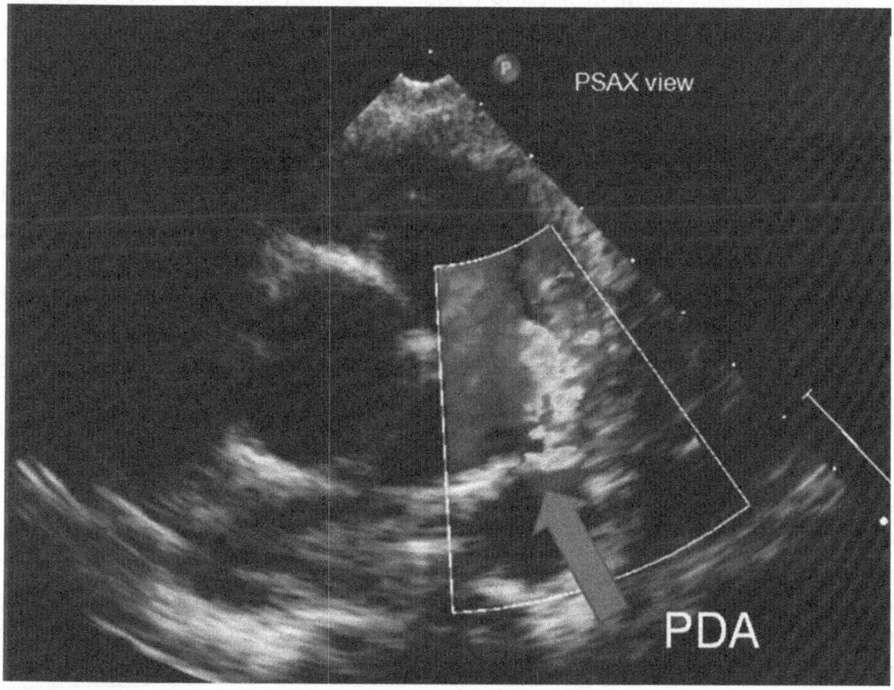

Fig. 21.5: Echo in parasternal short axis view (PSAX view) demonstrating a large PDA in color mode

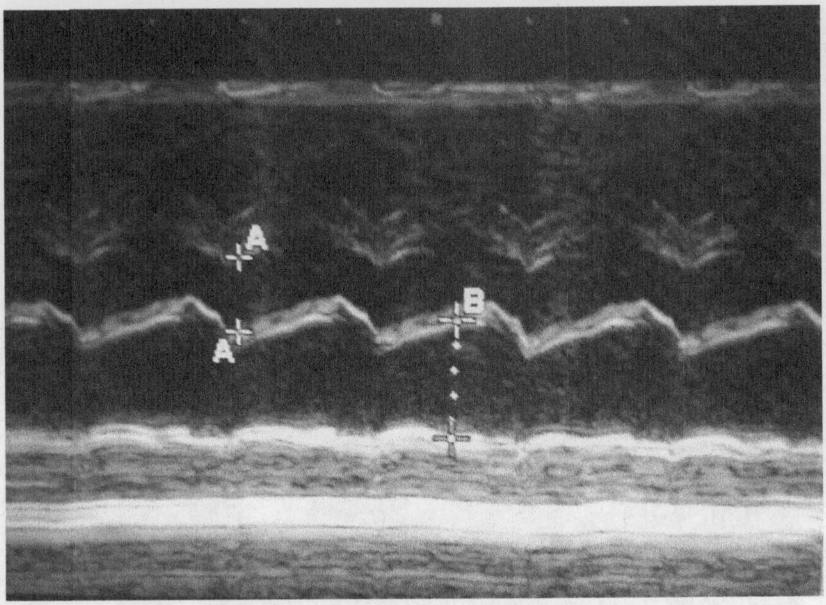

Fig. 21.6: M Mode echo of a preterm PDA patient demonstrating left atrial and aortic measurements. LA/AO ratio was calculated as 1.6 and patient was planned for pharmacological PDA closure

Let us take the case of PDA in infants recovering from lung disease. The respiratory distress syndrome (RDS) usually is evident within a few hours after birth and as it starts to improve after 3–4 days, early clinical evidence of a PDA appears. The ductus arteriosus is patent since birth and high pulmonary vascular resistance has prevented a detectable left-to-right shunt. As the pulmonary disease improves, PDA starts showing signs. Although as oxygenation increases and ductus arteriosus should constrict. However, most of these infants are quite immature, so a good constrictor response may not occur with improved oxygenation. Because recovery from the respiratory distress syndrome often is not continuously progressive but is intermittent with periods of deteriorating lung function, left-to-right shunting (and therefore the murmur) may be intermittent for several days. The murmur commonly disappears and reappears several times within short periods of time. Increasing precordial activity is a good clinical indication of the magnitude of shunting in these infants and increased heart rate, pulse pressure, and bounding pulses can present early. Crepts are unreliable a measure of left ventricular failure because they may be suppressed by positive pressure ventilation used in these infants. However, in those extubated, crepts may be heard. Apneic episodes are also common in this group. Deterioration in the ventilatory status of an infant recovering from respiratory distress syndrome is often a strong indication of a significant left-to-right shunt through a PDA. A chest X-ray will show the parenchymal changes of respiratory distress syndrome and increased pulmonary vascularity will be difficult to assess. Because many of the changes described may be due to deterioration resulting from underlying pulmonary disease, it is important to be able to assess the contribution to the clinical picture of a PDA. Echo is very helpful in such scenario. An increasing LA: Ao ratio will be produced by increasing left-to-right shunting, whereas a ratio that remains constant and within normal limits may indicate non cardiac causes of deterioration. Echo can also reliably document the size of PDA and dilation of LV to decide contribution of PDA.

In PDS associated with lung disease, many cases do show clinical evidence of a left-to-right shunt through the PDA, or fail to show improved respiratory status at an age when they should start to recover from the primary pulmonary disease. Failure to improve is manifested by the inability to wean the infant from ventilatory support. Murmurs may be difficult to hear. Changes in the ventilatory status may be due to progression of the primary pulmonary disease, and it is often difficult to separate left ventricular failure from increasing pulmonary problems. Increasing precordial activity, bounding pulses, and a widening arterial pulse pressure suggest the development of left-to-right shunting. The ECG and chest radiograph usually are not helpful, but as outlined above, Echocardiographic evaluation is diagnostic even before clinical signs are apparent.

Describe in short about aorto-pulmonary window and anomalous origin of branch pulmonary artery from aorta.

These uncommon defects can present in first month of life and the physiology is like a large post tricuspid left to right shunt (e.g., VSD/PDA).

Aorto-pulmonary window is a connection between ascending aorta and main pulmonary artery (Fig. 21.7). Mostly it is a large shunt and manifests in late neonatal period with CHF and PAH. Clinically features are not distinguishable from a Large VSD or PDA. Bounding pulses are seen due to arterial runoff into lungs.

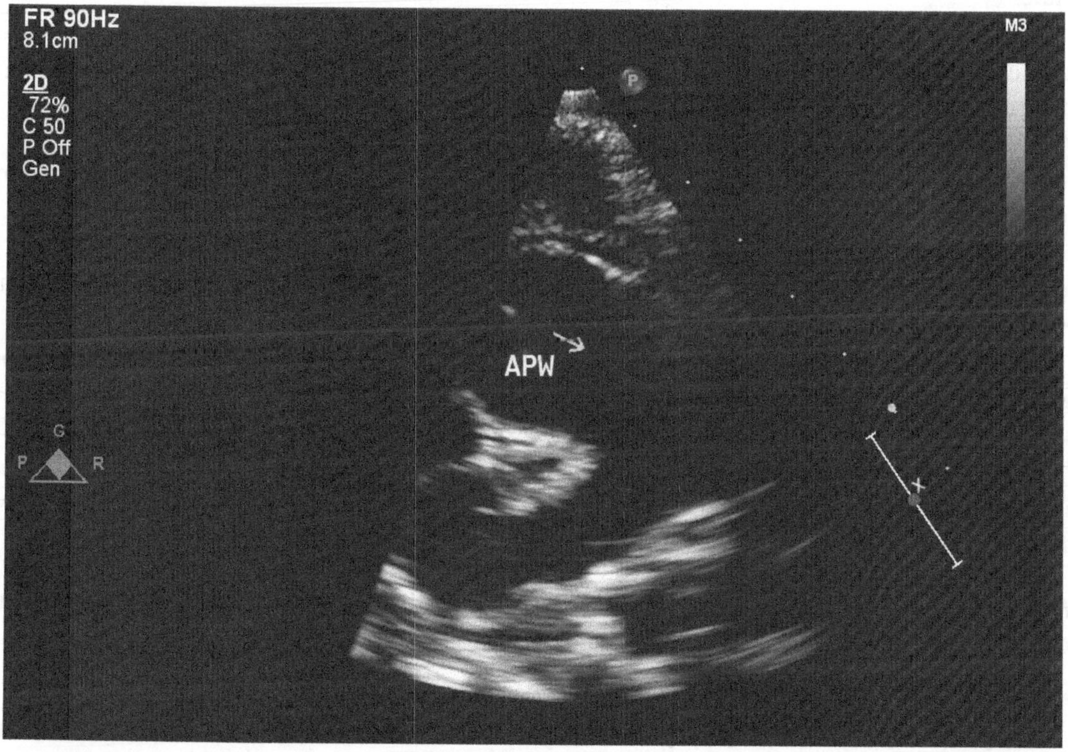

Fig. 21.7: A 20 days old neonate with complaints of feeding difficulty and tachypnea was found to have an ejection systolic murmur and Echo showed a large aorto-pulmonary window in high PSAX view

Anomalous origin of branch pulmonary arteries from Aorta is an uncommon disorder and characterized by features of flow from aorta into PA (similar to PDA) and clinical features are difficult to differentiate from PDA. Echo can confirm the diagnosis.

What are the manifestations of arteriovenous malformations (AVM) and how these are different from shunts?

The pathophysiology of AVM such as vein of Galen is high cardiac output failure due to high pulmonary blood flow. Abnormal arteriovenous malformation leads to excess blood flow to RA, RV and finally to Pulmonary arteries. Patients present with features of high pulmonary blood flow as in intracardiac shunts such as recurrent chest infections and failure to thrive.

More importantly, it is an obligatory shunt, that means, unlike intracardiac shunts, manifestations does not depend on fall in neonatal PVR and so can lead to early CHF even in Fetus or neonates.

What are the Regurgitant lesions presenting with CHF in neonatal period?

Severe forms of regurgitant lesions can present with CHF in neonatal period.

Pulmonary Regurgitation: Congenital forms of pulmonary insufficiency are commonly seen with absent pulmonary valve syndrome. There is significant RV overload in such cases leading to heart failure.

Tricuspid Regurgitation: Clinically significant tricuspid regurgitation can be seen in tricuspid valve disease (e.g., Ebstein anomaly, Endocarditis and dysplastic tricuspid valve) or secondary to overload of RV (e.g., PPHN, PS, TAPVC, systemic AV malformations).

Ebstein's anomaly (Tricuspid valve septal leaflets are apically displaced and teethered to Interventricular septum) mostly present in adulthood but severe forms of Ebstein anomaly can rarely present in neonates with CHF in association with SVT (due to dilated atria).

Right-sided endocarditis can be seen with long indwelling catheters. PPHN and PS lead to RV pressure overload. TAPVC and systemic AVM leads to volume overload of RV. RV pressure and volume overload can lead to dilatation of tricuspid valve and TR.

Aortic Regurgitation: A dilated aortic root with AR in Neonatal Marfan syndrome is frequently associated with aortic insufficiency and may cause left ventricular dilation and dysfunction. AR can also occur after balloon dilatation of stenosed aortic valve.

Mitral Regurgitation: Congenital mitral regurgitation leading to heart failure in the neonate is rare and is usually associated with other cardiac defects (as in Endocardial cushion defects), secondary to dilated cardiomyopathy or infarction of the papillary muscles (as in ALCAPA).

What are the treatable causes of LV dysfunction presenting in the neonatal period?

1. Hypertension–due to any cause, if uncontrolled, can lead to LV dysfunction.
2. Arrhythmias–Incessant Tachyarrhythmias can lead to LV failure and LV function rapidly reverses after control of arrhythmias. Similarly complete heart block with very low ventricular rate can lead to CHF and can be treated with pacemaker.

3. Left-sided obstructive lesions such as critical aortic stenosis and coarctation of aorta are amenable to therapeutic balloon dilatations or surgical repair.
4. ALCAPA (Anomalous left coronary artery from pulmonary artery).
5. Hyperthyroidism.
6. Hypocalcemia.

How does ALCAPA present in neonatal life and what are its diagnostic features?

Myocardial ischemia, as a result of anomalous origin of the coronary arteries, is an infrequent and potentially reversible cause of congestive heart failure in the neonate and infant.

In the fetus and early neonatal period, pulmonary artery pressure is high and left coronary artery perfusion is maintained from desaturated pulmonary flow. As pulmonary vascular resistance falls, pulmonary arterial pressure decreases leading to diminished left coronary artery perfusion which leads to myocardial ischemia and LV failure.

The earliest signs of heart failure include failure to thrive, tachypnea, wheezing, diaphoresis, and angina-like episodes that manifest as sudden inconsolability and pallor. ECG classically demonstrates ST segment elevation in the anterolateral leads and Q waves in leads I and avL (Fig. 21.8). Echo can demonstrate the origin of left coronary from pulmonary artery (Fig. 21.9).

What is the algorithmic approach to congenital heart disease?

Figure 21.10 presents an algorithmic approach to CHD.

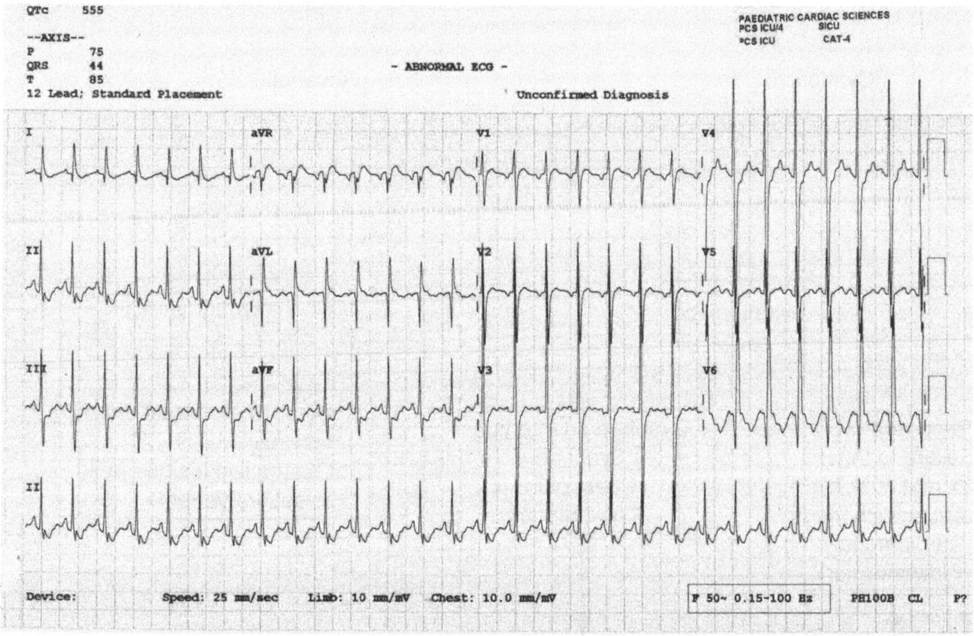

Fig. 21.8: ECG of a neonate with ALCAPA showing deep Q waves in leads 1 and avL and Echo confirmed the diagnosis of ALCAPA

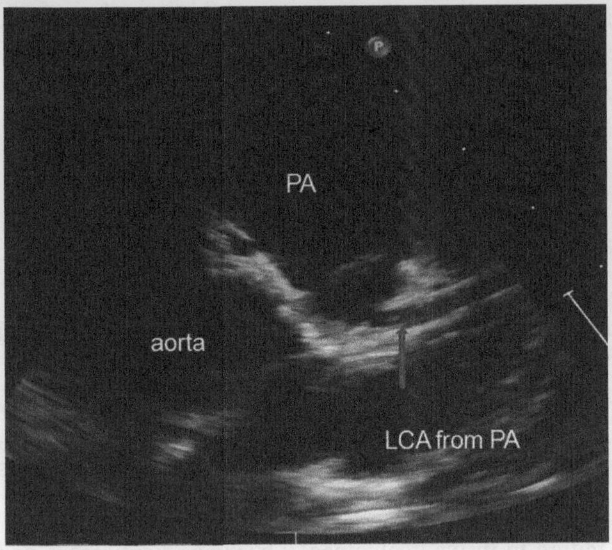

Fig. 21.9: ECHO in PSAX view showing origin of left coronary artery (LCA) from pulmonary artery (PA) confirming the diagnosis of ALCAPA

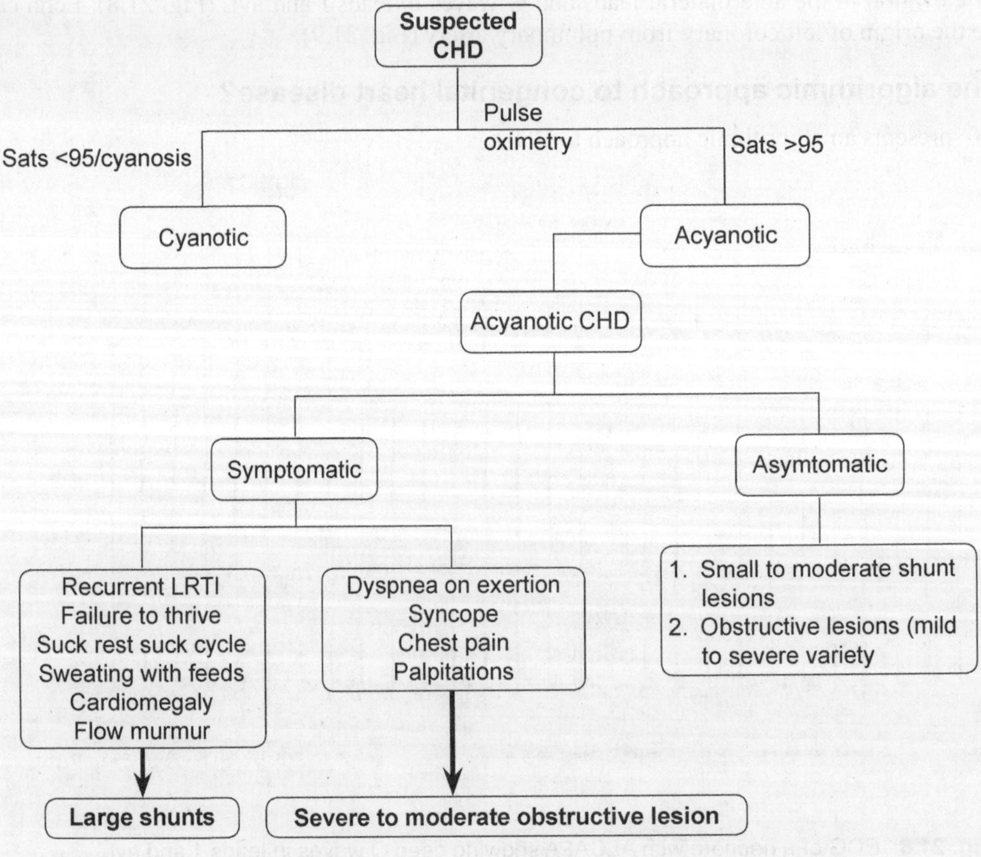

Fig. 21.10: Flowchart–Approach to congenital heart disease

CONCLUSIONS

Congenital heart disease can have varied presentation in neonatal period and early infancy. Presentation may vary from cyanosis, poor perfusion, tachypnea or overt CHF. A high index of suspicion is required for diagnosis. Pediatricians and neonatologists should be rapidly able to evaluate and participate in initial management of congenital heart disease.

TAKE HOME MESSAGES

- All neonates in heart failure should be evaluated for pulse oximetry and differential pulses to rule out a critical lesion.
- Obstructive and regurgitant lesions, systemic AV malformations and arrhythmias should be in the differential diagnosis of neonatal CHF presenting at birth or within first week of life in acyanotic cases.
- Shunt lesions present after 2–3 weeks of life when PVR falls, unless they are accompanied by associated defects like coarctation of aorta/valvular regurgitations or prematurity.

FURTHER READING

1. Abraham MR. *Congenital Diseases of Heart: Clinical Physiological Considerations*. 3rd edn. West Sussex: John Wiley 2009.
2. Fleiner S. Recognition and stabilization of neonates with congenital heart disease. *Newborn Infant Nurs Rev* 2006;6:137–150.
3. Krishnan US. Approach to congenital heart disease in the Neonate. *Indian J Pediatr* 2002;69:501–505.
4. Mc Connell ME, Elixson EM. The neonate with suspected congenital heart disease. *Crit Care Nurs Q* 2002; 25:17–25.
5. Warburton D, Rehan M, Shineboume EA. Selective criteria for differential diagnosis of infants with symptoms of congenital heart disease. *Arch Dis Child* 1981;56:94–100.
6. Yun SW. Congenital heart disease in newborn requiring early intervention. *Korean J Pediatr* 2011;54:183–191.

Chapter

22 Critical Cyanotic Congenital Heart Disease

Mridul Aggarwal, Raja Joshi, Neeraj Aggarwal, Reena Joshi

ABSTRACT

Critical congenital heart disease (CCHD) in neonates is a diagnostic and therapeutic challenge. It is important to diagnose it in time. No neonate with CCHD should be discharged undiagnosed. Planned and timely intervention always gives better outcome than operating on critical neonate in shock and organ failures. Diseases like d-Transposition of Great Arteries (d-TGA) or Total Anomalous Pulmonary Venous Connection (TAPVC) require single stage surgical correction while diseases like Pulmonary Atresias and single ventricle physiologies require planned multi-stage approach. Prostaglandin E1 (PGE1) is of great importance in resuscitation of neonates with CCHD. Management of CCHD requires coordination between various specialties for optimal outcome.

Key Words: Critical congenital heart disease (CCHD), Cyanosis, Prostaglandin, Pulse oximetry, Shock.

INTRODUCTION

The neonates with congenital heart disease (CHD) can have one of three possible presentations. First is critical CHD as cyanosis, shock or congestive heart failure. Other common possible way the CHD get detected is either during antenatal scan or during neonatal examination. It is of utmost importance to diagnose critical CHD early to ensure timely and optimum intervention.

CASE SCENARIO 1

A 4-day-old neonate presented to emergency room in a state of shock with poor pulses and altered sensorium. He had not passed urine for last 6 hours.

His abdomen was distended and liver enlarged. He was well when he had been discharged a day before.

CRITICAL CASE ANALYSIS

The case is presented here for two reasons: first for the disease and other for the reason how the neonate remained undiagnosed for 4 days.

A retrospective observation study published few years back from United Kingdom of all cases of CHD diagnosed by the age of 12 months in the northern health region of the UK for period of 7 years revealed that 1590 infants out of 300200 were diagnosed to have CHD (5/1000). Of the babies discharged home undiagnosed, 35% were diagnosed by 6 weeks of age and 57% by 3 months.

What this study suggested was that routine neonatal examination can miss disease as serious as hypoplastic left heart syndrome and pulmonary atresia. Thus, there is a need for modification in methodology of neonatal examination. A recent published article discussing strategy to detect critical CHD in newborn gives most emphasis on pulse oximetry screening of newborn at the time of discharge or before 48 hours. The study has suggested the protocol as well for the same (Fig. 22.1).

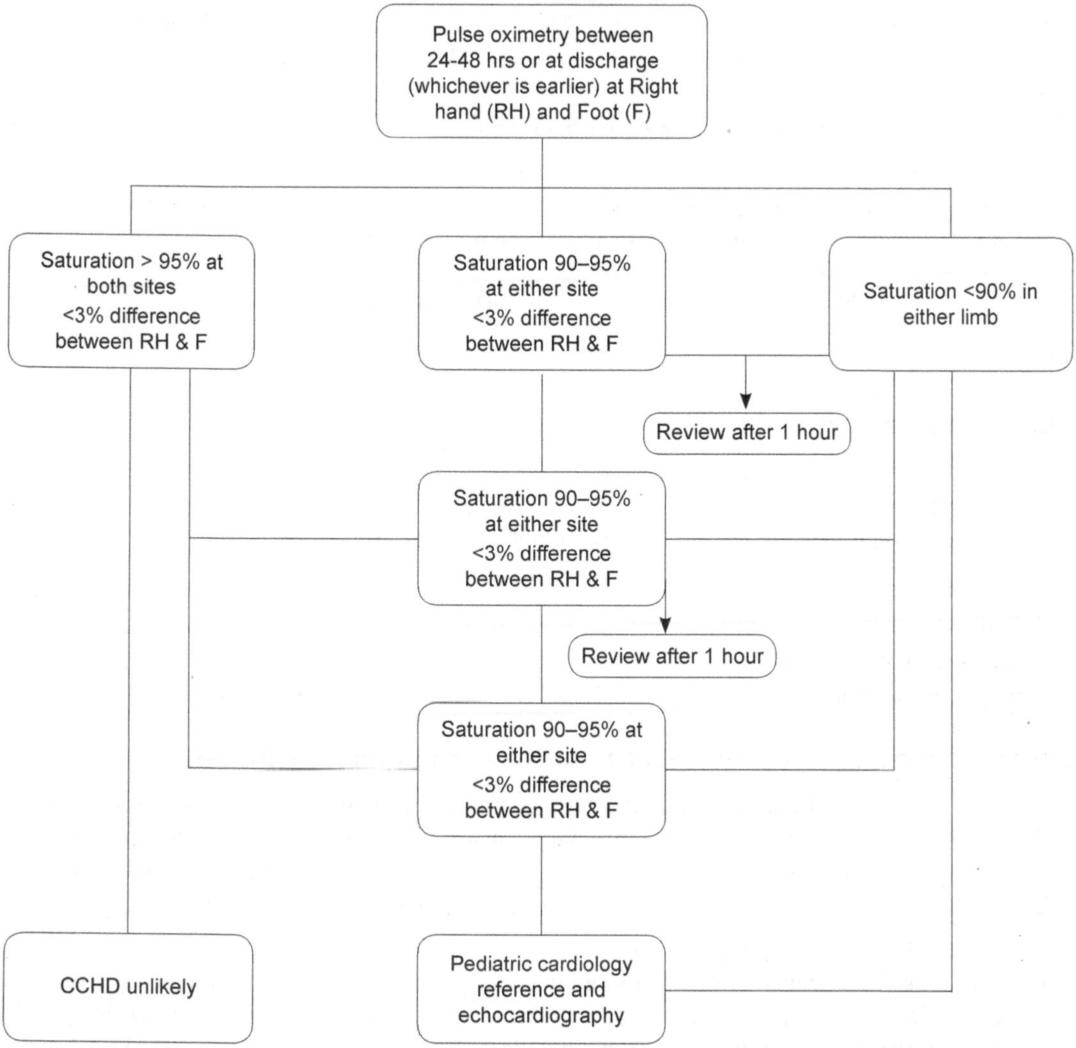

Fig. 22.1: Proposed protocol for pulse oximetry screening of newborn

INTERACTIVE TOPIC DISCUSSION

How can the diagnosis rate of congenital heart disease be improved during neonatal examination?

Routine pulse oximetry of all newborn infants before discharge is an effective tool to improve diagnostic rate of congenital cyanotic heart disease. Studies have found the sensitivity of pulse-oximetry monitoring to be 62.1% and the specificity to be 99.8% and the false-positive rate was 0.17% for critical cyanotic CHD. The cost involved is one tenth to one sixteenth of what is required for hearing screening. These studies have calculated that the savings in health care costs from the prevention of 1 case of complications of circulatory collapse resulting from an undiagnosed critical CHD may exceed the cost of screening of approximately 2000 newborns. The time consumed is also calculated as less than five minutes, which include explanation to parents as well as taking saturation.

What is the possible diagnosis in this case?

The index case here has one of the common presentations of critical CHD (Table 22.1); the circulatory collapse or shock. The presentation is usually suggestive of left sided obstructive lesion such as Hypoplastic left heart, critical aortic stenosis or Coarctation of aorta (Table 22.2).

Table 22.1: Presentations of critical congenital heart disease in neonates

1. Cyanosis
2. Shock
3. Congestive Heart Failure
4. Heart Murmur

Table 22.2: Left-side obstructive lesion presenting with shock in neonates

1. Coarctation of the aorta
2. Critical aortic stenosis
3. Hypoplastic left heart syndrome
4. Interrupted aortic arch

How to manage such cases before definitive diagnosis is made?

Management starts with the assessment and management of airway, breathing and circulation. If the breathing is irregular or shallow, baby should be intubated and mechanically ventilated. Intravenous access needs to be established followed by correction of glucose. If pediatric cardiac services are available then the logical next step is to get an echocardiogram done and get the final diagnosis.

Prostaglandin E1 (PGE1: Alprostadil) is a life-saving medication and should be present in all NICUs. PGE1 has been proven to open a closed ductus arteriosus especially during early neonatal life. Prostaglandin should be started in all neonates with suspected duct dependent cardiac lesion (Table 22.3). Although there are no criteria or guidelines described regarding, when to start PGE1 infusion pending echocardiogram but few possible clinical scenario suggesting urgent need for starting PGE1 are:

- Deep cyanosis (such as of SpO_2 <60–70%); or
- Sudden appearance of significant cyanosis without appropriate distress.
- Worsening cyanosis/SpO_2 with oxygen supplementation.
- Failed hyperoxia test.
- Absent or disappearing lower limb pulses in presence of good upper limb pulses.
- Sudden unexplained circulatory collapse with failed initial volume resuscitation.

Table 22.3: Duct-dependent lesions

Duct-dependent systemic circulation
1. Hypoplastic left heart syndrome
2. Coarctation of the aorta
3. Critical aortic stenosis
4. Interrupted aortic arch
Duct-dependent pulmonary circulation
1. Pulmonary atresia
2. Critical pulmonary stenosis
3. Critical pulmonary stenosis or pulmonary atresia with single ventricle physiologies
4. Severe Ebstein anomaly
Duct-dependent systemic and pulmonary circulations
1. Transposition of the great arteries (Parallel circulations with inadequate mixing at atrial or ventricle level)

Tables 22.4 and 22.5 detail the salient features of prostaglandin E1 therapy.

Table 22.4: Dosage of prostaglandin E1 (Alprostadil)

- Dose range–0.01–0.4 microgram/kg/min infusion
- Started at a dose of 0.05–0.1 µg/kg/min
- Increments of 0.05 microgram/kg/min every 5–10 minutes if there is no significant improvement in saturation
- Once the duct has opened, dose can be tapered to a maintain a target saturation
- Infusion should be maintained till definitive intervention or Echo rules out duct dependent cardiac lesion.

Table 22.5: Prostaglandin E1 infusion

- Preparation available: 1ml containing 500 mcg
- **Calculation**
  - 3 × wt × microgram/kg/min divided by concentration (mg) in 50 ml = flow rate in ml/hr
  - Or if we put all 1 ml (500 mcg) to 50 ml dextrose/NS then
  - For 0.1 mcg/kg/min = 0.6 ml × wt/hr (Infusion Rate)
  - e.g. for 3 kg @ 0.1mcg/kg/min = 1.8 ml/hr infusion rate

What is the definitive treatment in such cases?

Definitive surgical treatment depends on final diagnosis (Table 22.6).

Table 22.6: Management of left-side obstructive lesions

1. Hypoplastic Left Heart Syndrome • *First stage:* Norwoods Operation with Blalock–Taussig (BT shunt)–Emergency surgery • *Second stage:* Bidirectional Glenn Shunt–at the age between 4–8 months • *Third stage:* Fontan operation–after the age 3–5 years • Most of these kids needs heart transplant at later age due to failure of single right ventricle
2. Critical Coarctation of Aorta • Surgical coarctation of aorta repair • Balloon dilatation is done in cases where severe LV dysfunction is present or surgical correction is high risk due to hemodynamic instability
3. Critical Aortic Stenosis • Balloon Aortic Valvuloplasty (Fig. 22.2)

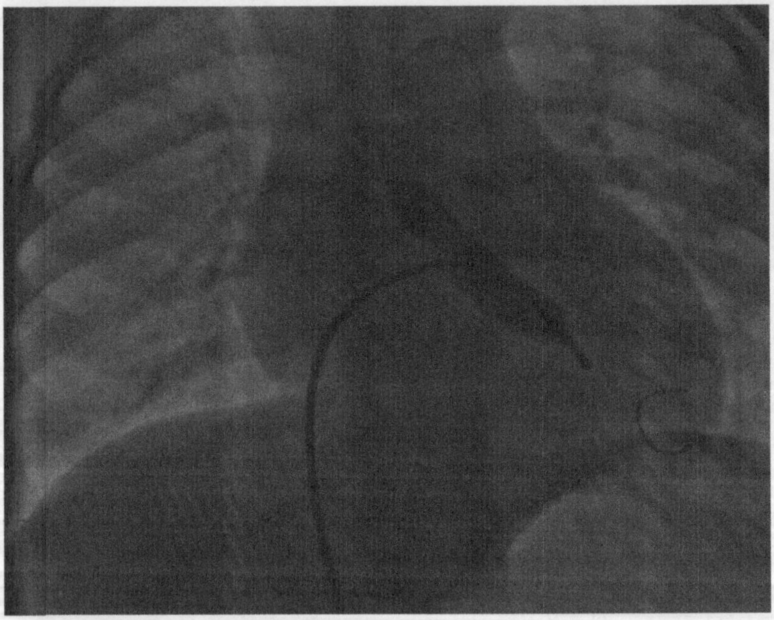

Fig. 22.2: Balloon aortic valvuloplasty (BAV). The picture shows inflated balloon across aortic valve and pacemaker lead in situ for elective pacing during BAV

Approach to management in such a case should be on the following lines:

- Airway, Breathing and Circulation (ABC) is to be prioritized.
- If severe respiratory distress: sedate, paralyze, intubate and mechanically ventilate.
- Intravenous access preferably central lines.
- Check and administer glucose and calcium as needed.
- Check ABG.
- Volume resuscitation.

- Prostaglandin infusion.
- Sepsis evaluation and empirical antibiotics pending culture reports is to be started.
- Transport to a facility for surgical or interventional management.

CASE SCENARIO 2

A normal neonate with his mother in postnatal ward was feeding well and was active. On 2nd day of life, parents alarmed the on-call pediatrician as they noticed bluish discoloration of lips. Baby was shifted to the nursery.

Vital measurement showed saturations of 70% and tachypnea but with only minimal distress.

Auscultation showed single S2 and soft systolic murmur. Baby was started on oxygen by hood but without improvement in saturations.

CRITICAL CASE ANALYSIS

This is a neonate with desaturation. It is important here to differentiate between a pulmonary, cardiac or CNS cause of desaturation. Once a neonate presenting with cyanosis early in life is not responding to oxygen supplementation, first important thing is to rule out respiratory causes and order a chest X-ray (Fig. 22.3). The hyperoxia test can help to differentiate between the three entities, i.e., cyanotic CHD, respiratory cause, and persistent pulmonary hypertension. If the echocardiography points to the diagnosis of duct-dependent cyanotic heart disease, PGE1 should be started and saturation maintained before definitive surgical procedure.

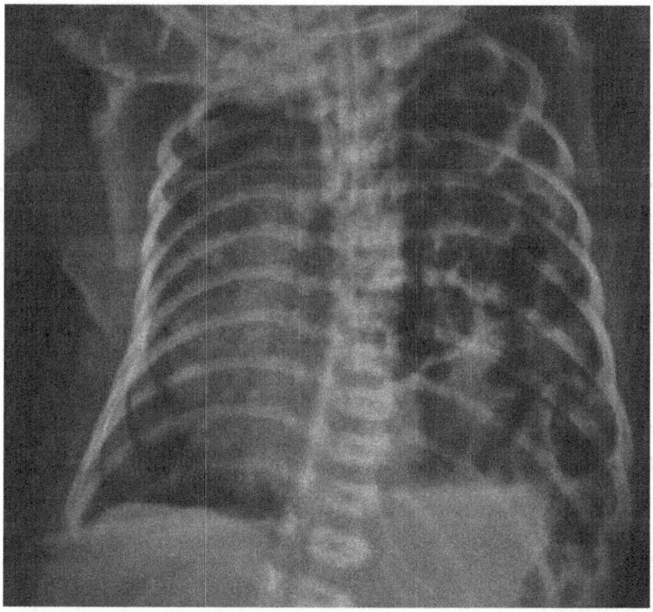

Fig. 22.3: Chest X-ray showing diaphragmatic hernia. In some cases cause of the desaturation is very obvious on chest X-ray

INTERACTIVE TOPIC REVIEW

What are possible differential diagnoses in this case?

Neonates presenting with cyanosis with decreased or normal pulmonary blood flow early in life belong to one of the three groups (Table 22.7).

Table 22.7: Cyanotic congenital heart disease presenting during early neonatal period

1. **Pulmonary Atresia**
   - With ventricle septal defect
   - With single ventricle, e.g., Tricuspid Atresia, DILV etc.
   - With intact ventricle septum
   - With transposition of great artery and VSD
   - With AV canal defect
2. **Critical Pulmonary Stenosis**
   - Isolated or with other defect similar to pulmonary atresia
3. **Transposition of Great Arteries (TGA)**

How should we manage neonate with cyanosis with normal or decreased pulmonary blood flow?

On echocardiography, once the diagnosis of duct dependent cyanotic heart disease is confirmed, the PGE1 should be started and saturation should be maintained before definitive surgical procedure.

Surgical Management plan in cyanotic CHD is presented in Table 22.8.

Table 22.8: Surgical management plan cyanotic CHD

Pulmonary Atresia
- Modified Blalock-Taussig (BT) shunt
- Further patient with possible two ventricle repair requires Rastelli Operation where conduit is used to establish RV to pulmonary artery continuity
- Patient of single ventricle physiology has to undergo Glenn and Fontan Operation route

Critical Pulmonary Stenosis
- Isolated critical PS require balloon dilatation of pulmonary valve (BPV)
- When associated with VSD or other; require modified BT shunt

Transposition of Great Arteries (TGA)
- If referred for surgery within first 3–4 weeks of life–Arterial Switch Operation (ASO)
- If referred late then Left Ventricle (LV) mass assessment require:
  - LV prepared–ASO
  - LV regressed–One of the following options
    - Rapid two staged ASO
    - ASO with ECMO support
    - Senning/Mustard (3–6 months)

What are the indications for Balloon Atrial Septostomy (BAS) (Fig. 22.4) in current era?

There are only few indications for BAS now in current era (Table 22.9). In case of TGA, BAS is used to improve mixing in parallel circulation. Usually now-a-days these babies are taken for arterial switch operation even within 48–72 hours. Only in cases where baby cannot be taken for early surgery as in case of septicemia or any other organ system failure on presentation, BAS can be done so that PGE1 can be stopped during the period baby is waiting for surgery.

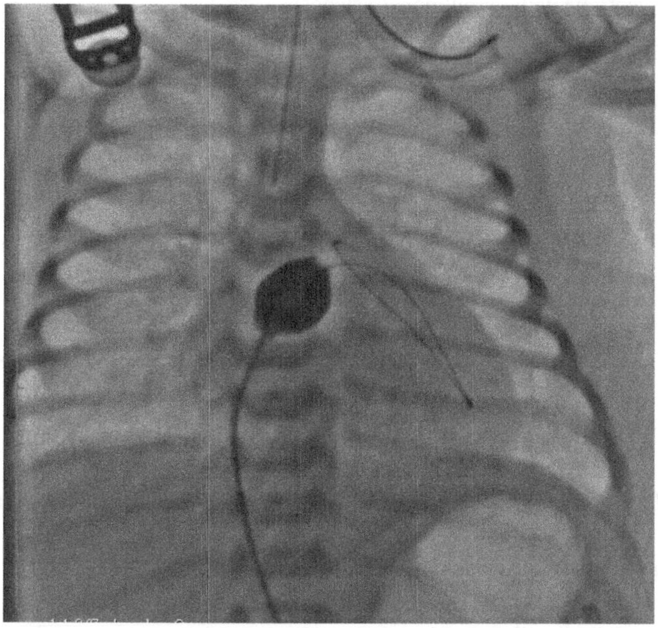

Fig. 22.4: Fluoroscopic picture of procedure Balloon Atrial Septostomy (BAS), is showing the balloon across interatrial septum in to left atrium over guiding wire

Table 22.9: Indications for balloon atrial septostomy

1. **To improve mixing between systemic and pulmonary circulation**
• TGA – where there is parallel circulation
2. **To decompress right atrium**
• Tricuspid atresia with restrictive inter-atrial septum
3. **To decompress left atrium**
• Mitral atresia with restrictive inter-atrial septum

Some cyanotic congenital heart disease can present with sign and symptoms of congestive heart failure (CHF). If the patient also has signs of venous congestion on chest X-ray, usually suggests obstructed TAPVC, a surgical emergency. Management of these neonates includes initial management in line of congestive heart failure treatment which includes use of oxygenation, diuretics and inotropes.

What are the possible differential diagnoses in this case?

The CHDs present with cyanosis with signs of CHF are listed in Table 22.10.

Table 22.10: Cyanotic CHD presenting as congestive heart failure (CHF)

1. Total anomalous pulmonary venous connection (TAPVC)
2. Truncus arteriosus
3. Transposition of great arteries with large VSD
4. Double outlet right ventricle without pulmonary stenosis
5. Single ventricle physiology without pulmonary stenosis

What is definitive management in neonate with cyanosis and congestive heart failure?

The definitive treatment depends on final diagnosis (Table 22.11).

Table 22.11: Management of cyanotic CHD with increased pulmonary blood flow

1. **Total Anomalous Pulmonary Venous Connection (TAPVC)**
   - Obstructive type – Emergency surgery
   - Non-obstructive type – As soon as possible beyond the neonatal period
2. **Truncus Arteriosus** – Total repair using RV to PA conduit
   - Uncontrolled CCF – Early surgery
   - Controlled CCF – Surgery by 6–12 weeks
3. **Transposition of Great Arteries with Large VSD** – Arterial switch operation with VSD closure between 1 and 2 months
4. **Double Outlet Right Ventricle without pulmonary stenosis**
   - Managed in line of large VSD or TGA-VSD depending on anatomy
5. **Single Ventricle Physiology without pulmonary stenosis**
   (a) **First stage:** Pulmonary Artery Banding between age of 3 and 6 weeks.
   (b) **Second stage:** Bidirectional Glenn Shunt–at the age between 4 and 8 months.
   (c) **Third stage:** Fontan operation–after the age 3–5 years.

CONCLUSIONS

Critical cyanotic CHD in newborn belongs to one of the three-symptom complex. Initial management of these neonates depends on the symptom complex before definitive diagnosis can be made. Prostaglandin E1 is life-saving in case of suspected duct-dependent lesion. Systematic assessment of newborn and appropriate management contribute to achieving optimum outcome.

TAKE HOME MESSAGES

- No newborn baby should be discharged without cardiac evaluation.
- Because existing screening methods still miss up to 30% of cases, the addition of pulse oximetry screening (which increases detection to over 90%) should be encouraged.

Contd...

Contd...

- Judicious use of prostaglandin (PGE1) helps in resuscitation in critical CHD and should be accessible to all nurseries.
- Appropriate timing of intervention in managing cyanotic congenital heart disease is vital.
- Most of the babies with single ventricle physiology can be managed well with good longevity.

FURTHER READING

1. de-Wahl Granelli A, Wennergren M, Sandberg K, *et al.* Impact of pulse-oximetry screening on the detection of duct-dependent congenital heart disease: A Swedish prospective screening study in 39,821 newborns. BMJ 2009;338:a3037 *Available at: https://www.google.co.in/search?q=de-Wahl+Granelli+A,+Wennergren+M,+Sandberg+K,+et+al.+Impact+of+pulse-oximetry+screening+on+the+detection+of+ductependent+congenital+heart+disease:+A+Swedish+prospective+screening+study+in+39,821+newborns.+BMJ+2009%3B338:a3037&gws_rd=cr,ssl&ei=Nr_nV66nA8vpvATTiYKgDw Accessed on: 25 September 2016.*
2. Ewer AK, Middleton LJ, Furmston AT, *et al.* (For PulseOx Study Group). Pulse oximetry screening for congenital heart defects in newborn infants (PulseOx): A test accuracy study. *Lancet* 2011;378(9793): 785–794.
3. Kemper AR, Mahle WT, Martin GR, *et al.* Strategies for implementing screening for critical congenital heart disease. *Pediatrics* 2011;128: e1259–1267.

Chapter

23 Neonatal Arrhythmias

Poonam Singh, Anup Thakur

ABSTRACT

Identification and treatment of arrhythmias in newborns is challenging and differs from older children. Natural history of arrhythmias presenting in the neonates is often dramatically different. The chapter describes normal electrocardiogram (ECG) of newborn and common neonatal rhythm disturbances with their management.

Key Words: Bradyarrhythmias, Heart blocks, Long QT syndrome, Neonatal arrhythmias, Supraventricular tachycardia (SVT), Tachyarrhythmias, Wolf-Parkinson-White syndrome.

INTRODUCTION

Diagnosis of arrhythmias is challenging in the neonatal period. Normal heart rate may vary markedly depending on the level of activity. Clinical features often overlap with sepsis and normal heart rate varies greatly from that of the older children.

Diagnosing rhythm disturbances in the neonatal period begins with knowledge of healthy newborn electrocardiogram (ECG). All pediatricians and neonatologists should be well-versed in interpreting normal and abnormal rhythm. Early diagnosis and treatment of rhythm disorders is life saving.

CASE SCENARIO

The 15 days male presented with complaints of running nose and cough for 2 days followed by rapid breathing, restlessness, irritability and refusal to feed for 1 day.

Physical examination

Baby was irritable with heart rate of 260/min, respiratory rate of 88/min, poor pulses, cold peripheries, mottled and ashen colored appearance.

Blood pressure was unrecordable.

Cardiac auscultation revealed marked tachycardia and no audible murmur.

Contd...

Contd...

Liver was palpable 7 cm below the right costal border.

Investigations

Sepsis screen was unremarkable.

Electrolytes were normal.

ECG showed heart rate of 278/min, absent P waves, narrow QRS complexes (<0.08 sec) and fixed RR interval.

Diagnosis

Supraventricular tachycardia (SVT) with congestive cardiac failure (critically ill infant).

Treatment given

Immediately synchronized cardioversion was done, 0.5 J/kg resulting in restoration of sinus rhythm.

Outcome

Once the baby reverted to sinus rhythm, maintenance therapy with propranolol was started.

CRITICAL CASE ANALYSIS

Clinical presentation of this baby closely resembles that of sepsis. However, there are clinical pointers to the diagnosis of SVT such as tachycardia with heart rate more than 180/min, features of congestive heart failure and ECG showing narrow QRS complexes (<0.08 sec) with fixed RR interval.

The infant was critically ill with signs of hemodynamic compromise in the form of poor pulses, cold peripheries and nonrecordable BP.

Treatment of narrow complex tachycardia begins with assessment of hemodynamic status. In a critically ill infant, synchronized cardioversion is indicated. Stable patients are managed by vagal maneuvers with or without adenosine.

If these measures fail in a stable infant, electrical cardioversion is an option.

INTERACTIVE TOPIC DISCUSSION

What are the normal neonatal ECG parameters?

In normal sinus rhythm, every beat originates in the sinus node. The P wave is generated as atrial depolarization occurs. There is a brief delay from slow conduction in the atrioventricular (AV) node to optimize ventricular filling, shown by the isoelectric PR segment. Electrical conduction to the ventricles occurs at high speed via the His–Purkinje system to allow near-synchronous ventricular contraction and produces the QRS complex. Ventricular repolarization takes place more slowly and is shown by the T wave. Only after repolarization is complete, can the next depolarization occur. Normal sinus rhythm in ECG is characterized by upright P waves in leads I and aVF, followed by narrow QRS complexes.

ECG is the gold standard for identifying problems with heart rate and regularity. Interpretation of ECG should take into account the normal values of various ECG parameters in neonatal period. Normal ECG and various waves and intervals are delineated in Figure 23.1. Normal values are described in Table 23.1.

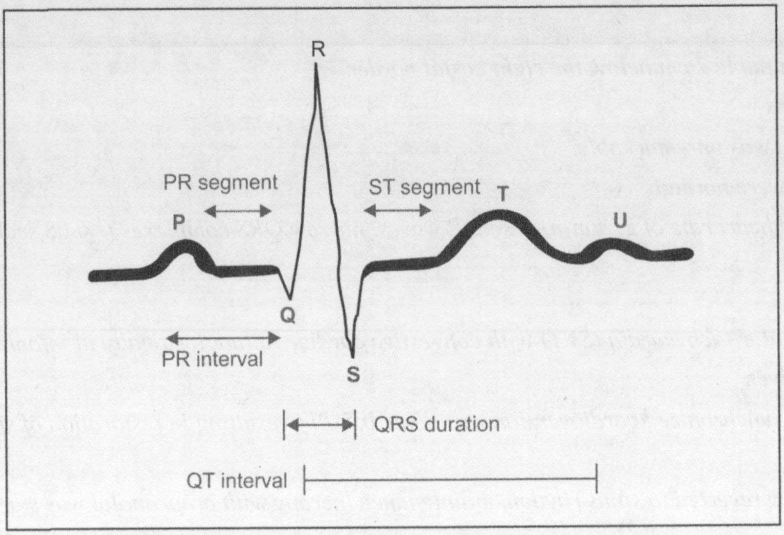

Fig. 23.1: Waves and intervals of ECG in lead II

Table 23.1: Normal values of ECG parameters in newborns

Parameter	Normal range	Events in the heart during intervals and comments
Heart rate	Average: 120–160/min Range: 90–230/min	• Sinus arrhythmia is normal variation in heart rate with respiration.
PR interval	70–140 msec	• Measured from onset of the P wave to the Q or R wave in lead II. • Atrial depolarization and conduction through AV node.
QRS axis	Term: 55–200° Preterm: 65–174°	–
QRS duration	20–80 msec	• Ventricular depolarization and atrial repolarization. • Range described is measured in lead V5.
QTc interval	Mean on postnatal day: 4–400 ± 20 msec	• Ventricular depolarization plus ventricular repolarization. • Begins from onset of the QRS complex to the end of the T wave, is measured best in leads II, V5 and V6. • As QT interval varies with heart rate so corrected, QTc interval is calculated by Bazett's formula: $QTc = QT(sec)/\sqrt{RR}$ (preceding RR interval in seconds). • Physiologic prolongation of QTc occurs by 2 months of age (mean QTc, 410 msec), with return to a mean of 400 msec by 6 months of age.
ST interval		• Ventricular repolarization (during T wave). • In the first postnatal week, T waves vary substantially but are usually positive (upright) in lead V1. • After the first postnatal week, the T wave typically is negative (downgoing) in lead V1 and positive in V5 and V6.

What are the types of rhythm disorders in neonates?

Rhythm disturbances can be broadly classified into tachyarrhythmia or bradyarrhythmias. They can be benign or life threatening. Symptomatic neonatal arrhythmias are rare. Supraventricular tachycardia (SVT) is the most common among them. Ventricular arrhythmias are often secondary arising to metabolic disturbances. Hence, they are potentially treatable.

Depending upon the site of origin, rhythm disorders are classified as in Table 23.2.

Table 23.2: Classification of common arrhythmias in neonates

Tachyarrhythmia	Bradyarrhythmia
Sinus tachycardia	Sinus bradycardias
Atrial tachycardia • Atrial flutter • Atrial fibrillation • Multifocal atrial tachycardia	Heart blocks • First degree • Second degree • Third degree
Conduction system arrhythmia • Wolff-Parkinson-White syndrome • Concealed accessory pathways • AV nodal re-entry tachycardias • Permanent junctional reciprocating tachycardia	
Ventricular tachycardia	

What is sinus tachycardia and how does it differ from supraventricular tachycardia?

Sinus tachycardia in neonate denotes heart rate more than normal for gestation and age. It is usually secondary to some other systemic problem. ECG criteria for sinus tachycardia are normal P wave axis, gradual onset and termination, and rates less than 230 beats per minute. Causes of sinus tachycardia include:

- Fever
- Pain
- Hypoxia
- Cardiac failure
- Drugs: Isoproterenol, dobutamine, xanthine therapy
- Under-sedation in paralyzed infants supported by mechanical ventilation
- Hyperthyroidism.

In supraventricular tachycardia, the heart rate is usually more than 230/min. It manifests as a narrow QRS complex (<0.08 sec) with P waves visible on a standard ECG in only 50–60% of the cases. It is detectable with a transesophageal lead in most patients. Differentiation from sinus tachycardia is difficult. If the rate is >230 beats/min with an abnormal P-wave axis, sinus tachycardia is not likely. The heart rate in SVT tends to be unvarying. In sinus tachycardia the heart rate varies with changes in vagal and sympathetic tone. Vagal maneuvers and other methods of converting supraventricular tachycardia fail to terminate sinus tachycardia.

What are the mechanisms of tachyarrhythmia?

The two main mechanisms of tachyarrhythmia include: Re-entry and increased automaticity.

- Re-entry as a mechanism to result in tachyarrhythmia requires fulfillment of three conditions:
  (a) Presence of an anatomically distinct conducting pathway.
  (b) Unidirectional conduction block must occur in the re-entrant pathway allowing subsequent reversed conduction in that segment.
  (c) There must be an area of conduction delay in the re-entry circuit sufficient to allow recovery of all components of the circuit before the arrival of the next wave of activation.

The circuit is constituted by the accessory pathway, atrium, AV node, and ventricle. This is shown in Figure 23.2. The peculiar feature of re-entrant tachycardias is that they have a tendency to have an abrupt onset and cessation and they can be terminated with direct current cardioversion which is of no utility in cases of abnormal rhythm resulting from increased automaticity.

- Increased automaticity: Spontaneous depolarization of the conduction system occurs beyond SA node as in ectopic focus.

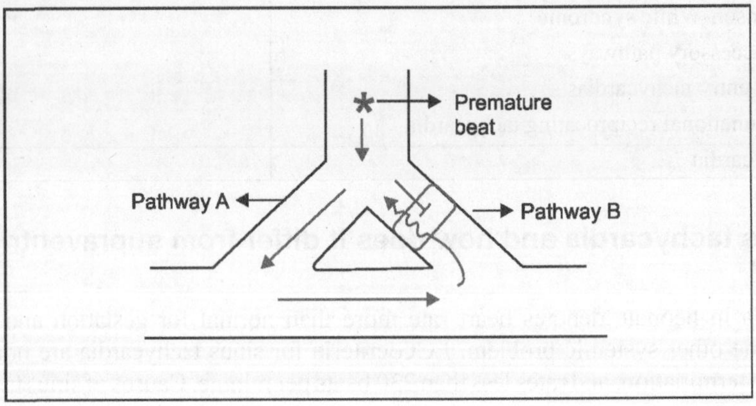

Fig. 23.2: Diagram showing re-entry phenomena. In re-entry, electrical signals generated from an appropriately timed premature beat find pathway B refractory, resulting in conduction block in this limb of the circuit. Meanwhile, conduction down pathway A proceeds unimpeded and subsequently the signal is conducted back via pathway B which has recovered leading to circus like movement

What is SVT and what are its mechanisms?

The most common life-threatening arrhythmia of the newborn is supraventricular tachycardia. SVT is defined as narrow complex tachycardia that requires atrial tissue or AV node as an integral part of arrhythmia substrate. In the neonate, SVT of 12–24 hours duration usually results in heart failure.

What are clinical manifestation of SVT?

The diagnosis of SVT in a newborn may be difficult because of the normally more rapid heart rate in infancy. Infants may be stable or hemodynamically unstable presenting with cardiac failure or shock. Infants usually present with poor feeding, tachypnea and irritability, with heart rates of 200–300 beats/min. These babies are often misdiagnosed as septic and SVT can be overlooked.

Depending upon the mechanism SVT can be of following three types:

1. **AV Reciprocating Tachycardia (AVRT):** AVRT uses a bypass tract which facilitates re-entry. Conduction may be orthodromic or antidromic. Orthodromic conduction means there is antigrade conduction through AV node and retrograde through accessory pathway. Reverse is true for antidromic conduction.

   Depending upon the direction of transmission across accessory pathway SVT of AVRT type can be further classified into two:

   (i) **The Concealed Accessory Connection:** This accessory pathway allows only unidirectional retrograde electrical conduction from ventricle to the atria. Such pathways can only mediate orthodromic re-entry. As these pathways do not disturb electrical transmission during sinus rhythm so during routine ECG they remain "concealed" or invisible.

   (ii) **The Wolf-Parkinson-White Accessory Connection:** This may either be able to conduct bidirectionally [Wolff-Parkinson-White (WPW) syndrome] or retrograde only (concealed accessory pathway). Wolff–Parkinson–White (WPW) syndrome describes the combination of ventricular pre-excitation in sinus rhythm with paroxysmal tachycardia. The most common arrhythmia seen in WPW syndrome is orthodromic AV re-entry tachycardia, but antidromic re-entry and atrial fibrillation also can occur.

   The typical electrocardiographic features of the Wolff-Parkinson-White syndrome are seen when the patient is not having tachycardia (in sinus rhythm). The hallmark of pre-excitation seen in WPW is a short PR interval and a widened QRS with slow early activation – the delta wave (Fig. 23.3).

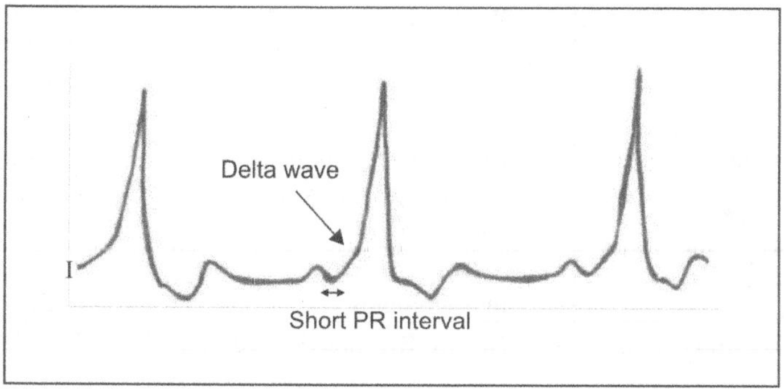

Fig. 23.3: ECG showing pre-excitation as short PR interval and a widened QRS with slurred upstroke–Delta wave

2. **AV Nodal Re-entrant Tachycardia (AVNRT)** involves the use of two pathways within the AV node one fast and other slow. This involves re-entry using functional equivalent of an extra-connection within AV node. Neonatal AVNRT more commonly is associated with other cardiorespiratory problems (e.g., congenital diaphragmatic hernia, congenital heart disease, sepsis) and is uncommon in an otherwise healthy infant.

3. **Ectopic or Automatic Tachycardias:** Atrial and junctional ectopic tachycardias are more commonly associated with abnormal hearts (cardiomyopathy) and in the immediate post-operative period following surgery for congenital heart disease.

List the ECG characteristics of common forms of tachyarrhythmia.

ECG characteristics and salient features of tachyarrhythmia are enlisted in Table 23.3.

Table 23.3: Types and characteristics of various tachyarrhythmia

Tachyarrhythmia	ECG characteristics	Comments
Ectopic atrial tachycardia 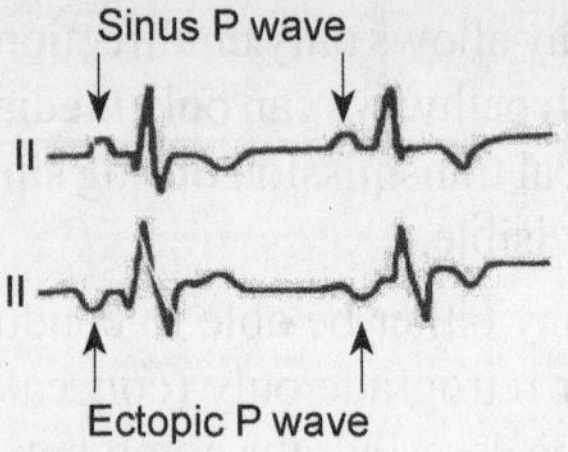	• Abnormal P wave axis. • P wave precedes QRS. • Variable rate. • "Warm up" (rate gradually increases over first several beats).	• Abnormal automaticity is most likely. • May be incessant. • May not respond to cardioversion. • Can lead to tachycardia induced cardiomyopathy.
Atrial flutter 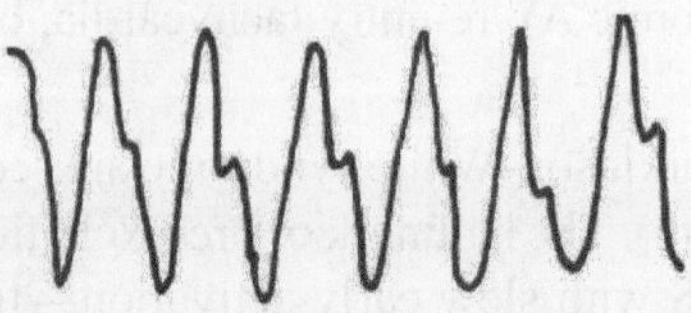	• Atrial rate up to 500 beats/min in newborn. • Sawtooth flutter waves. • Variable AV conduction is common. • Distinguished from atrial tachycardia by absence of an isoelectric period between P waves.	• Diagnosis is suspected from ventricular rate and confirmed by adenosine which increases the AV block to unmask the flutter waves. • Sinus rhythm is restored by transesophageal overdrive pacing or synchronized DC cardioversion (0.5–1 J/kg). • Recurrence is rare so prophylactic medication is not required.
Multifocal atrial tachycardia 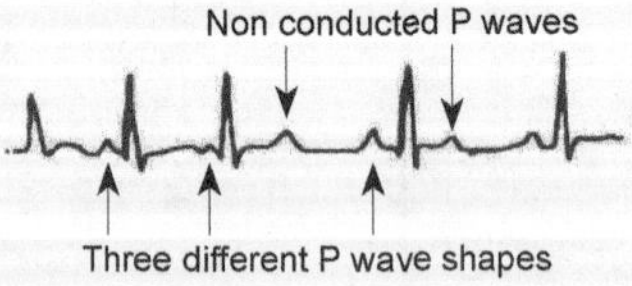	• Irregularly irregular heart rate as many P waves are not conducted. • Multiple different P wave morphologies. • No two RR intervals are same.	• If heart rate is normal and infant is asymptomatic no treatment is required. • Spontaneous resolution occurs in weeks or months following which medication can be withdrawn.
Atrioventricular re-entry tachycardia (Orthodromic) 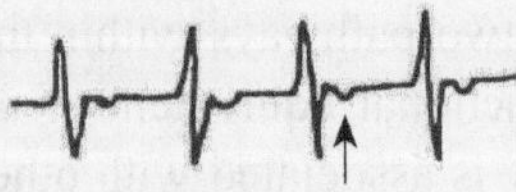	• P wave follows QRS typically on upstroke of T wave.	• Most common form of neonatal SVT. • Adenosine sensitive.
Atrioventricular re-entry tachycardia (Antidromic) 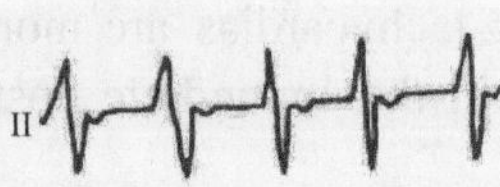	• Superior P wave axis (inverted in lead II and aVF).	• Pre excitation (delta wave) and short PR interval is seen post-termination in WPW. • Adenosine sensitive.

Contd..

Contd..

Atrioventricular nodal re-entry tachycardia 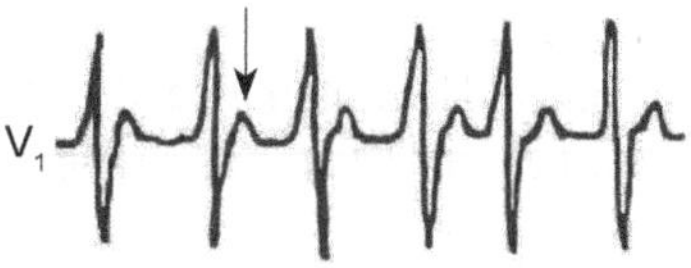	• P wave usually not visible superimposed on QRS. • Produces a small positive deflection at the end of the QRS in lead V1, which looks a bit like an r' wave.	• Adenosine sensitive.
Permanent junctional reciprocating tachycardia 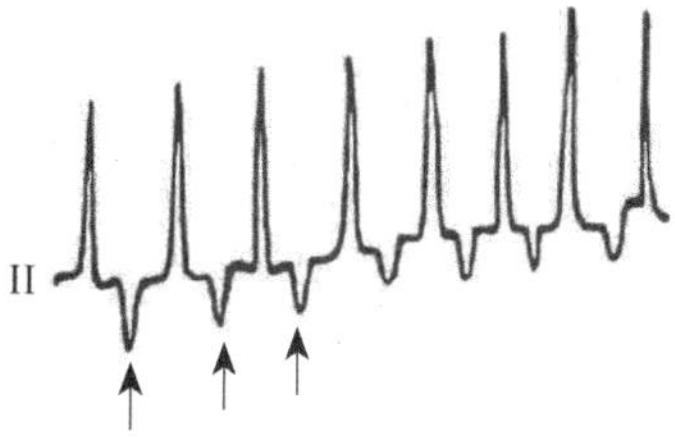	• Inverted P waves in II, III, aVF appear to precede QRS complex. • P waves are characteristically deeply inverted in leads II, III and aVF.	• Incessant, slower rate than others–about 200 beats/min. • Typically restarts after electrical cardioversion or adenosine. • Maintenance antiarrhythmics such as Flecainide always required. • Early catheter ablation may be required. • Can lead to tachycardia induced cardiomyopathy.
Ventricular tachycardia 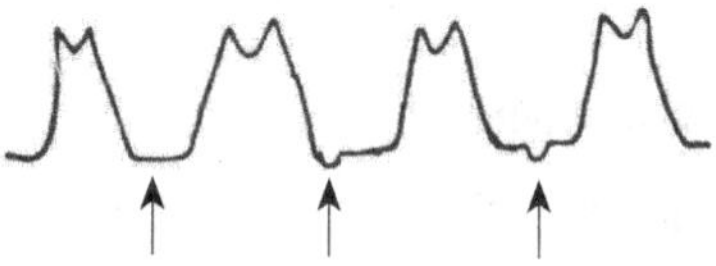	• Wide QRS complexes. • P wave may be dissociated from QRS complex. • "Capture" or "fusion" beats diagnostic.	• Rare in neonates. • VT is defined as an arrhythmia with three or more consecutive beats originating in the ventricles usually at a rate of 120/min or more. • Broad complex QRS always treated as VT unless proved otherwise. • Not terminated by adenosine.
Ventricular fibrillation 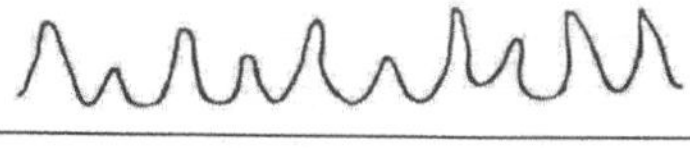	• Chaotic irregular rhythm.	• Rare in neonates. • Consider long QT syndrome or Brugada syndrome.

What is the management of SVT?

Any baby presenting with narrow QRS complex tachycardia is managed as a case of SVT. Management begins with hemodynamic assessment of the infant. SVT can be managed as per categorizes discussed below:

1. **Symptom Free or Mildly Affected Infants:** These babies are picked up during routine clinical examination or by the parents. Some symptom-free neonates do not require short- or long-term treatment. In cases with poor activity during episode or when there is an increased risk for prolonged arrhythmia, long-term treatment is necessary.
2. **Seriously Ill Infants:** These babies have features of congestive cardiac failures like tachypnea, sweating, poor feeding, hepatomegaly, rales in the chest, gallop rhythm and cardiomegaly on

chest X-ray with recordable BP and are conscious. These infants may be stable or unstable depending on the stage of congestive cardiac failure.

3. **Critically Ill Infants:** Rapid heart rates result in critically low blood pressure, non-palpable pulses, altered sensorium or complete loss of consciousness.

   Treatment of SVT includes termination of tachycardia paroxysm and maintenance therapy. Interventions for termination are illustrated in Figure 23.4 for reverting SVT to sinus rhythm in an infant depending upon the hemodynamic status.

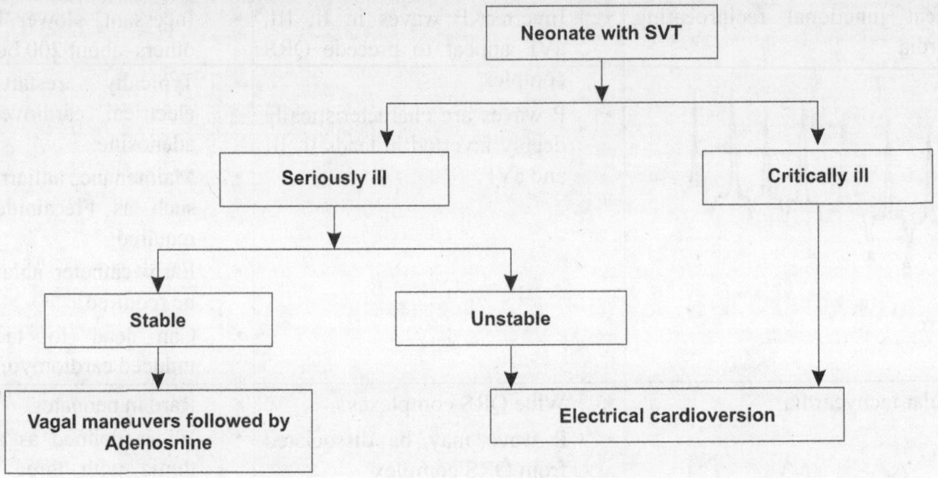

Fig. 23.4: Treatment options for reverting SVT to sinus rhythm

How does vagal stimulation help to terminate an attack of SVT and how to elicit vagal maneuvers in neonates?

Acetylcholine liberated at vagal endings by stimulating reflex vagal discharge depresses conduction in the atrial musculature and AV node. The increase in the degree of AV block, abruptly lowers the ventricular rate by blocking atrial impulses to the ventricle. Vagal maneuvers should be tried with i/v line in place and should not be continued for more than 5 minutes before trying other modalities in a seriously ill baby. Various maneuvers which can be tried include:

- Elicit gag with nasogastric tube.
- Elicit diving reflex by placing a bag filled with ice over the face and ears for 15 seconds.

Carotid massage or orbital pressure application should not be done in neonates.

What is the dose and route of administration of adenosine for SVT?

Adenosine is the drug of choice for SVT where AV node is part of re-entry circuit. Adenosine causes a temporary AV nodal conduction block and interrupts re-entry circuit that involve the AV node. The drug has a wide safety margin because of its short half life of 10 seconds. Adenosine should be given only intravenously as close to the heart as possible followed by rapid saline flush to promote drug delivery to central circulation.

Dose: 100 mcg/kg, given by rapid IV infusion (not in umbilical artery). Repeated as 200 mcg/kg and then 400 mcg/kg if no effect is seen. When given by rapid IV injection, onset of effect is seen in 7 or 8 seconds. AV blockade is brief.

The neonate should be under continuous ECG monitoring during therapy. This may show termination of SVT or may unmask other arrhythmias.

What are the factors associated with adenosine failure in terminating SVT?

Adenosine failure may be due to:

(a) Inadequate dosage or too slow administration of the drug.

(b) The mechanism being atrial tachycardia; as adenosine blocks the AV node, it may reveal atrial flutter or atrial tachycardia as the cause of the problem.

(c) The mechanism being VT.

In such circumstances, options are other anti-arrhythmics like amiodarone, esmolol, procainamide or cardioversion.

Discuss the long-term management of SVT.

Choice of long-term anti-arrhythmic drugs is based on the severity of the presentation and the mechanism of the tachycardia, in particular the presence/absence of delta wave (pre-excitation).

Maintenance Therapy

- For mildly symptomatic babies with adenosine sensitive tachycardia that reverted easily maintenance therapy can be omitted.
- For an infants presenting frequent attacks with circulatory collapse, or in whom cardioversion was difficult, beta blockers (propanolol 0.5 mg/kg PO every 6 hours) are used. Digoxin is used only if there is no evidence of pre-excitation in sinus rhythm in the dose of 5 mcg/kg PO every 12 hours after initial load.

About 40% of newborns who have a treated episode of SVT do not have another episode when treated with anti-arrhythmics for a minimum of 1 year after the first episode. If SVT persists beyond 1 year, spontaneous resolution is unlikely. Transcatheter ablation of the accessory pathway is of limited use in neonates for the concerns like perforation, AV block and damage to the coronary arteries. Ablation is reserved for life-threatening, medically refractory cases.

What is the management of wide complex tachycardia?

Most infants with wide QRS tachycardia have ventricular tachycardia rather than supraventricular tachycardia with an aberration. Because it may be nearly impossible to differentiate the two in neonates with ECG, patients with wide QRS tachycardia are treated as if they have ventricular tachycardia. Wide complex tachycardia with collapse is treated with electrical cardioversion. In patients who are not seriously ill and cardioversion can be deferred, procainamide would be a good choice because it is effective both for ventricular and supraventricular arrhythmias. Lidocaine can be used if the diagnosis of ventricular tachycardia is certain.

Describe cardioversion in brief.

Defibrillation is non-synchronized random administration of shock during a cardiac cycle. Cardioversion is a synchronized administration of shock during the R waves or QRS complex of a cardiac cycle. During defibrillation and cardioversion, electrical current travels from the negative to the positive electrode by traversing myocardium. It depolarizes all of the heart cells simultaneously. This interrupts and terminates abnormal electrical rhythm. This, in turn, allows the sinus node to resume normal pacemaker activity.

Paddle size: Small paddles those used for direct delivery to epicardial surface of heart in older patients intraoperatively are appropriate for neonates.

Interface: The electrode-chest wall interface is part of self adhesive pad, in contrast, electrode gel must be applied liberally on manually applied paddles. Saline soaked pads, ultrasound gel and bare paddles should not be used.

Paddle Position: Place manual paddles over the right side of upper chest and the apex of the heart (to the left of the nipple over the left lower ribs) so the heart is between the two paddles.

Energy Dose: Initial dose is 0.5–1.0 J/kg.

Indications: Synchronized cadioversion is done for SVT and VT whereas for VF cardioversion is used in asynchronous mode.

Describe an algorithm for identifying tachycardias.

A sequential analysis of the ECG helps to classify the tachyarrhythmia. An easy approach is to look for

1. QRS complex rate, regularity, and width followed by
2. The relation of the P wave to the QRS
3. P-wave morphology

Figure 23.5: Provides an algorithm to tachyarrhythmia.

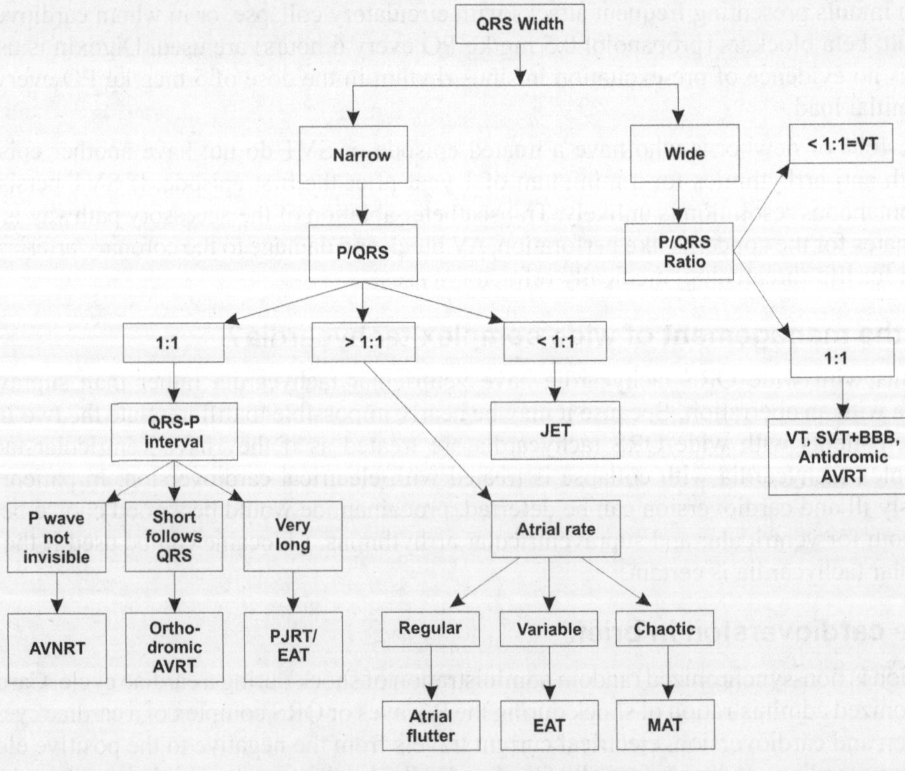

Fig. 23.5: Approach to tachyarrhythmia

What are the causes of bradycardia in neonates?

Newborn cardiac innervation has vagal dominance predisposing to episodic sinus bradycardia. Sinus bradycardia is characterized by regular slow atrial rate with normal P waves and 1:1 conduction. Pathologic causes of sinus bradycardia include hypoxia, acidosis, increased intracranial pressure, abdominal distention, hypoglycemia, apnea of prematurity and drugs such as digoxin and propranolol.

Describe different types of heart blocks.

Heart block is basically of following three types:

1. **First-degree AV Block:** First degree heart block is characterized by prolonged PR interval but all the atrial impulses are conducted to the ventricle.
2. **Second-degree AV Block:** It is further classified into 2 types:

   Mobitz Type I (Wenckebach Type): In this variant, the PR interval increases progressively until a P wave is not conducted. In the cycle following the dropped beat, the PR interval normalizes. Mobitz type is usually due to a functional suppression of AV conduction and it can usually be reversed with catecholamines or with vagolytic agents. It has better prognosis as compared to type II block.

   Mobitz Type II: There occurs intermittent non conducted P waves without prolongation of PR interval. This conduction defect is less common but has more potential to cause syncope and may be progressive. One specific form of second-degree block requires immediate attention: the form of 2:1 conduction seen in infants with markedly prolonged QR intervals. 2:1conduction in such infants is an important risk factor for the development of torsades de pointes and sudden death. Mobitz type II is usually due to failure of conduction at the level of the His-Purkinje system as a result of structural damage to the conducting system.
3. **Third-degree AV Block (Complete Heart Block):** No impulses from the atria reach the ventricles so that AV dissociation occurs with regular R-R intervals and regular P-P intervals. The atrial rate is usually greater than the ventricular rate, and P waves that occur well after the T wave have no effect on the R-R interval.

What are the clinical scenarios leading to complete heart block in a neonate? Discuss congenital heart block in neonate associated with maternal collagen vascular disease.

Conditions associated with complete heart block in a neonate include congenital, surgically induced, or acquired. Complete Heart Block can occur in association with congenital heart disease such as dTGA, following surgical correction or acquired due to myocarditis.

Complete heart block in the absence of structural heart defect is associated with collagen vascular diseases of the mother. Maternal SS-A/Ro and SS-B/La antibodies made as a result of maternal systemic lupus erythematosus, rheumatoid arthritis, dermatomyositis, or Sjogren's syndrome disrupt the developing fetal heart conduction system, leading to second-degree AV block or complete heart block. It can be seen as early as 16–28 weeks' gestation, with an incidence of approximately 1:20,000 live births. The risk of sudden cardiac death in an infant who has complete AV block is greatest when the heart rate averages less that 55 beats/min, and this is generally an indication for dual-chamber pacemaker implantation. Recent studies have shown a risk for the late development of dilated cardiomyopathy in children who have congenital AV block due to maternal auto antibodies, and therefore, these infants should have regular cardiac follow-up throughout childhood.

What are long QT syndromes? Mention drugs that can prolong QT interval.

Congenital long QT syndromes (LQTS) are genetic disorders of sodium and potassium channels resulting in prolongation of ventricular repolarization and QT interval. The rhythm disorder associated with this condition is polymorphic VT also called as torsades de pointes. The estimated incidence is about 1 per 10,000 births but variable penetrance makes precise assessment difficult. This arrhythmia may be asymptomatic if brief and self-limited, but if sustained beyond several seconds, usually results in ventricular fibrillation.

Genetics: More than 400 different mutations have been identified in 10 LQTS susceptibility genes, including genes that encode for subunits of sodium, potassium and calcium voltage-gated ion channels. Genotype may predict clinical presentation for example, LQT1 events are usually stress induced, whereas events in LQT3 often occur during sleep. LQT3 has the highest probability for sudden death, followed by LQT2 and then LQT1.

Clinical Features: LQTS may be detected during ECG done for other reasons. It may be one of the causes for sudden infant death. LQTS gene variants have been found in 9.5% of SIDS victims. Other manifestations include syncope provoked by exercise, fright, or a sudden startle, seizures, aborted cardiac arrest, or sudden death. Some babies are diagnosed when ECG is done due to history of syncope (especially with stress), and a familial history of either LQTS or unexplained sudden death.

Diagnosis: Diagnosis of LQTS depends on accurate measurement of QT interval which is best measured in lead II and V5 because these leads usually have an upright T wave with a distinct end. The QT interval varies with heart rate, becoming shorter at higher heart rates; so corrected QT interval for heart rate called as QTc is calculated. The mean QTc on the fourth postnatal day is 400 ± 20 msec, with an upper limit of normal (2 standard deviations above the mean, 97.5%) of 440 msec. Therefore, in 2.5% of healthy newborns, the QTc is expected to be greater than 440 msec. The more prolonged the QTc, the greater the likelihood that it is clinically significant. In healthy infants, there is physiologic prolongation of the QTc by 2 months of age (mean QTc, 410 msec), with return to a mean of 400 msec by 6 months of age. Mild QTc prolongation (≤470 msec) may occur following stressful labor or delivery but usually resolves within 48–72 hours. Q-T interval of >0.47 sec is highly indicative, whereas a Q-T interval of >0.44 sec is suggestive.

Infants are screened for LQTS with an ECG due to a family history. Such screening should be delayed until the infant is 6–8 weeks of age because modest QT interval prolongation is relatively common (2.5%) among healthy infants and may cause undue family concern.

Treatment: Treatment of LQTS includes the use of β-blocking agents at doses that blunt the heart rate response to exercise. If drug therapy causes profound bradycardia then pacemaker needs to be implanted. Those who are unresponsive to β-blockers and experienced cardiac arrest, an implantable cardiac defibrillator is indicated. β-blocking agents are not effective in patients with LQT3, hence implantable cardiac defibrillator is indicated.

Common drugs used in neonatal period which can prolong QT interval are mentioned in Table 23.4.

Table 23.4: Drugs that can prolong QT interval

Antibiotics	Erythromycin, Azithromycin, Trimethoprim/Sulfamethoxazole
Antifungals	Fluconazole, Itraconazole
Antihistamines	Astemizole, Terfenadine
Antipsychotics	Haloperidol, Risperidone, Chlorpromazine
Antiarrhythmics	Quinidine, Procainamide, Disopyramide, Amiodarone, Sotalol
Diuretics (Through K^+ Loss)	Furosemide, Ethacrynic Acid, Bumetanide
Promotility agents	Cisapride
Dyselectrolytemia	Hypokalemia, Hypocalcemia, Hypomagnesemia

What are salient details of drugs recommended for neonatal arrhythmias?

These are listed along with their dosage and special comments in Table 23.5.

Table 23.5: Antiarrhythmic drugs used in arrhythmias in neonates

Drug	Dosage	Special comments
Esmolol	50–500 mcg/kg/min.	• Monitor pulse, blood pressure. • Contraindicated in congestive heart failure. • Do not give with verapamil.
Procainamide	10–15 mg/kg IV over 30–45 min.	• Can cause hypotension. • Continuous blood pressure monitoring is essential.
Digoxin	10 mcg/kg IV as initial load; second dose in 6 hours and third at 24 hours.	• Do not use in hypokalemia or if toxic reaction to digoxin is suspected.
Adenosine	Start IV dose of 100 mcg/kg; double dose repeatedly until effect is seen, to maximum of 400 mcg/kg.	• Contraindicated in pre-existing second- and third-degree AV block without pacemaker. • Use with caution in severe asthma; half-life is 10 sec in serum. • Occasionally induces atrial fibrillation.
Amiodarone	5 mg/kg IV over 15–30 min or as 5 separate 1 mg/kg aliquots.	• Given by central line diluted in D_5W. • Can cause gasping syndrome in infants due to benzyl alcohol.
Propranolol	0.25–1 mg/kg PO every 6 hours.	• Observe for wheezing and symptoms of hypoglycemia.
Atenolol	0.5–2 mg/kg/day PO divided every 12 hours.	–
Sotalol	2–8 mg/kg/day PO divided every 8 hours.	• Torsade de pointes is likely with hypokalemia.

CONCLUSIONS

Rhythm disorders can have variable presentation in neonatal period. All pediatricians and neonatologists should be able to interpret ECG in neonates and identify arrhythmias. Appropriate and timely management of such neonates is life saving with good long-term outcomes in most of the cases.

TAKE HOME MESSAGES

- High index of suspicion is required to diagnose rhythm disorder in neonates.
- Tachyarrhythmia can be either narrow QRS complex or broad QRS complex tachycardia.
- Narrow QRS tachycardia more than 230/min should raise the suspicion of SVT.
- Narrow QRS tachycardia in a critically ill, unstable seriously ill baby and broad complex tachycardia is treated with electrical cardioversion.
- For a seriously ill baby with SVT and stable hemodynamic status, adenosine is the drug of choice.
- Most important bradyarrhythmia in newborn is complete heart block occurring in the setting of maternal systemic lupus erythematosus. Treatment is conservative except when heart rate decreases to 55 beats/min. requiring pacemaker implantation.

FURTHER READING

1. Kothari DS, Skinner JR. Neonatal tachycardias: An update. *Arch Dis Child Fetal Neonatal Ed* 2006;91:F136–F144.
2. Long WA, Frantz EG, Henry GW, Freed MD, Brook M. Evaluation of newborns with possible cardiac problems. In: Taeusch HW, Ballard RA (eds): *Avery's Diseases of the Newborn*, 7th edn. Noida; Harcourt Asia 2000:711–763.
3. Stacy A, Killen S, Fish FA. Fetal and Neonatal Arrhythmias. *NeoReviews* 2008;9;e242–252.
4. Tanel RE, Rhodes LA. Fetal and neonatal arrhythmias. *Clin Perinatology* 2001;28:187–207.
5. Van Hare G F. Neonatal arrhythmias. In: Martin RJ, Fanoroff AA, Walsh MC (eds): *Fanaroff and Martin's Neonatal-Perinatal Medicine: Diseases of the Fetus and Infant,* 9th edn. New York: Elsevier 2010:1277–1289.
6. Walsh EP. Clinical approach to diagnosis and acute management of tachycardias in children. In: Walsh EP, Saul JP, Triedman JK (eds). *Cardiac Arrhythmias in Children and Young Adults with Congenital Heart Disease.* Philadelphia: Lippincott Williams and Williams 2001:103–104.

Chapter

24 Acute Renal Failure in the Newborn

Monica Dutta, Elizabeth Bell, Michael Davidson

ABSTRACT

Acute kidney injury, is defined as a serum creatinine > 1.5 mg/dL regardless of age or urine output with normal maternal renal function. It is a common problem, occurring in 25% of neonates needing intensive care for one or the other reason. It may be anuric, oliguric and nonoliguric. Around 85% cases are of prerenal type and only 15% intrarenal and postrenal types. Presence of risk factors renders a neonate more vulnerable to ARF. Treatment is dictated by the type of renal failure.

Key Words: Acute kidney injury, Acute renal failure, Risk factors, Serum creatinine.

INTRODUCTION

Acute kidney injury, earlier termed acute renal failure, is a common problem, occurring in 1/4th of neonates needing intensive care for one or the other reason. Around 85% cases are of prerenal type and only 15% intrarenal and postrenal types. Left untreated, mortality is very high. Even with appropriate treatment, a consideerrable morbidity and mortality is a rule.

CASE SCENARIO

A preterm baby (35 weeks), aged 3 days and weighing 1.4 kg failed to pass urine until 72 hours of birth. Then, the urine output started but in drops only. Mother was a known diabetic on therapy.

Investigations: *BUN 32 mg/dL, Serum creatinine 1.9 mg/dL.*

Urine osmolality 380 mOsmol/kg water

Urine sodium 68 mEq/L

Urine/plasma creatinine ratio 12

Fractional excretion of sodium 2.8%

Renal failure index (RFI) 3.3

Contd...

Contd...

A diagnostic fluid challenge with normal saline, 5 ml/kg IV bolus twice followed by furosemide, 1 mg/kg showed no response.

Impression: *Intrinsic renal failure.*

At this stage imaging studies showed no evidence of any anatomical lesion or malformation of the kidneys. Radionuclide scanning showed poor renal parenchymafunction. The overall impression was as "acute tubular necrosis".

Therapy: *Since response to conservative measures for intrinsic renal failure proved of not much help, he was subjected to peritoneal dialysis which proved life-saving.*

Subsequently, he was put on renal feeding formula with low renal solute and phosphorus.

CRITICAL CASE ANALYSIS

Though all healthy neonates pass urine by 48 hours, this neonate did not pass urine for 72 hours. The risk factors for acute renal failure in this neonate included prematurity, very low birthweight, and maternal diabetes. Investigations left no doubt about the diagnosis of "acute renal failure". Absence of any anatomical cause or lesion and poor renal parenchymal function, the moist likely diagnosis was "acute tubular necrosis". That it was "intrinsic" type was confirmed by the diagnostic fluid challenge. In the wake of poor response to conservative therapy, eventually he had to be placed on renal replacement therapy in the form of peritoneal dialysis which proved life-saving.

INTERACTIVE TOPIC DISCUSSION

How is ARF defined?

ARF is defined as a serum creatinine > 1.5 mg/dL regardless of age or urine output with normal maternal renal function.

Why is it replaced by the new semantic, "Acute kidney injury"?

Acute renal failure denotes a sever renal dysfunction. The new term carries under its umbrella even mild renal dysfunction.

What is anuric, oliguric and non-oliguric ARF?

Anuric ARF means absence of urinary output by 24–48 hours of age.

Oliguric ARF means urine output < 1 ml/kg.

Nonoliguric ARF means output > 1 ml/kg.

Is it possible to have ARF with normal urine output?

Yes, in asphyxiated infants.

What should be the normal urine output in healthy neonates?

1–3 ml/kg/h.

What is the pathophysiology of prerenal failure, the most common ARF?

Decreased renal blood flow/perfusion, regardless of the cause, is the fundamental factor causing poor renal function. Dehydration, hemorrhage, septic shock, CCF, PDA, and NEC are its common causes. However, even RDS, hypoxia, CHD, hypoalbuminemisa, perinatal asphyxia, ECMO/ECLS, hypotension, and drugs (indomethacin, ACE inhibitors, ibuprofen, phenylaphrine ophthalmic drops) can cause ARF.

Can maternal medication also cause it?

Indeed, it can. Such medication includes NSAIDs, ACE inhibitoirs and COX2 inhibitors.

Which structural kidney conditions can cause intrinsic renal failure?

Acute renal tubular necrosis is the most common. Others include congenital anomalies, vascular lesions, infections and exogenous toxins.

What about postrenal failure?

Any condition that causes obstruction of urinary outflow after the kidneys have produced it may cause postrrenal failure. The conditions include posterior urethral valve, urethral stricture, meatal stenosis, bilateral bladder-neck obstruction, neurogenic bladder, blocked urinary drainage catheter, megaureter and prune belly syndrome.

Are there any risk factors for ARF?

Definitely, presence of risk factors renders a neonate more vulnerable to ARF. These factors include:

- Dehydration
- Asphyxia
- Sepsis
- Nephrotoxic drugs
- Prematurity
- VLBW
- CHD undergoing pulmonary bypass
- ECMO/ECLS
- Maternal diabetes.

What is the usual clinical presentation?

The neonate may present with:

- Decreased (oliguria) or absent urine output (anuria).
- *Potter facies:* Suggest renal agenesis.
- *Abdominal mass:* May be distended bladdere, hydronephrosis, polycystic kidney, tumor.
- *Prune belly syndrome:* Hypoplastic abdominal wall muscles, cryptorchidism, dilated upper urinary tract.
- *Meningocele:* Neurogenic bladder.
- *Pulmonary hypoplasia:* Severe oligohydramnios in utero.
- *Urinary ascites:* Posterior urethral valve, severe upper urinary tract obstruction.

Whereas oliguria or anuriua are an essential feature of ARF others may or may not be present.

There may well be a history of maternal diabetes, oligohydramnios, and renal dysplasia or agenesis urinary, or tract disease in family members.

Any situation where ARF may occur without presence of oliguria or anuria?

Asphxiated neonates may have normal urine output in spite of ARF.

How to establish the diagnosis?

The first step in diagnosis is urtheral catheterization to measure volume of retained urine of monitor output. A 5 F or 8 F feeding tube is good enough for this purpose.

The laboratory tests are listed in Table 24.1.

Table 24.1: Laboratory investigations in ARF

Blood Indices		
BUN Blood urea nitrogen 15–20 indicates dehydration or renal insufficiency. *Creatinine* In healthy neonates serum creatinine varies from 0.5 to 1.0 mg/dL (highest at day 1 and lowest at day 7); in LBW neonates, up to 1.5 mg/dL. In ARF, higher the value, more is the loss of renal function. It is said that if serum creatinine doubles up, 50% of renal function is lost.		
Urinary Indices		
	Prerenal	**Intrinsic**
Urine osmolality (mOSmol/kg/water)	>400	<400
Urine sodium (mEq/L)	31 ± 19	63 ± 35
Urine plasma creatinine ratio	29 + 16	10 ± 4
Fractional excretion of sodium	<2.5	> 2.5
Renal failure index	< 3	> 3.5
Platelet count Thrombocytopenia is a feature of sepsis and renal vein thrombosis. **Serum potassium** In renal insufficiency, it has a tendency to increase. **Biomarkers** • Serum and urinary crystatic C level for calculating glomerular filtration rate. • Plasma and urinary neutrophil gelatinase-associate lipcalion (NGAL) levels. • Serum and urinary interleukin (IL)–187 levels. • Urinary albumin – t-creatinine ratio (ACR).		

What is diagnostic fluid challenge in diagnosis?

It consists in giving an IV bolus of 5–10 ml/kg of normal saline or colloid solution. If there is no response, repeat once. If still no response, give furosemide, 1 mg/kg IV. If no response and there is no evidence of obstruction above the level of bladder, intrinsic renal failure stands nearly confirmed.

Any precaution for this challenge?

The infant must not have CCF or clinical volume overload.

Can imaging studies be useful?

Abdominal X-ray may show spina bifida, absent sacrum (pointing to neurogenic bladder) displaced bowel loops (pointing to space-occupying mass).

Abdominal ultrasonography for identifying hydronephrosis, dilated ureters, abdominal masses, distended bladder, renal vein thrombosis.

Radionucleotide scanning is helpful in assessing function of renal parenchyma.

What are the components of general management?

1. Replacement of insensible fluid losses (50–70 ml/kg/day in preterm and 30 ml/kg/day in term) plus fluid output from urine and GIT.
2. Strict intake and output chart.
3. Frequent weighing.
4. Serum sodium and potassium monitoring with replacement of losses.
5. Protein restriction to < 2 gm/kg/day. Breast milk is fair enough to achieve this.
6. Administration of aluminium hyroxiode as a phosphate binder.
7. IV calcium replacement using calcium gluconate to safeguard from tetany.
8. Supplementation with chronic oral bicarbonate to combat mertabolic acidosis.

What are the major components of definitive treatment?

Treatment is dictated by the type of renal failure.

In prerenal failure, most critical therapy lies in providing volume to enhance and restore renal perfusion and to treat the cause of such a failure.

In postrenal failure, therapeutic thrust is in bypassing the cause (usually an obstruction) employing a bladder catheter or bu percutaneous nephrostomy drainage. The decision about the choice would depend on the level of obstruction.

In intrinsic renal disease, this first initiative should be discontinue nephrotoxic drug(s) or at least reduce the dose.

Furosemide, 1–2 mg/kg/dose, assists in increasing urine output and fluid management.

Low dose dopamine may be of value in enhancing renal perfusion.

It is advisable to monitor for hypertension, hyponatremia, hyperkalemia, hyperphosphatemia, hypocalcemia, and metsabolic acidosis.

Renal feeding formula, providing low renal solute and phosphorus, may be given.

What about the renal replacement therapy?

Undoubtedly renal replsacement therapy in the form of hemodialysis, peritoneal dialysis or hemofiltration is indicated when conservative measaure prove ineffective.

Finally, won't it be crucial to surgically remove the obstruction?

Of course, surgical intervention has got to be carried out to relieve obstruction as soon as feasible.

What are the factors that contribute to mortality?

- Hemodynamic instability
- Multiorgan failure
- Hypotension and shock
- Mechanical ventilation requirement
- Dialysis
- Vasopressor use.

CONCLUSIONS

A large majority of the cases of neonatal kidney injury, defined as serum creatinine > 1.5 mg/dL, are of prerenal type. Hemodynamic instability, multiorgan failure, hypotension and shock, mechanical ventilation requirement, dialysis and vasopressor use, etc. add up to morbidity and mortality. Early recognition and appropriarte treatment are mandatory for good outcome. In prerenal failure, most critical therapy lies in providing volume to enhance and restore renal perfusion and to treat the cause of such a failure. In postrenal failure, therapeutic thrust is in bypassing the cause (usually an obstruction) employing a bladder catheter or by percutaneous nephrostomy drainage. In intrinsic renal disease, this first initiative should be to discontinue nephrotoxic drug(s) or at least reduce the dose.

TAKE HOME MESSAGES

- Acute kidney injury occurs in 25% of neonates in NICU for one or the other reason.
- It is defined as a serum creatinine > 1.5 mg/dL regardless of age or urine output with normal maternal renal function.
- It may be **anuric, oliguric and nonoliguric ARF.**
- A vast majoirity of cases are of prerenal type, remaining of intrarenal and postrenal types.
- Presence of risk factors renders a neonate more vulnerable to ARF.
- Treatment is dictated by the type of renal failure.
- Factors contributing to morbidity and mortality include hemodynamic instability, multiorgan failure, hypotension and shock, mechanical ventilation requirement, dialysis and vasopressor use.

FURTHER READING

1. Askenazi DJ, Ambalavanan N, Goldstein SL. Acute kidney injury in critically ill newborns: What do we know? What do we need to learn? *Pediatric Nephrol* 2009;24:265–274.
2. Gomella TL, Cunningham MD, Eyal FG. *Neonatology,* 7th edn. New Delhi: McGraw Hill 2013.
3. Koralkar R, Ambalavanan N, Levitan EB, *et al*. Acute kidney injury reduces survival in very low birth weight infants. *Pediatr Res* 2011;69:354–358.
4. Sharma H, Kulkarni A. Neonatal acute kidney injury. In: Gupte S, Gupte SB, Gupte M (eds): *Recent Advances in Pediatrics (Special Vol 25: Perspectives in Neonatology)*. New Delhi: Jaypee 2014:257–271.

Chapter

25 Bleeding Neonates

Rajib Chatterjee

ABSTRACT

Disorders of coagulation present with increasing frequency in NICUs due to physiologically decreased levels of most procoagulant and anticoagulant proteins. Maternal medication and state of health also affects the normal hemostatic mechanisms adversely. Inherited and acquired disorders of coagulation present in the neonatal period often with life-threatening bleeding. Nearly all significant bleeding disorders in neonates can be identified using simple screening tests. Timely recognition with proper approach to diagnosis and management can prevent avoidable morbidity and mortality.

Key Words: Bleeding, Coagulation tests, Hemostasis, Hemostatic system, Intracranial hemorrhage, Vitamin K.

INTRODUCTION

Disorders of coagulation with or without obvious bleeding are relatively common in the neonatal period. Coagulation proteins are synthesized by the fetus from the 5th week of gestation onwards. Levels gradually rise during fetal life but do not reach adult values until several months after birth, even in term babies. Thus "normal values" in neonates vary not only with gestational age but also postnatal age. Coagulation proteins do not cross the placenta, or do so only in very small amounts, and therefore, need to be synthesized by the fetus. However fetal coagulation factor synthesis can be affected by maternal medication and state of health. Blood platelet counts at birth in term and preterm neonates are within the normal adult range. Though in vitro studies show impaired function of neonatal platelets in term and preterms, bleeding problems associated with abnormal platelet function are rare in neonates. Thus, the hemostatic system can be easily overwhelmed.

Defects in the coagulation proteins (vitamin K dependent factors) in platelet numbers or function or in the fibrinolytic pathway are associated with an increased risk of bleeding. In contrast, defects in the naturally occurring anticoagulants (protein C) or in the vessel wall (damage from vascular catheters) are associated with thrombosis. However in many cases, both pro and anticoagulant abnormalities occur simultaneously (DIC).

Reports suggest intracranial hemorrhage (ICH) after spontaneous vaginal delivery at a rate of 1 per 1900, whereas rate of ICH in vacuum-assisted deliveries is 1 per 860. In addition 15–30% patients with inherited bleeding disorders present in the neonatal period.

CASE SCENARIO

A female neonate weighing 3000 gm delivered to a primigravida mother by forceps application presenting for admission to SCNU at 28 hours age with significant swelling on head.

A thorough history supplemented with referral notes from obstetrician mentions prolonged second stage of labor followed by difficult forceps application for extraction of fetal head in delivering the baby who had cried soon after birth. Since, the swelling on the head was larger on 2nd DOL referring doctor thought it prudent to send the baby to our institute.

Maternal history revealed regular ANC, uneventful pregnancy, no history of medications (phenobarb, phenytoin), no history suggestive of TORCH, and no history of PROM. Referral note failed to mention any medication given to baby, however, conveyed baby was breast-fed.

Examination: *Baby appeared well, sleeping comfortably, having breast-fed recently passed urine and meconium. Vitals stable. Swelling on right parietal region of the head measuring 10 cm in length, tense, slightly fluctuant, non-tender, non-pulsatile, non-transilluminant (Fig. 25.1) with unremarkable examination of neck, spine and back. Clinical jaundice visible over face with pink palms and soles Kramer zone I. Per-abdomen examination revealed liver 2 cm and spleen 1 cm palpable.*

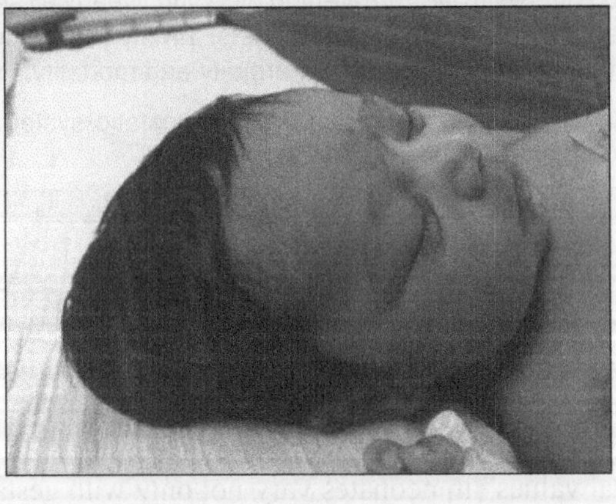

Fig. 25.1: Extensive right parietal cephalohematoma in neonate (birth trauma due to forceps delivery)

Investigations: *All relevant test were normal, except:*

- *PT and APTT: prolonged.*
- *Serum bilirubin 17 mg/dL (day 5).*
- *CT scan on day 8: Linear non-depressed fracture.*

Impression: *Clinical Impression: FT/AGA female Vertex presentation with Forceps delivery with Cephalohematoma. Possibility of underlying HDN (hemorrhagic disease of the newborn) since referral note fails to mention Vitamin K administration.*

Contd...

Contd...

Treatment and Hospital Course: Prolonged PT and APTT suggest the diagnosis of HDN due to Vitamin K deficiency. Inj Vitamin K was administered 2 mg IV immediately. FFP 10 ml/kg was infused slowly over 2 hours.

Exaggerated physiological jaundice was treated with phototherapy and PRBC.

CT scan on Day 8 revealed Linear non-depressed fracture. Serial Neurosonography was normal.

On Day 10 examination revealed vitals stable, alert, active, feeding, reflexes normal. Baby discharged on exclusive breast feeding with an advise for follow-up on day 14 to evaluate clinical activity, change in size of cephalohematoma, etc.

Follow-up at 3 months was advised to detect any dislocation of lens of eye.

CRITICAL CASE ANALYSIS

There was no difficulty in diagnosing right-sided parietal cephalhematoma in this otherwise normal looking baby with the backdrop of application of forceps during delivery. Other differentials, i.e., caput succedaneum and subgaleal hemorrhage were unlikely (Figs. 25.2 and 25.3). The issue needing sorting was whether cephalhematoma was a consequence of just the birth trauma or a part of a bleeding disorder. Since information about administration of vitamin K was not forthcoming, the possible contribution of vitamin K deficiency (hemorrhagic disease of the newborn) was considered. All relevant investigations turned to be normal, except PT and APTT which were prolonged, again suggesting diagnosis of HDN. He was, therefore, given vitamin K, 2 mg IV. FFP 10 ml/kg was infused slowly over 2 hours. For rising serum bilirubin (17 mg/dL on 5th day), diagnosed as exaggerated physiological jaundice, phototherapy and PRBC were given with good outcome.

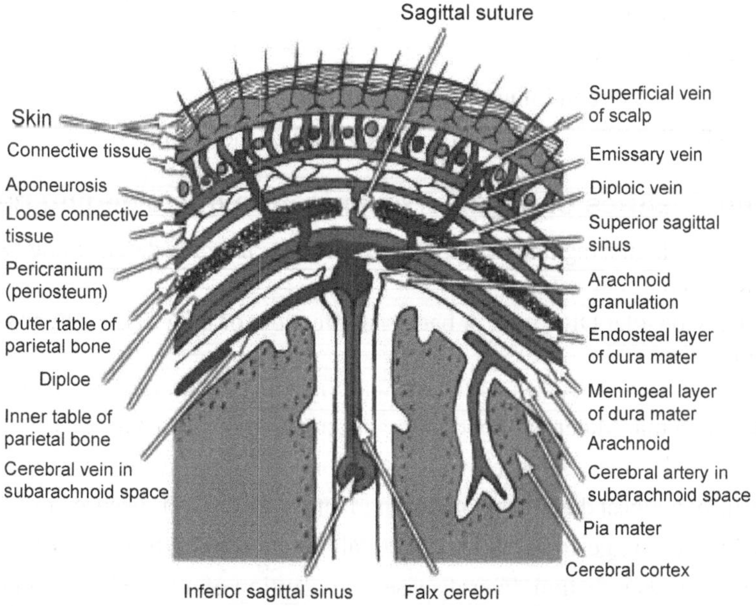

Fig. 25.2: Layers of the scalp and cranium

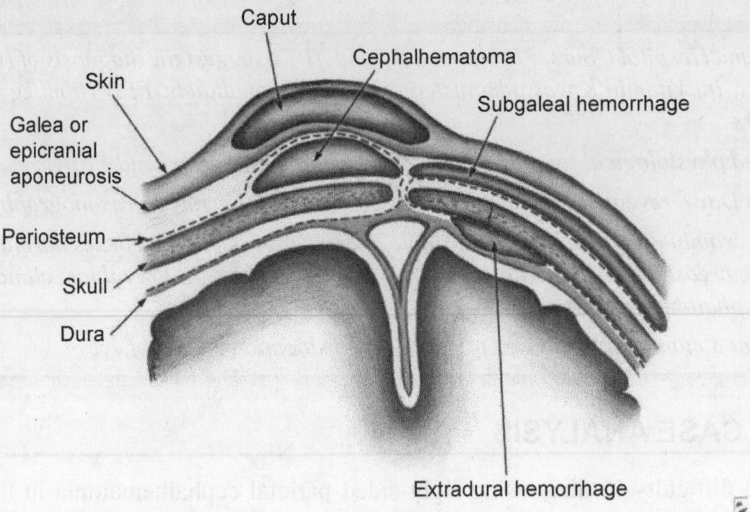

Fig. 25.3: Location of caput, cephalohematoma and subgaleal hemorrhage

INTERACTIVE TOPIC DISCUSSION

What is the approach to diagnosis of bleeding in neonates in terms of history?

The following points should particularly be borne in mind:

- Family history of excessive bleeding or clotting.
- Maternal medications (aspirin, phenytoin).
- Pregnancy and birth history.
- Maternal history of birth of an infant with a bleeding disorder.
- Any illness, medication, anomalies or procedures done to the infant.

What are salient features of physical examination in a bleeding neonate?

The crucial decision in diagnosing and managing the bleeding neonate determining whether the baby is sick or well (Table 25.1):

(i) *Sick infant:* Consider DIC, viral or bacterial infection, or liver disease hypoxic/ischemic injury may lead to DIC.

(ii) *Well infant:* Consider vitamin K deficiency, isolated clotting factor deficiency, or immune thrombocytopenia. Maternal blood in the infant's GIT will not cause symptoms in the infant.

(iii) Petechiae, small superficial ecchymosis, or mucosal bleeding suggests a platelet problem.

(iv) Large bruises suggest deficiency of clotting factors, DIC, liver disease or vitamin K deficiency.

(v) Enlarged spleen suggests possible congenital infection or erythroblastosis.

(vi) Jaundice suggests infection, liver disease or resorption of a large hematoma.

(vii) Abnormal retinal findings suggest infection.

Table 25.1: Differential diagnosis of bleeding in the neonate

Clinical evaluation	Laboratory studies			Likely diagnosis
	Platelets	PT	PTT	
"Sick"	D-	I+	I+	DIC
	D-	N	N	Platelet consumption (infection, necrotizing enterocolitis, renal vein thrombosis)
	N	I+	I+	Liver disease
	N	N	N	Compromised vascular integrity (associated with hypoxia, prematurity, acidosis, hyperosmolality)
"Healthy"	D-	N	N	Immune thrombocytopenia, occult infection, thrombosis, bone-marrow hypoplasia (rare), or bone marrow infiltrative disease
	N	I+	I+	Hemorrhagic disease of newborn (vitamin K deficiency)
	N	N	I+	Hereditary clotting factor deficiency
	N	N	N	Bleeding due to local factors (trauma, anatomic abnormalities); qualitative platelet abnormalities (rare); Factor XIII deficiency (rare)

PT = prothrombin time; PTT = partial thromboplastin time; D- = decreased; I+ = increased; DIC = disseminated intravascular coagulation; N = normal.

Name Various Laboratory Tests

1. Apt test
2. Peripheral blood smear
3. Platelet count
4. Prothrombin time (PT)
5. APTT
6. Fibrinogen
7. D-Dimer assays
8. Specific Factor Assay
9. *Bleeding times:* Abandoned.
10. *Platelet function:* PFA 100 may be useful as a screening test for vWD or platelet dysfunction in some settings, but confirmatory specific assays are required for positive tests.

What is the clinical presentation of hemophilia A in neonates?

Boys (5%) with hemophilia born in countries with a good standard of health care suffer from intracranial hemorrhage in the neonatal period, probably due to a slow expansion of a small subdural hemorrhage associated with delivery. Less common sites are subgaleal collections, post-circumcision, bleeding from venous or arterial puncture sites, and prolonged bleeding from umbilical cord. Hemorrhage into major organs such as liver, spleen or lungs are much less common and hemarthroses are rare.

How hemophilia A diagnosed?

Blood sample (either cord blood or peripheral blood) shows a prolonged or a very prolonged APTT with a normal PT, TT, platelets and fibrinogen. The diagnosis is then established by measurement of factor VIII clotting activity, which is always reduced in hemophilia (all other coagulation factors including von Willebrand anigen are normal). Clinically, the severity of the disease is classified according to the level of factor VIII activity: levels of < 2% (i.e., <0.02 IU/ml) are classified as severe disease, 2–10% (0.02–0.1 IU/ml) as moderate and >10% (>0.1 IU/ml) as mild. Family history would prompt prenatal diagnosis by mutational analysis of the factor VIII gene on a chorionic villus biopsy in the first trimester.

How should a neonate with hemophilia A be managed?

Acute management of the bleeding neonate with hemophilia requires intravenous administration of recombinant factor VIII. If absolutely necessary, FFP or cryoprecipitate (15–20 ml/kg) may be used for major hemorrhage if there is significant delay. The usual treatment dose of factor VIII in neonates is 50–100 units/kg intravenously twice a day. Since the half life of factor VIII is shorter in children than in adults, more frequent dosing or a continuous factor VIII infusion may be required. The dose should be adjusted by monitoring plasma factor VIII activity to achieve factor VIII levels of 100% (1.0 IU/ml). Treatment is continued for 2 weeks in case of ICH.

Venepuncture should be performed with great care while arterial avoided. Lumbar puncture only if essential with factor VIII cover. Fibrin glue is useful in circumcision associated bleeds.

Once the baby is ready for discharge parents should be provided guidance and counseling for future life through hemophiliac centers.

What are the current guidelines for prenatal management and delivery of prenatally diagnosed hemophilia A?

Significant hemorrhage can occur whatever be the mode of delivery. Vaginal delivery can be safe if no difficulties are anticipated, however, vaccum extraction should be avoided because of risk of subgaleal hematoma and cephalohematomas. Cord blood should be taken for a coagulation screen and factor VIII level to confirm the diagnosis. Oral vitamin K should be given at birth because the IM route should be avoided due to risk of hematoma formation. Role of prophylactic factor VIII administration following difficult delivery to reduce risk of ICH with significant sequelae undoubtedly beneficial is of concern only due to risk of inhibitor formation leading to problems in later life. Routine NSG for all newborns known or suspected to have haemophilia is recommended though may miss peritentorial bleeds which MRI can pick up, advised as indicated.

How can one distinguish hemophilia A from B?

Clinically indistinguishable and both cause prolonged APTT, so only option is demonstrating a low factor IX level. Factor IX is low in Vitamin K deficiency and liver disease but accompanied by deficiency of other Vitamin K dependent factors. It is recommended to check factor IX levels at 6 weeks and 6 months age.

How should a neonate with hemophilia B be managed?

As in case of factor VIII deficiency. Treatment of bleeding is with recombinant factor IX concentrate. The usual dose is 100 units/kg intravenously once daily, and treatment should be monitored to achieve a factor IX level of 80–100 % (1.0 IU/ml). As for hemophilia A, treatment for ICH should continue for at least 2 weeks.

What is the presentation and management of von Willebrand (vWD) disease in neonates?

The vWD disease is caused by quantitative or qualitative defects in vWF. It is the commonest inherited bleeding disorder, affecting around 1% of the population. There are several types of vWD, each of which has different clinical and genetic characteristics, but only two forms of the disease present in the neonatal period.

Type 2b vWD is autosomal dominant and presents with thrombocytopenia usually without bleeding.

Type 3 vWD is the most severe form of the disease, autosomal recessive and presents similar to hemophilia, as levels of both vWF and factor VIII are low. The diagnosis is made by measuring both factor VIII and vWF followed by determining the pattern of vWF multimers. Clinical clues are the presence of hemophiliac pattern of bleeding in girls or families without X-linked inheritance and a poor response to factor VIII concentrates. Type 3 vWD is currently treated with intermediate purity factor VIII (Hemate P).

What is the presentation and management of Factor XIII deficiency in neonates?

Rare autosomal recessive disorder in which routine diagnostic coagulation screen is normal. It usually presents clinically with delayed bleeding from the umbilical cord during the first 3 weeks of life. Intracranial haemorrhage has been reported in up to 30% of neonates with homozygous factor XIII deficiency. The diagnosis is made by measuring clot solubility in 5M urea solution as screening test followed by a specific factor XIII assay; molecular tests for the common mutations are also available. The treatment of bleeding associated with factor XIII deficiency is factor XIII concentrate; cryoprecipitate (10 ml/kg) can be used prior to establishment of the diagnosis or where the specific concentrate is unavailable. Infants with homozygous factor XIII deficiency have a lifelong risk of ICH, hence current guidelines recommend monthly factor XIII to reduce this risk.

What are the other inherited coagulation factor deficiencies?

A number of rare coagulation deficiencies may present in neonates with bleeding or unexplained prolongation of coagulation tests. The majority is autosomal and so a history of parental consanguinity is relatively common. Factor VII deficiency can produce a very severe bleeding disorder with a high incidence of ICH. In some cases factor VII has been shown to cross the placenta and in this way delay hemorrhage in severe factor VII deficiency until after birth. Recombinant factor VIIa is now available to treat this disorder but must be given at frequent intervals as it has a very short half life. Factor XI deficiency is most frequent in Askenazi Jews and presents in a similar way to hemophilia. There are a number of rare congenital fibrinogen disorders including dysfibrinogenemias and hypo/afibrinogenemia.

They may present with umbilical stump bleeding but other sites of bleeding are extremely unusual in neonates. One of the commonest inherited causes of an isolated prolonged APTT in a healthy baby with no signs of bleeding is factor XII deficiency; despite what is often a markedly prolonged APTT, affected individuals have no clinically apparent bleeding disorder throughout life.

What is vitamin K dependent/deficiency bleeding (VKDB)?

Levels of active forms of the vitamin K dependent procoagulant factors (factors II, VII, IX and X) and of the natural anticoagulants protein C and protein S are physiologically low at birth. There are many reasons for this Vitamin K is essential for gamma carboxylation of these proteins, which converts them to their active form: placental transfer of vitamin K is insufficient to build up adequate stores in the neonate; breast milk has low vitamin K content and bacterial vitamin K synthesis is lacking in the sterile neonatal gut. In neonates, vitamin K deficiency can lead to hemorrhagic disease of the newborn (HDN) now more commonly referred to as vitamin K deficiency bleeding (VKDB) and classified as early, classical and late according to age of presentation.

Define three types of VKDB based on age of onset.

Early VKDB: Presents within 24 hours age, with severe hemorrhage, including ICH and GIT bleed. It is caused by severe in utero deficiency of vitamin K usually due to maternal medication (oral anticoagulants, anticonvulsants and antituberculous therapy) that interferes with vitamin K.

Classical VKDB: Presents after 24 hours till 168 hours (7 days) of life in babies who have not received prophylactic vitamin K at birth. Risk is increase in breastfed babies and those with poor oral intake. It can be prevented by a single IM of 1mg at birth.

Late VKDB: Presents between week 2 to 8 after birth; sometime up to 6 months of life. Characteristic presentation is of sudden ICH in an otherwise well breastfed term baby or in babies with liver disease (biliary atresia) or malabsorptive states. Late VKDB in healthy breastfed babies can be prevented by a single IM dose of vitamin K during this age period while the others need weekly supplementation for prolonged periods.

In all forms of VKDB, clotting studies show a prolonged PT with normal platelets and fibrinogen. In severe deficiency the APTT may also be prolonged. In view of a typical history further diagnostic tests are unnecessary and the correction of PT following administration of vitamin K confirms the diagnosis. If doubt remains, factor assay of vitamin K dependent factors and of the inactive form of factor II (decarboxyprothrombin: PIVKA II) can be used to confirm diagnosis.

How should different VKDBs be managed?

Treatment of VKDB depends on the severity of the bleeding. In mild cases, vitamin K (1 mg) which should be given IV or SC (not intramuscularly because of the risk of hematoma), should suffice as this increases the levels of active vitamin K dependent coagulation factors within a few hours. In severe bleed, vitamin K dose varies from 2–5 mg IV. Additionally, FFP may be given.

What is the pathophysiology of disseminated intravascular coagulation (DIC) in the newborn?

The pathophysiology of DIC is complex and not fully understood (Fig. 25.4). The main precipitants of DIC in neonates are associated with severe hypoxia, and/or acidosis and include peripartum hemorrhage, severe birth asphyxia, meconium aspiration and sepsis. The process seems to be triggered by release of TF and cytokines from damaged endothelium and/or monocytes, which results in widespread activation of the coagulation cascade with subsequent consumption of clotting factors and a combination of thrombotic and hemorrhagic manifestations.

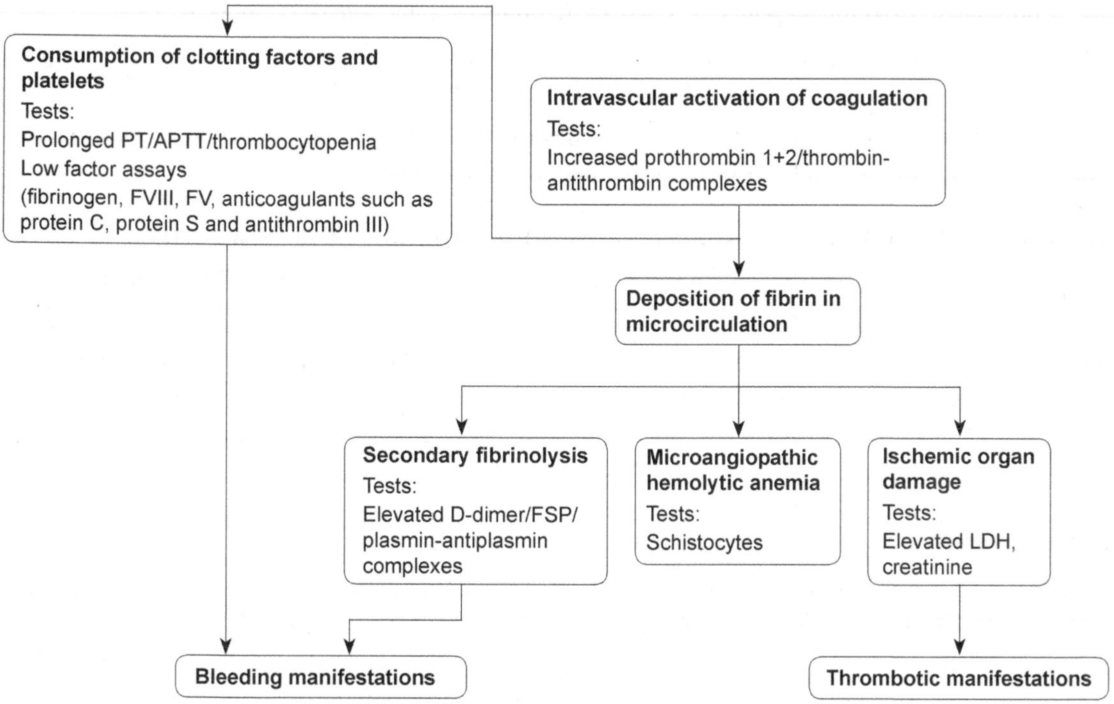

Fig. 25.4: Pathophysiology of DIC

What is the presentation of DIC?

Clinically, DIC is seen in sick neonates and presents with generalized bleeding, including pulmonary hemorrhage and oozing from venepuncture sites. The usual pattern of coagulation abnormalities in DIC is prolongation of the PT, APTT and TT together with low platelets and fibrinogen.

What are the important steps in management of DIC?

The most important aspect of management of DIC is treatment of the underlying cause. Blood product replacement is indicated for the treatment of clinical bleeding. FFP is a good source of procoagulant proteins as well as protein C, protein S and antithrombin; cryoprecipitate contains higher concentration of factor VIII and fibrinogen and is useful when fibrinogen levels are low. Aim of management should be to maintain platelet count above $30 \times 10^9/l$ and the fibrinogen >1gm/l. Recombinant actor VIIa is used in a dose of 100 μg/kg when bleeding is unresponsive to above.

What are the other acquired coagulation disorders?

Other causes of acquired coagulopathy in neonates include liver disease, metabolic disorders (hyperammonemia), ECMO, consumptive coagulopathy with thrombocytopenia secondary to giant hemangioendothelioma (Kasabach-Merritt syndrome).

What is neonatal thrombocytopenia?

Thrombocytopenia (platelet count $<150 \times 10^9/l$) is common in neonates is common in preterms whereas *severe thrombocytopenia* (platelet count $<50 \times 10^9/l$) is common in sick neonates.

It presents in two *clinical patterns*: *Early* (< 72 hours age) and *late* (>72 hours age).

Early thrombocytopenia caused by reduced megakaryocytosis usually mild, self limiting and resolves within 10 days. Early severe thrombocytopenia is due to NAIT.

Late thrombocytopenia is due to increased destruction and reduced production of platelets more often severe, due to sepsis and NEC, requiring platelet transfusion.

What are the common causes of thrombocytopenia in the newborn?

Common *causes* of *early thrombocytopenia* (within 72 hours age) are: placental insufficiency (pre-eclamptic toxemia, IUGR, DM), NAITP, birth asphyxia, perinatal infection (GBS, E.coli, and L. monocytogenes), congenital infection (CMV, toxoplasmosis, rubella, coxsackie virus), maternal auto-immune (ITP, SLE), severe Rh HDN, thrombosis (renal vein, aortic), aneuploidy (trisomies: 21, 18, 13).

Common *causes* of *late thrombocytopenia* (beyond 72 hours age) are: LO Sepsis, NEC, congenital infection, maternal autoimmune, Inherited congenital (TAR, Wiskott-Aldrich).

What is neonatal alloimmune thrombocytopenia?

This is the platelet equivalent of HDN and alloimmune neutropenia. NAITP affects 1:1000 pregnancies, is frequently severe and occurs in the first pregnancy in almost 50% of cases. Thrombocytopenia may present in the first few days of life or prenatally (20 weeks) referred to as FAIT. The thrombocytopenia results from transplacental passage of maternal platelet specific antibodies to human platelet antigens (HPAs), which the mother lacks but which the fetus inherits from the father. In 80% of case these are anti-HPA-1a antibodies and in 10–15% anti–HPA-5b. Main clinical problem is ICH with long-term neurodevelopmental sequelae in survivors. Affected neonates may present with seizures, petechiae or incidental but severe thrombocytopenia. Diagnosis is by demonstrating platelet antigen incompatibility between mother and baby either serologically or by PCR. Affected infants should be transfused with HPA compatible platelets. In an emergency, random donor platelets can be used till compatible become available. If there is ongoing severe thrombocytopenia and/or hemorrhage despite HPA compatible platelet transfusions, IV IgG (total dose 2 gm/kg) over 2–5 days is often useful in ameliorating thrombocytopenia until spontaneous recovery occurs 1–6 weeks after birth.

What is neonatal autoimmune thrombocytopenia?

This is secondary to transplacental passage of maternal autoantibodies in maternal idiopathic thrombocytopenic purpura and less often, systemic lupus erythematosus, which affects 1–5/10,000 pregnancies. Affected infants usually develop mild thrombocytopenia, rarely severe which has risk of ICH and hence treated with IV IgG.

Platelet transfusions are given in dose of 10–20 ml/kg since higher doses are neither effective nor safer.

What should be the algorithmic approach to a bleeding neonate?

Figure 25.5 presents an algorithmic stepwise approach to bleeding neonates.

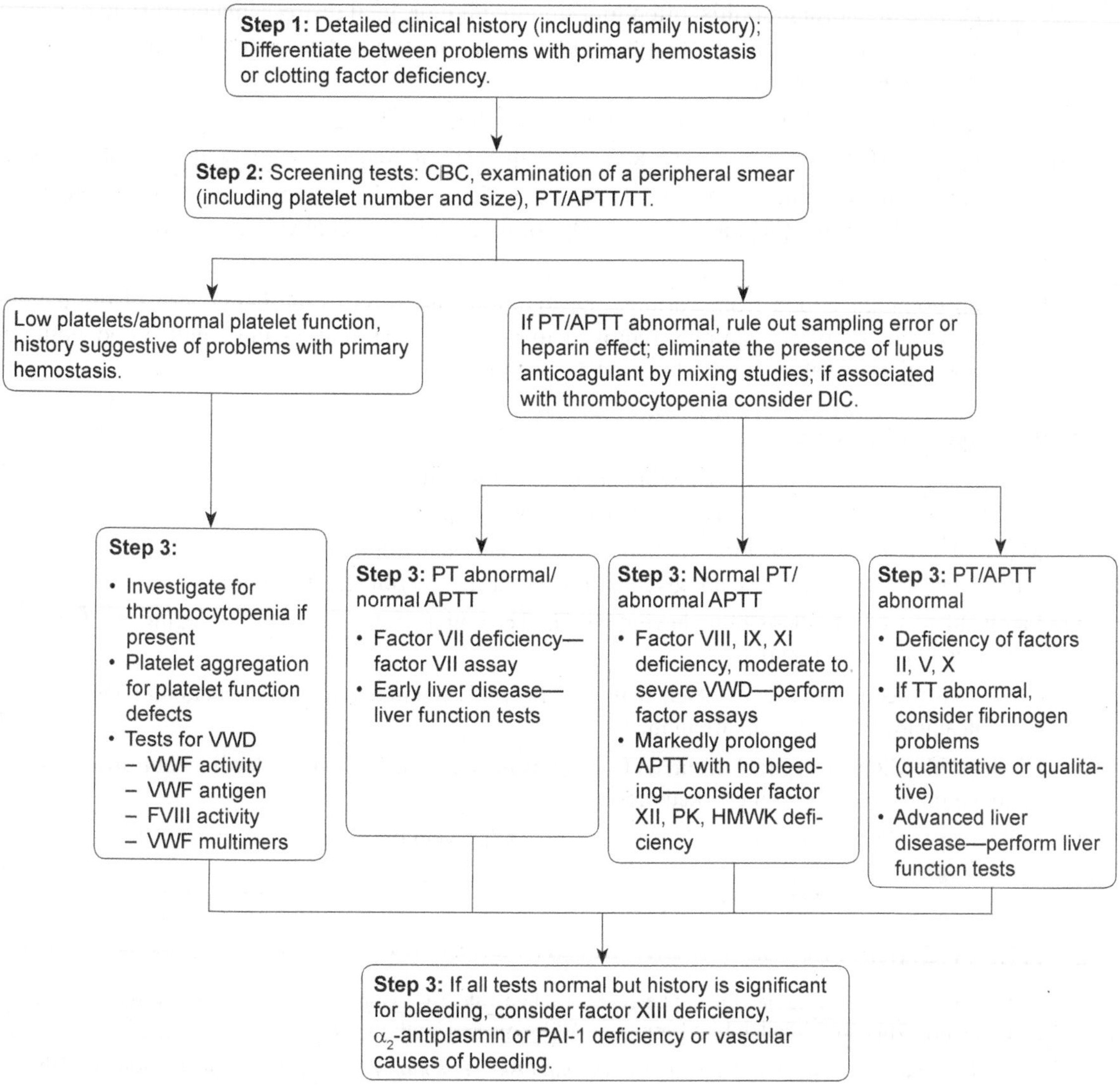

Fig. 25.5: Algorithmic approach to a bleeding neonate

CONCLUSIONS

It is common to encounter disorders of coagulation present the NICU due to physiologically decreased levels of most procoagulant and anticoagulant proteins, the most common disorder being the hemorrhagic disease of the newborn (HDN), now renamed vitamin K-dependent bleeding (VKDB).

Clinical evaluation of a bleeding neonate includes:

(a) Maternal history with particular reference to mode of delivery including instrumentation (e.g., vacuum, forceps) risks for sepsis, e.g., PROM, triad of fever, tachycardia and uterine tenderness suggestive of choriamnionitis, often foul smelling liquor, fetal distress, maternal state of health requiring medication (phenytoin, phenobarbital) autoimmune disease, need of maternal blood counts and urine reports.

(b) Family history of bleeding disorder or previous affected sibling.

(c) Neonatal evaluation: First step is the look of the neonate whether well or ill. Then in terms of gestation, birthweight, sex, postnatal age and evidence of birth trauma, e.g., bruises, petechiae, abnormal abdominal (hepatosplenomegaly) or flank masses (renal vein thrombosis) suggestive of DIC.

(d) When obtaining blood from various investigations attention to the hematocrit of the patient and volumes of blood samples removed to avoid exsanguinating the small blood volume. Interpretation of values with references to gestation.

TAKE HOME MESSAGES

- Disorders of coagulation present with increasing frequency in NICUs due to physiologically decreased levels of most procoagulant and anticoagulant proteins.
- Maternal history of medication (anticonvulsants, antituberculosis) OR the neonatal history of missed medication (vitamin K not given at birth) bearing on etiological diagnosis.
- Family history of previous sibling having inherited coagulation disorder OR the lacking of a family history can be a new mutation.
- Concealed bleeding may reveal itself with seizures (ICH), jaundice (cephalohematoma) and shock (subgalealhematoma). Not all are innocuous.
- Obvious bleeding in aspirate from GIT of neonate may not be a real bleeding but swallowed maternal blood at birth from cracked nipple.
- Follow up of bleeding neonate for ICH is important to prevent or minimize catastrophic long-lasting neurodevelopmental sequelae.

FURTHER READING

1. Abdulhayoglu E. Birth trauma. In: Cloherty JP, Eichenwald EC, Hansen AR, Stark AR (eds): *Manual of Neonatal Care,* 7th edn. Philadelphia: Lippincott Williams and Wilkins 2012:63–73.
2. Orkin SH, Nathan DG, Ginsburg D, *et al. Nathan and Oski's Haematology of Infancy and Childhood,* 7th edn. Philadelphia: Saunders 2009.
3. Singh M. *Care of the Newborn*, 8th edn. New Delhi: Sagar 2015.
4. Stoll BJ, Kliegman RM: Nervous system disorders. In: Kligman RM, Stanton BF, St Geme III JW, Schor NF (eds): *Nelson Textbook of Pediatrics,* 20th edn. London: Elsevier, 2016.

Chapter

26 Hemorrhagic Disease of the Newborn

Bashir A Charoo, Asif Ahmed

ABSTRACT

A newborn baby may have bleeding due to vitamin K deficiency, which results in a decreased level of vitamin K dependent coagulation factors II, VII, IX and X. This disorder may present within 24 hours after birth or there may be a delayed presentation. The condition is easily preventable by administering vitamin K to all neonates. However, late hemorrhagic disease of newborn may lead to serious intracranial hemorrhages with resultant complications, including diabetes insipidus. HDN is easily preventable by administering vitamin K to all neonates immediately after birth.

Key Words: Diabetes insipidus, Hemorrhagic disease of the newborn (HDN), Intracranial hemorrhage, Late hemorrhagic disease of the newborn, Vitamin K, Vitamin K dependent bleed.

INTRODUCTION

Hemorrhagic disease of the newborn, now redesignated "vitamin K deficiency bleeding", is bleeding secondary to inadequate activities of vitamin K dependent coagulation factors (Factor II, VII, IX, X) that is correctable by vitamin K replacement. It is classified as early (onset < first 24 hours), classical (onset first 24 hours – 7 days) and late (after 7 days). Most cases of late HDN are seen up to 12 weeks of age. Recently, upper age limit has been extended to 6 months. HDN is easily preventable by administering vitamin K to all neonates right at birth.

CASE SCENARIO

A 26-day-old male neonate, born premature at 36 weeks of gestation with a weight of 2.7 kg, in at home (the delivery had been conducted by a trained birth attendant), presented with history of refusal of feeds for last one day.

On examination, the child had frank bleed from nose and rectum, signs of severe dehydration, though there was no history of gastroenteritis or recurrent vomiting.

He was seen to have a urine output of 9 ml/kg/h. Within 12 hours, the child developed seizures.

Contd...

Contd...

The initial investigations showed a normal hemogram, kidney function tests, serum potassium and blood sugar. Initial serum sodium of 161 mEq/dl and a deranged coagulogram (PT 24 sec against control of 12 sec. aPTT of 49 sec against a control of 24 sec).

Neuroimaging showed right basal ganglia venous infarction with hemorrhagic transformation with evidence of intraventricular extension of the hemorrhage.

Serum osmolality was increased and urinary osmolality was decreased in the patient.

A diagnosis of hemorrhagic disease of newborn (HDN) with intracranial bleeding with diabetes insipidus was made and the child was treated with vitamin K and his fluid and electrolyte status was taken care of. He was given anticonvulsants for the seizures.

CRITICAL CASE ANALYSIS

There was no difficulty in clinically reaching the diagnosis of late hemorrhagic disease of the newborn in view of the clinical manifestations of bleeding from different sites in this premature neonate. What was of added interest was the manifestations and investigations consistent with diagnosis of diabetes insipidus due to intracranial bleeding which is known to occur but is rare as a complication of HDN.

INTERACTIVE CASE DISCUSSION

What is hemorrhagic disease of newborn?

It is a bleeding disorder occurring in neonates due to deficiency of vitamin K. It occurs in 1 out of every 200–400 neonates who do not receive vitamin K prophylaxis. Vitamin K is required for carboxylation of various proteins in body since it is an essential co-factor for γ-glutamyl carboxylase enzymatic activity that catalyses the γ-carboxylation. Coagulation factors II, VII, IX and X are also dependant on this vitamin K mediated carboxylation for their activity. A deficiency of vitamin K in neonates leads to deficient levels of fully functional coagulation factors II, VII, IX and X and manifests as bleeding.

What are the various types of HDN based on presentation?

The HDN may be early, classic or late.

Early HDN: This usually presents within first 24 hours of life. It may be seen in infants born to mothers taking anticonvulsants or antitubercular drugs. These babies can have serious intracranial, intrathoracic and intra-abdominal bleeds. These can be prevented by administering vitamin K to mothers during last 2 to 4 weeks of pregnancy.

Classic HDN: This usually presents from day 2nd to day 7th of life. It typically occurs in neonates who do not receive vitamin K prophylactically after birth. The bleeding commonly occurs in the gastrointestinal tract, umbilicus, skin, nose, surgical sites (i.e., circumcision), and, rarely, in the brain. Sometimes the classic HDN may even present later in the first month of life. The condition can be easily treated with vitamin K.

Late HDN: It usually presents from second to 12th week of life, but may sometimes be seen even as late as 6th month of life. It usually occurs in exclusively breastfed babies, since breast milk is deficient in vitamin K. These children usually have underlying cholestatic diseases like biliary atresia or other conditions like abetalipoproteinemia. Intracranial hemorrhage is the most common manifestation of late HDN, but gastrointestinal, cutaneous, mucosal, epistaxis and injection site bleeds are also seen.

What is the pathophysiology of vitamin K deficiency in neonates?

There is very limited transplacental transfer of vitamin K during pregnancy. The vitamin K stores in neonatal liver are very low. The levels of vitamin K in breast milk are also very low (1–4 μg/l against a recommended dietary intake of 1 μg/kg/day. In a breastfed baby, the gut is initially colonized by Lactobacillus, which does not produe vitamin K unlike Bacteroides species which colonize in the gut later. All these factors lead to a deficiency of vitamin K in the neonates who are breastfeeding.

What is the differential diagnoses for HDN?

Von Willebrand disease: These patients do not respond to vitamin K and usually present later.

Disseminated intravascular coagulopathy: These patients are very sick and also have thrombocytopenia.

Hereditary clotting factor deficiencies: These patients do not respond to vitamin K. They usually present later.

What investigations are required for diagnosing HDN?

An initial work up consists of prothrombin time (PT), activated partial thromboplastin time (aPTT), platelet count and fibrinogen levels. PIVKA level, which will establish vitamin K deficiency, is usually unavailable in routine laboratories and is available only in research labs. The low levels of vitamin K are indirectly established by clinical response to vitamin K.

What is management for HDN?

The disease can be usually prevented by intramuscular vitamin K, 1mg, administered after birth to a neonate. The disease is treated by slow intravenous infusion of 2 5 mg of vitamin K_1. More serious bleeds, especially in patients with extreme prematurity or underlying liver disease, may be treated with infusion of fresh frozen plasma (FFP), infused at rate of 10–20 ml/kg, a protein complex concentrate, 50 units/kg, or recombinant factore VIIa, 100 mcg/kg.

Is parenteral vitamin K safe?

Yes, by and large.

Doesn't it enhance incidence of cancer?

At one time question was raised about its routine use in neonates in the wake of suspicion of increased cancer risk. However, well-planned studies have ruled out such a risk.

What about oral vitamin K?

One recommendation favors oral vitamin K as an alternative, 2 mg at birth followed by 1 mg every week for 12 weeks. Whether this regimen is as effective as parenteral vitamin K remains doubtful.

CONCLUSIONS

Though HDN is a preventable disease, late HDN is likely to have serious complications that may culminate in death. Late HDN usually presents between 2–12 weeks but may manifest as late as 6 months of life. Incidence of ICH is high in these infants. Predisposing factors include exclusive breastfeeding with no or inadequate administration of vitamin K after birth, alabsorption, cholestatic jaundice, cystic fibrosis, biliary atresia, $alpha_1$-antitrypsin deficiency etc. Complications include diabetes insipidus.

TAKE HOME MESSAGES

- Vitamin K deficiency results in a decreased level of vitamin K dependent coagulation factors II, VII, IX and X.
- HDN may present within 24 hours after birth or there may be a delayed presentation.
- HDN is easily preventable by administering vitamin K to all neonates.
- Late HDN may lead to serious intracranial hemorrhages with resultant complications, including diabetes insipidus.

FURTHER READING

1. American Academy of Pediatrics Committee on Fetus and Newborn. Controversies concerning vitamin K and the newborn. *Pediatrics* 2003;112(1 Pt 1):191–192.
2. Alatas FS, Hayashida M, Matsuura T, Saeki I, Yanagi Y, Taguchi T. Intracranial Hemorrhage Associated with Vitamin K-deficiency Bleeding in Patients with Biliary Atresia: Focus on Long-term Outcomes. *J Pediatr Gastroenterol Nutr* 2012;54:552–527.
3. Clarke P, Shearer MJ. Vitamin K deficiency bleeding: The readiness is all. *Arch Dis Child* 2007;92:741–743.
4. Gomella TL, Cunningham MD, Eyal FG. *Neonatology: Management, Procedures, On-call Problems, Diseases and Drugs*. New Delhi: McGraw Hill/Lange 20013.
5. Ozdemir MA, Karakukcu M, Per H, Unal E, Gumus H, Patiroglu T. Late-type vitamin K deficiency bleeding: experience from 120 patients. *Childs Nerv Syst* 2012;28:247–251.
6. van Hasselt PM, de Koning TJ, Kvist N, *et al*. Prevention of vitamin K deficiency bleeding in breastfed infants: Lessons from the Dutch and Danish biliary atresia registries. *Pediatrics* 2008;121:e857–863.

Chapter

27 Rhesus Isoimmunization

Susanta Kumar Badatya, Pankaj Garg

ABSTRACT

Rhesus antigen is one of the antigen system on red blood cells. These antigens can lead to hemolytic disease of the newborn when there is incompatibility between maternal and fetal antigen expression. Rh incompatibility manifestation may range from fetal hemolysis to gross hydrops fetalis and recurrent fetal losses. Surveillance for incompatibility should be started early in pregnancy and antibody prophylaxis should be offered appropriately in Rh negative pregnancy. If there is documented isoimmunization, fetal monitoring and interventions should be carried out to prevent hydrops in the child.

Key Words: Anti D antibody, Indirect Coomb's test (ICT), Middle cerebral artery peak systolic velocity (MCA-PSV), Rhesus antigen.

INTRODUCTION

Rh isoimmunization is one of the pathological phenomenons which depict immunological interaction between fetus and maternal blood group. Rh system is one of the antigen systems on RBC surface. Transplacental passage of Rh D-positive fetal blood into the maternal circulation could trigger the production of antibodies against fetal cells. This leads to production to antibodies that is again transferred in subsequent pregnancy to cause fetal RBC hemolysis, leading to effect ranging from anemia to hydrops. Understanding the pathophysiology will help to diagnose and intervene timely to prevent isoimmunization which is discussed below.

CASE SCENARIO

A 28-year-old G3P1L1A1 mother with O negative blood group came on routine antenatal checkup at 6 weeks of gestation and had Indirect Coomb's Test (ICT) positive. Mother had not received anti-D in previous pregnancies and her first baby had history of neonatal jaundice requiring exchange transfusion. Mother was followed with antibody titre every 4 weeks and underwent Doppler studies at 24 weeks to look for middle cerebral artery (MCA) flows. USG was not suggestive of hydrops.

Contd...

Contd...

Based on deranged MCA flows, cord hematocrit was done, which was 7 g/dL. Mother underwent two intrauterine transfusions. Baby was delivered at 35 weeks of gestation and was found to have O positive blood group and cord bilirubin level of 7 mg/dL and hematocrit of 30%. Baby was managed for hyperbilirubinemia with one exchange transfusion and intensive phototherapy for 5 days. Mother received anti-D postnatally. Baby was discharged on day 6 of life and parents were counseled for follow-up after 48 hours.

Key Words: *Anti-D, Coomb's test, Exchange transfusion, Hyperbilirubinemia, Intensive phototherapy, Intrauterine transfusions, Rhesus isoimmunization, Rh incompatibility.*

CRITICAL CASE ANALYSIS

This is a clinical profile of a case of Rh isoimmunization. The history of first baby being affected with no history of anti-D prophylaxis suggest possible Rh sensitization in previous pregnancy. ICT titre determination as done in this case becomes important to know the risk of developing Rh isoimmunization in this pregnancy. Doppler study done in this case is important noninvasive tool to check for degree of fetal anemia. Intrauterine transfusions and postnatally double volume exchange transfusion remain modality of therapy for anemia and hyperbilirubinemia resulting from isoimmunization.

INTERACTIVE TOPIC DISCUSSION

What do we understand by the term, *Rhesus isoimmunization?* What are the different red blood cell antigens?

Rhesus isoimmunization means presence of antibodies against the rhesus antigen present on the red blood cell. This is named rhesus antigen as this antigen resembles antigen present in rhesus monkey's RBCs.

As per Fisher–Race nomenclature, Rh gene complex antigen system is represented with the presence of three genetic loci, each with two major alleles. Three of the most concerning antigens in pregnancy-the Rh (D), Rh (Cc) and Rh (Ee) antigens are on chromosome 1 (1p36.1). The antigens produced by these alleles originally were identified by specific antisera and have been lettered C, c, D, E, and e. No specific antiserum has been found for "d" antigen and use of the letter "d" indicates the absence of an evident allelic product. Anti-C, anti-c, anti-D, anti-E, and anti-e designate specific antibodies directed against their respective antigens. An Rh gene complex is described by the three appropriate letters. Eight gene complexes are possible (listed in decreasing order of frequency): CDe, cde, cDE, cDe, Cde, cdE, CDE, and CdE. Genotypes are indicated as pairs of these gene complexes, such as CDe/cde. Similarly, other common antigens include Kell, Duffy, and Lewis.

What are the various reasons for fetal isoimmunization?

As feto-maternal interface is not an absolute barrier, sufficient **feto-maternal hemorrhage** before birth or at delivery leads to B lymphocyte clones in mother recognize the foreign red cell antigen. The initial production of IgM is short-lived and is followed by a rapid change to an IgG response. After the initial antigenic exposure, memory B lymphocytes can recognize the appearance of red cells containing the putative antigen in a subsequent pregnancy. As IgM antibodies cannot cross-placental barrier it does not cause Rh isoimmunization in the same pregnancy. But in subsequent antigen exposure, the response for IgG production is increased and the anti-D antibodies cross placenta and then bind to the antigen. This causes Rh isoimmunization.

The minimal amount of fetal blood needed to cause alloimmunization is estimated to be 0.25 ml. The greatest risk occurs at the time of delivery when that risk is approximately 17%. ABO incompatibility of the mother and fetus in pregnancy with Rh sensitization (mother O; father A, B, or AB) will reduce the sensitization risk to 2%.

Causes of fetomaternal hemorrhage and Rh isoimmunization in turn are listed in Table 27.1.

Table 27.1: Conditions causing fetomaternal hemorrhage and Rh isoimmunization

Antenatal period	Intrapartum	Postpartum period
Ectopic pregnancy	Cesarean sections	Inadvertent Rh positive Blood transfusion
Placental abruption	Manual removal of placenta	
Feto-maternal hemorrhage	Feto-maternal hemorrhage Blood transfusion	
Abdominal trauma		
Spontaneous abortion		
Amniocentesis		
Chorionic villus sampling		
External cephalic version		
Fetal blood sampling		
Placenta previa with bleeding		

What are the various investigations required to be done in Rh negative woman who comes for prenatal counseling?

Investigations planned for an Rh negative mother who comes for antenatal care depends upon her sensitization status. For first conception, following investigations are planned:

1. **Initial maternal antibody screen** is to be done, if positive then to look for its significance for causing hemolytic disease of newborn. Most commonly it is Anti-D antibody, but cases may present with Anti E, Anti c, anti kell antibody etc.
2. **Determination of antibody titre** is the next investigation. A critical titer is that titer which poses a significant risk for severe erythroblastosis fetalis and hydrops. In most centers, this is between 1:8 and 1:32. When there is a history of a previously affected fetus or neonate, serial titer assessment is inadequate for surveillance of fetal anemia. As variation in titer results from different laboratories is common, so titers should be obtained in the same laboratory when monitoring a patient, and a change of more than one dilution during serial monitoring is significant.

3. **Determination of partner's genotype:** As D antigen is dominant and baby inherits its allele for D antigen from father, determination of zygosity of paternal D antigen is helpful. If the paternal phenotype is D antigen positive with a homozygous genotype, then the baby has a 100% chance of being rhesus-D antigen positive and therefore at risk, because homozygotes always pass the rhesus-D antigen to their offspring. Fetuses from rhesus-D positive fathers who are heterozygous for the D gene have a 50% chance of being rhesus-D negative. But paternal zygosity could only be determined with around 95% certainty.
4. **Determination of fetal blood group:** Fetal blood group can be determined to rule out if the fetus is at risk when father is heterozygous for D antigen. Invasive methods such as amniocentesis, chorionic villus sampling or fetal blood sampling may be used. Amniocentesis seemed to be the safest and most reliable of these methods. It is usually carried out after 12 weeks' gestation, and amniocytes are used to obtain the fetal genotype using PCR. This technique is associated with a false–positive rate of up to 1.5%.
5. **Cell-free fetal DNA analysis (cff DNA):** By non-invasive prenatal testing (NIPT), fetal rhesus-D status can be reliably determined by PCR analysis of cell-free fetal DNA from maternal plasma or serum. This enables women to avoid invasive procedures for fetal genotype determination. Testing has proved to be very accurate (94–97%), with high sensitivity and specificity. This test can be performed after 8 weeks onwards.
6. **Tests for predicting fetal anemia at risk infants for hydrops:** Ultrasonography is useful for obtaining serial middle cerebral artery peak systolic velocity (MCA-PSV) values through targeted ultrasounds, and excluding the presence of hydrops. Cordocentesis is used to determine level of fetal anemia to decide for intrauterine transfusions. Ancillary invasive procedure like amniocentesis to determine ΔOD450 and to predict risk of fetal anemia as per various charts, e.g., Liley chart are other tests that can be used to predict fetal anemia.

How is an Rh negative pregnancy followed?

- **First Pregnancy**

Once blood typing reveals Rh negative status, routine investigation and strict follow up is required to screen for isoimmunized fetus. Once an antibody reported to cause HDFN has been detected in an initial maternal antibody screen, a titer should be obtained to assess the amount of antibody present. If the value remains below a critical value (1:32 for anti-D and most other antibodies; 1:8 for anti-Kell), titers are obtained every 4 weeks until approximately 24 weeks' gestation, and then every 2 weeks thereafter. Paternal blood is drawn to determine if the patient's partner is positive for the involved red cell antigen and to investigate his zygosity. DNA techniques are employed in the case of RhD; for other antigens, serology is used to determine the paternal genotype. In cases of a heterozygous paternal genotype for Rh D, cff DNA is used to determine the fetal Rh D status. For other red cell antigens, amniocentesis is performed after 15 weeks' gestation to determine the fetal antigen status. If the paternal blood typing is negative for the involved red cell antigen, further maternal and fetal monitoring is not required as long as paternity is ensured. When the patient's partner is unavailable for testing or paternity is in question, cff DNA allows accurate assessment of the fetal Rh D status. A homozygous paternal phenotype or genotype indicates an antigen-positive fetus and negates the need for off DNA or amniocentesis for fetal typing.

If fetus is Rh antigen positive and maternal screen is positive for antibodies, Doppler assessment of the MCA is performed serially at 1 to 2-week intervals starting at around 24 weeks' gestation. An MCA-PSV (Peak systolic velocity) greater than 1.5 MoM (multiple of median) is an indication for cordocentesis for fetal hematocrit determination and intrauterine transfusion if needed. Antenatal testing for fetal well being with non stress test or biophysical profile should be initiated after 32 weeks' gestation. Induction by 38 weeks' gestation should be considered.

- **Previously Affected Fetus or Infant**

  If the patient has a new partner and there is a history of a previous sibling loss related to hydrops fetalis, a previous need for IUT, or a previous need for neonatal exchange transfusion; paternal red cell typing and zygosity testing should be undertaken. In the case of a partner who tests negative for the involved red cell antigen with ensured paternity, no further testing is necessary. A complicated previous pregnancy with the patient's same partner should result in a referral to a tertiary care center with experience in the management of severely alloimmunized pregnancies. In these cases, maternal titers are not predictive of the degree of fetal anemia. If fetus is antigen-positive as tested by cell free fetal DNA or amniocentesis, serial MCA-PSV testing should begin at as early as 16 weeks of gestation and repeated every 1 to 2 weeks.

Timing of Delivery

Prior to introduction of the direct intrauterine transfusions, fetuses with isoimmunization were routinely delivered by 32 weeks' gestation. As experience with intrauterine transfusions (IUT) became widespread, most experienced centers now perform the final IUT up to 35 weeks' gestation with delivery anticipated at 37–38 weeks. Finally, the administration of maternal oral phenobarbital may be considered in the 7–10 days before delivery. This has been proposed to induce hepatic maturity to allow improved conjugation of bilirubin.

What is the principle of fetal doppler flows of middle cerebral artery and its relation with fetal anemia? How do they help in the management? What are the limitations?

The objective of Doppler flow studies is to detect physiologic compensatory changes in the fetal circulation that would be associated with mild to moderate anemia. As anemia progresses, both right and left ventricular outputs increase up to 45% with the heart rate remaining unchanged leading to increased stroke volume. Anemia leads to decreased viscosity and increased stroke volume resulting in increased flow. If the given fetal blood vessel cross-sectional area also remains unchanged, then applying Poiseuille's law (blood velocity is directly proportional to flow), we know that blood velocity is also increased. Middle cerebral artery was selected as cerebral arteries respond rapidly to hypoxemia by increasing blood flow velocity to maintain cerebral perfusion. It is easy to identify the artery with low inter-observer and intra-observer variability. Measurements can be initiated at as early as 16–18 weeks' gestation and should be performed weekly. Moderate or severe anemia (hemoglobin below 0.65 MoMs) was predicted by values of peak systolic velocity in the fetal middle cerebral artery above 1.5 times the median for gestational age with a sensitivity of 100% and false-positive rate of 12%.

Limitation: Studies have suggested that there is a higher false-positive rate after 34–35 weeks of gestation. Therefore, relying on MCA peak systolic velocity to either exclude or suspect fetal anemia is not recommended after 36 weeks. In addition, as with any new technology, the measurements must be done by a practitioner specifically trained to perform Doppler for measurement of peak systolic velocity in the fetal middle cerebral artery.

What is anti-D? When is it given antenatally in an Rh negative pregnancy? What are the indications? What is the dose and how is the dose decided?

Anti-D is pool of passive immunoglobulins consisting of IgG antibodies which are polyclonal antibody products derived from human plasma. These are administered by either the intravenous or the intramuscular route. All current products undergo micropore filtration to eliminate viral transmission.

American Association of Blood Banks (AABB) recommends that a repeat antibody screen be obtained before antenatal Rh immunoglobulin (RhIG) administration, even though the incidence of alloimmunization before 28 weeks is very low. Severe maternal sensitization does occasionally occur before 28 weeks and by not performing the antibody screen, opportunity to detect a potentially salvageable anemic fetus is lost. It is, therefore, prudent to repeat the antibody screen. The maternal blood sample can be drawn at the same office visit as the RhIG injection. Repeat dosing should be done after 12 weeks of first dose, i.e., at 40 weeks if she has not delivered yet.

Indications

Indications of anti-D are listed in Table 27.2.

Table 27.2: Indications of anti-D in Rh isoimmunisation

Indications of Anti-D	
Antepartum indication	**Postpartum indication**
• Spontaneous abortion/IUFD • Therapeutic abortion • Chorionic villus sampling • Ectopic pregnancy • Amniocentesis • Percutaneous umbilical blood sampling • Abruptio placenta/placenta previa • Antepartum vaginal bleeding • External cephalic version • Trauma • Pregnancy (28 weeks' gestation and ≤72 h postpartum)	• Delivery • Fetomaternal hemorrhage with Rh positive fetus

Dose

Antenatal Administration: After the initial screen at the first prenatal visit, a repeat Rh-D antibody screen is done at 24–28 weeks. If the antibody screen is negative, 300 μg of anti-D immune globulin is administered at that gestational age and then again within 72 hours of delivery if the neonate is Rh-D positive. 300 μg of RhIG should be administered within 72 hours of delivery if umbilical cord blood typing reveals an RhD-positive infant.

Suggested doses of anti-D immune globulin for a first-trimester induced or spontaneous abortion, amniocentesis, or chorionic villus sampling, and first-trimester ectopic pregnancy are 50 μg of anti-D immune globulin.

Three hundred micrograms of anti-D immune globulin will suppress the immune response of 30 ml of fetal blood or 15 ml of packed D-positive red blood cells. Dose of 50 μg of RhIG is effective until 12 weeks' gestation because of the small volume of red cells in the fetoplacental circulation. From logistic standpoint, stock of this dosage of RhIG is not kept, therefore, a standard dose of 300 μg is often given.

In ongoing pregnancies when RhIG is administered in the first or second trimester for one of these indications, a repeat dose should still be given at 28 weeks' gestation. Alternatively, if the antenatal dose was given in the late second trimester (e.g., at 22 weeks for suspected placental abruption), the dose should be repeated 12 weeks later (i.e., at 34 weeks' gestation in that example).

Calculation of Actual Dosage

As per AABB recommendation, all Rh negative deliveries should be screened for fetomaternal hemorrhage. A Kleihauer-Betke stain or fetal cell stain using flow cytometry is performed. AABB standards indicate that the percentage of fetal blood cells should then be multiplied by a factor of 50 (based on a standard blood volume of 5 l for all pregnant women) to determine the volume of the fetomaternal hemorrhage. This is then divided by 30 to determine the number of vials of RhIG to administer. If the calculation results in a fraction of a unit of 0.5 or greater, the number of vials required is rounded up to the higher whole integer.

What is hydrops fetalis and its consequences?

Hydrops fetalis is defined as the presence of excessive fluid in two or more of the following spaces: abdominal ascites, pleural effusion, pericardial effusion, skin edema, polyhydramnious, or placentomegaly as per the following criteria to define excessive fluid collection by ultrasonography.

Hydrops fetalis is caused by three main mechanisms: anemia, hypoproteinemia and cardiac failure. Approximately 50% of fetuses with non-immune hydrops fetalis die in utero, and about half of the live born infants survive. Fetal hydrops is a medical emergency for which detailed and comprehensive ultrasound examination and early identification of any treatable causes is important.

Table 27.3 lists the USG criteria for hydrops fetalis.

How to manage a baby delivered to Rh isoimmunized mother?

Whenever an Rh isoimmunized mother is delivering, following steps to be observed.

The steps to be followed include:

1. Keep cross-matched (with mother's blood) blood ready before induction of labor.

Table 27.3: USG criteria for hydrops

Parameter	Criteria
Ascites	Echolucent rim encompassing entire fetal abdomen in the transverse view
Pleural effusions	Unilateral or bilateral visualization of lung border
Pericardial effusion	Nonphysiologic fluid ≥ 2 mm
Skin edema	Subcutaneous edema ≥ 5 mm
Polyhydramnios	Single deepest fluid pocket ≥ 8 mm or AFI ≥ 25 cm
Placentomegaly	Placenta ≥ 6 cm thickness

2. Clamp cord immediately.
3. Keep cord at least 2–3 cm long for possible catheterization.
4. Collect cord blood for blood group, hemoglobin, reticulocyte count, bilirubin and direct agglutinin test.
5. Preparation for exchange transfusion may be needed soon after birth.

Immediate postnatal management targets achieving hemodynamic stability depending upon hydropic status of baby. If baby is hemodynamically unstable, urgent ultrasonogrpahy and chest X-ray can be done to detect presence of pleural effusion, pericardial effusion or ascites. These fluid accumulations should be drained immediately to achieve good perfusion and ventilation. Then immediate partial exchange can be done using packed RBCs.

Non-hydropic baby and stable hydropic baby can be followed for cord blood parameters to decide for intervention for hyperbilirubinemia and anemia.

- **Indication of Exchange Transfusion**
  - Cord bilirubin >4.5 mg/dL and cord hemoglobin is <11 g/dL.
  - Rising bilirubin > 1 mg/dL/hour despite of phototherapy.
  - Hemoglobin level between 11 and 13 mg/dL and bilirubin level is rising > 0.5 mg/dL/hr despite of phototherapy.
  - Age specific bilirubins rising above cut off levels of exchange transfusion.
- **Indication of Intravenous Immunoglobulin:**

  Rising bilirubin nearing exchange transfusion in case of Coomb's test positive cases

  Dose: 500–1000 mg/kg, may be repeated if required.

Finally, what should be the algorithmic approach to Rh negative pregnancy?

Figure 27.1 presents the algorithmic approach to Rh negative pregnancy.

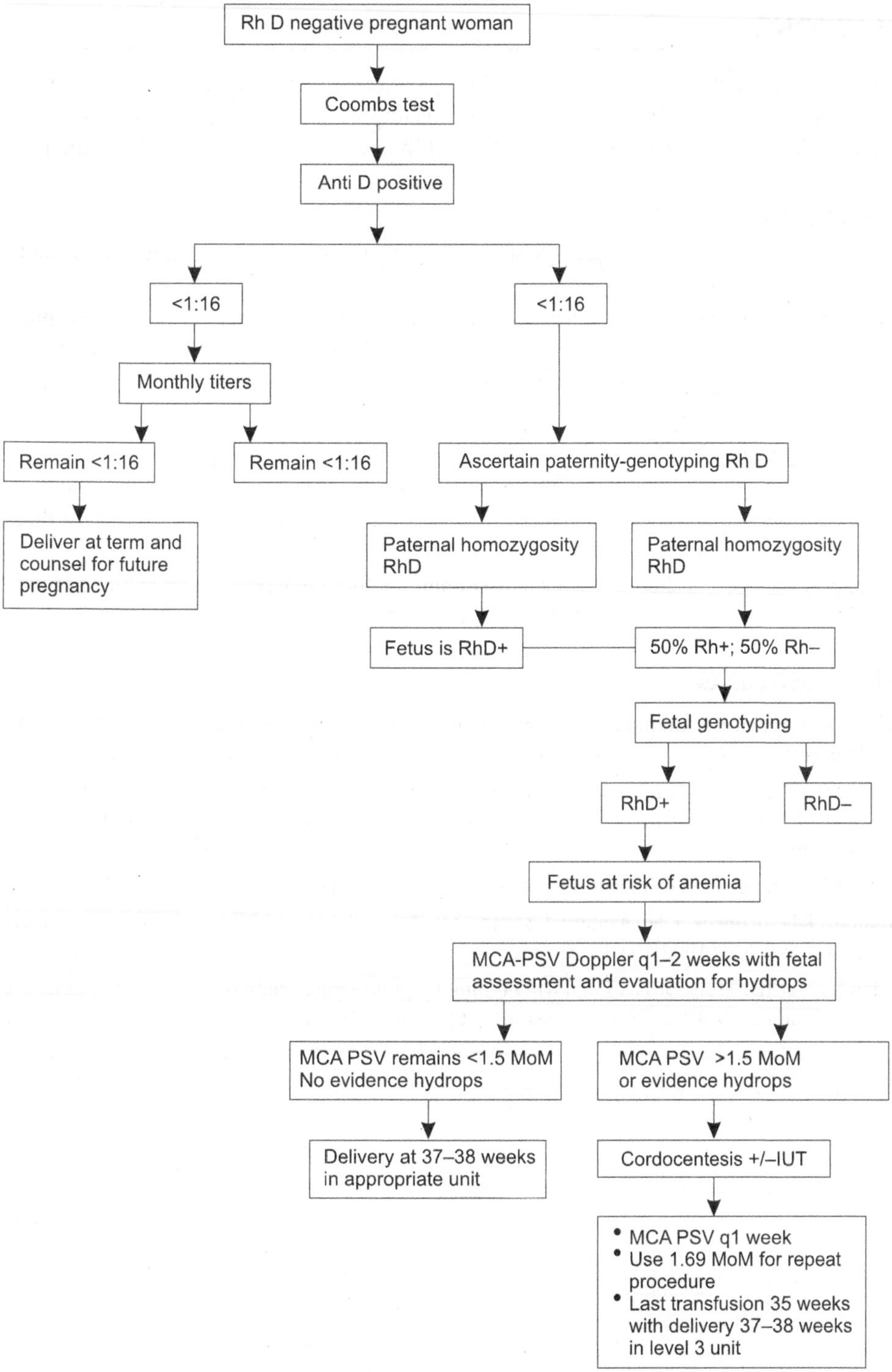

Fig. 27.1: Flowchart for approach to Rh negative pregnancy

CONCLUSIONS

It is common to have antenatal and postnatal complications in Rh isoimmunization if there is ongoing hemolysis. So supervision of Rh negative pregnancy is important to screen for potential complication and timely intervention. Use of Doppler studies is useful in assessing degree of fetal anemia noninvasively.

TAKE HOME MESSAGES

- Supervision of Rh negative pregnancy should be done to rule out Rh isoimmunization and potential complications if any.
- Rh isoimmunization is usually seen in second or third pregnancies, but is also possible in primigravida mother when there is prior sensation in form of blood transfusion or prior missed abortion.
- Initial maternal antibody screen is to be done, if positive then to look for its significance for causing hemolytic disease of newborn.
- Determination of fetal genotype for Rh blood group should be done to determine risk of sensitization.
- Serial documentation of antibody titres helps in advising tests to determine fetal anemia.
- Uses of non-invasive tests like Doppler of MCA vessel have made it easy to pick of threshold for intrauterine transfusions.
- Postnatally all mothers should receive anti-D immunoglobulin depending upon blood group of baby.

FURTHER READING

1. Dahlke JD, Magann EF. Immune and nonimmune hydrops fetalis. In: Martin RJ, Fanaroff AA, Walsh MC (eds): *Fanaroff and Martin's Neonatal Perinatal Medicine*, 10th edn. Philadelphia: Elsevier 2015:1434–1459.
2. Gregory MLP, Martin CR, Cloherty JP. Neonatal hyperbilirubinemia. In: Cloherty JP, Eichenwald EC, Hansen AR, Stark AR (eds): *Manual of Neonatal Care,* 7th edn. Philadelphia: Lippincott Williams and Wilkins 2012:304–309.
3. Moise KJ Jr. Management of rhesus alloimmunization in pregnancy. *Obstet Gynecol* 2002;100:600–611.
4. Nicolaides KH, Rodeck CH. Maternal serum anti-D antibody concentration and assessment of rhesus isoimmunization. *BMJ* 1992;304:1155–1156.
5. Van den Veyver IB, Moise Jr KJ. Fetal RhD typing by polymerase chain reaction in pregnancies complicated by rhesus alloimmunization. *Obstet Gynecol* 1996;88:1061–1071.

Chapter

28 Polycythemia in the Newborn

Abhishek Chopra, Neelam Kler

ABSTRACT

Polycythemia is defined as increased hematocrit >65%. It is commonly seen in babies born small for gestational age or infant of diabetic mother. Polycythemia can lead to various complications like hypoglycemia, respiratory distress and hyperbilirubinemia. Asymptomatic polycythemia with hematocrit less than 75% should be managed initially by increasing fluid/feed intake. Partial exchange transfusion should be done in asymptomatic babies polycythemia with hematocrit >75% or symptomatic polycythemia.

Key Words: Hematocrit, Hyperbilirubinemia, Hypoglycemia, Infants of diabetic mothers, Partial exchange transfusion (PET), Polycythemia, Respiratory distress, Small-for-gestation age (SGA).

INTRODUCTION

Polycythemia (or more accurately, erythrocythemia), an abnormal rise of the circulating red blood cell (RBC) mass, is seen frequently in newborns. Polycythemia of the neonate was first mentioned in the Bible. In the 1970s, there were a number of case reports and small series of infants with symptoms that were thought to be secondary to an elevated hematocrit and blood viscosity. The abnormal rise in hematocrit increases the risk of hyperviscosity, microcirculatory hypoperfusion and multisystem organ dysfunction.

CASE SCENARIO

A baby weighing 1680 gm was born to the mother with pregnancy-induced hypertension at 37 weeks. Baby was shifted to nursery in view of being small for gestational age. He was started on paladi (cup) feeds. Blood sugar monitoring was done.

Hematocrit (Hct) sent at 2 hours of life was 70%. At 2 hours of life baby also became tachypneic and had hypoglycemia (blood sugar 20 mg/dL).

He was started on glucose infusion @ 6 mg/kg/min. He became euglycemic at glucose infusion of 10 mg/kg/min. Partial exchange transfusion was done for symptomatic polycythemia with normal saline.

Since hematocrit decreased to 56% and respiratory distress settled, glucose infusion was tapered over next 24 hours and the baby started on breastfeeding.

CRITICAL CASE ANALYSIS

This baby, small for gestational age (weight less than 10th centile for age on Fenton's chart) was shifted to nursery for monitoring. Being at high risk for polycythemia, hematocrit was monitored at 2 hours of life. Hematocrit was 70%. Baby developed respiratory distress and hypoglycemia, the two common complications due to polycythemia. Hence, baby had symptomatic polycythemia for which partial exchange transfusion was done with normal saline. Both these complications resolved with correction of polycythemia after partial exchange transfusion.

INTERACTIVE TOPIC DISCUSSION

What is polycythemia?

Polycythemia is defined as hematocrit more than 65% when obtained from large, freely flowing peripheral vein. Polycythemia occurs due to increased RBC cell mass while plasma volume can be normal, decreased or increased. Hematocrit value normally peaks at 2 hours of life, remains at plateau for 2 hours and then drops slowly over next 12–18 hours and by 24 hours achieves value similar to that at birth.

What is hyperviscosity? What's its relationship with polycythemia? Can they be used interchangeably?

Viscosity is the magnitude of internal friction in a fluid, as measured by the force per unit area resisting uniform flow. Hyperviscosity is defined as values beyond 3 standard deviation. Many factors affect viscosity of blood such as plasma proteins, RBC deformability, WBC, fibrinogen, platelets, blood pH and blood vessel size. Hematocrit remains primary determinant in neonate. Hyperviscosity causes blood flow to be sluggish and thus symptoms due to impairment of tissue oxygenation. In clinical practice, hematocrit is measured and not viscosity. But polycythemia and hyperviscosity cannot be used interchangeably.

What is the incidence of polycythemia? Which babies should be screened for polycythemia?

The incidence of polycythemia is 1.5–4% of all live births. The incidence is higher among both small-for-gestational age (SGA) and infant of diabetic mother. The incidence of polycythemia is 1% among term SGA infants as compared to 2% in term AGA infants.

Screening should be done in following high risk babies:

1. Small-for-gestational-age (SGA) babies.
2. Larger of the monochorionic twins.
3. Infant of diabetic mothers.
4. Beckwith-Wiedemann, Trisomy 13, 18, 21.

Screening should be done at 2 hours of age. Capillary hematocrit measurements are unreliable and highly subject to variations in blood flow and are significantly higher than venous hematocrit. Two methods of hematocrit estimation are capillary centrifuge and automated hematology analyzer. Values obtained from centrifuge are higher than that of hematology analyzer. Most of available data in literature is from centrifuged hematocrit.

What are the triggering factors of polycythemia?

1. **Chronic Fetal Hypoxia:** Fetal and intrauterine factors can cause chronic fetal hypoxia which results in increased fetal erythropoiesis, RBC mass and hematocrit. Conditions such as maternal diabetes, pregnancy induced hypertension, fetal hyperthyroidism and maternal smoking cause chronic fetal hypoxia.
2. **Acute Fetal Hypoxia:** Perinatal asphyxia and acute fetal hypoxia can also result in polycythemia. Acute intrauterine hypoxia can cause shift of blood from placental compartment to fetus resulting in polycythemia.

Polycythemia is also seen in babies with Beckwith-Wiedemann syndrome and in babies with Trisomy 13, 18 and 21. Cause of polycythemia in these conditions is not known.

What are the clinical features of polycythemia?

- **CNS:** Poor feeding, lethargy, hypotonia, apnea, tremors, jitteriness, seizures, cerebral venous thrombosis.
- **Cardiorespiratory:** Cyanosis, Tachypnea, congestive heart failure, cardiomegaly, increased pulmonary vascular resistance.
- **Renal:** Decreased Glomerular filtration rate, decreased sodium excretion, renal vein thrombosis, hematuria, proteinuria.
- **Others:** Thrombocytopenia, poor feeding, hyperbilirubinemia, persistent hypoglycemia, hypocalcemia, testicular infarcts, necroterizing enterocolitis, disseminated intravascular coagulation.

How should babies with asymptomatic polycythemia be managed?

Asymptomatic infants: Those babies whose central hematocrits are between 65% (0.65) and 75% (0.75) should be monitored closely and aggressively hydrated with adequate enteral intake or with intravenous fluids. The hematocrit should be reassessed in 12–24 hours and plasma glucose, bilirubin along with cardiorespiratory status should be monitored. If the hematocrit decreases or remains stable and the patient remains asymptomatic, monitoring should be continued for a further 24–48 hours. Partial exchange transfusion (PET) should be performed in asymptomatic babies with hematocrit above 75%.

What are the indications of partial exchange transfusion? Which fluid should be used?

Symptomatic infants: The recommended therapy for symptomatic infants is hemodilution by PET. However before considering PET, the infant should be evaluated for any other cause for the observed symptoms. Following formula is used to calculate amount of blood (fluid) that needs to be exchanged:

$$\text{PET} = \frac{\text{Circulating blood volume (80–90 ml/kg)} \times \text{observed hematocrit} - \text{desired hematocrit (55\%)}}{\text{Observed hematocrit}}$$

In our case, amount of blood (fluid) calculated was

$$80 \times 1.8 \times (70 - 55)/55 = 39 \text{ ml.}$$

Fluid type: Two systematic reviews have been performed by De Waal, *et al.* (2006) and Dempsey and Barrington (2005). Both these reviews concluded that crystalloid solutions are as effective as colloid solutions for PET. In addition, crystalloid have no risk of transmission of blood borne diseases or anaphylaxis, they are easy available and less expensive. Hence, crystalloid solutions (example normal saline) should be used as a standard solution for PET.

What is the best algorithmic approach to polycythemia?

Figure 28.1 provides an algorithmic approach to polycythemia.

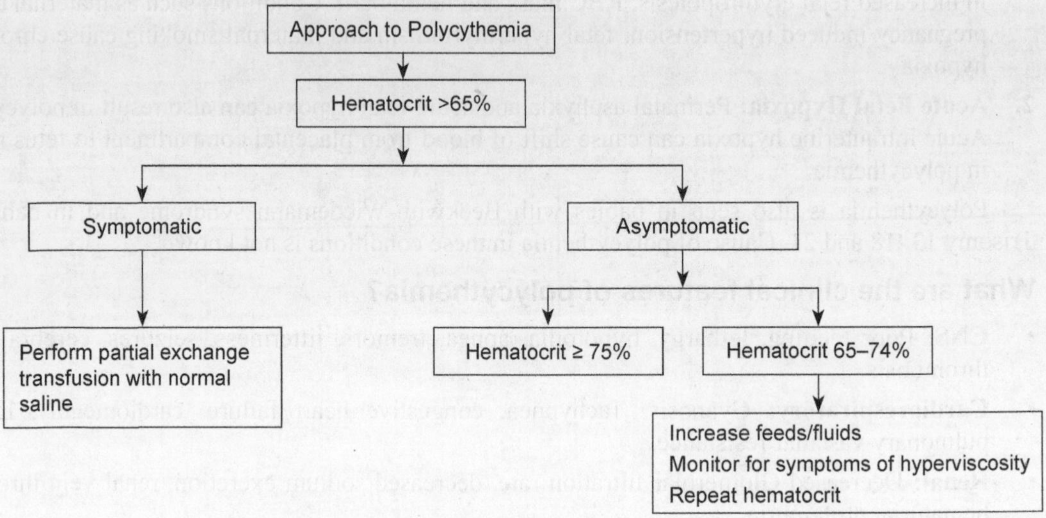

Fig. 28.1: Algorithmic approach to polycythemia

CONCLUSIONS

Polycythemia is a common problem in SGA babies and infants of diabetic mothers. These babies should have their hematocrit closely monitored for hyperviscosity syndrome. Partial exchange transfusion should be done with crystalloids in symptomatic babies if hematocrit is above 65% and in asymptomatic babies with hematocrit more than 75%.

TAKE HOME MESSAGES

- Polycythemia is defined as hematocrit more than 65%.
- Clinical manifestations are due to hyperviscosity which is not measured in clinical practice.
- Babies with polycythemia are at high risk for various complications.
- Partial exchange transfusion should be performed in symptomatic babies and in asymptomatic babies with hematocrit above 75%.
- Normal saline should be used as fluid for partial exchange transfusion.

FURTHER READING

1. de Waal KA, Baerts W, Offringa M. Systematic review of the optimal fluid for dilutional exchange transfusion in neonatal polycythaemia. *Arch Dis Child Fetal Neonatal Ed* 2006;91:F7–10.
2. Dempsey EM, Barrington K. Crystalloid or colloid for partial exchange transfusion in neonatal polycythemia: a systematic review and meta-analysis. *Acta Paediatr* 2005;94:1650–1655.

3. Ramamurthy RS, Brans YW. Neonatal polycythemia: Criteria for diagnosis and treatment. *Pediatrics* 1981; 68:168–174.
4. Rosenkrantz TS, Oh W. Cerebral blood flow velocity in infants with polycythemia and hyperviscosity: Effects of partial exchange transfusion with Plasmanate. *J Pediatr* 1982;101:94–98.
5. Rosenkrantz TS, Philipps AF, Skrzypczak PS, Raye JR. Cerebral metabolism in the newborn lamb with polycythemia. *Pediatr Res* 1988;23:329–333.
6. Wood JL. Plethora in the newborn infant associated with cyanosis and convulsions; a review of postnatal erythropoiesis. *J Pediatr* 1959;54:143–151.

Chapter

29 Congenital Diaphragmatic Hernia

Alpana Prasad

ABSTRACT

Congenital diaphragmatic hernia (CDH) is a neonatal emergency in the delivery room with a normal appearing infant not responding to resuscitation, if it has not been diagnosed by antenatal sonography.

Endotracheal intubation with gentle ventilation, followed by orogastric decompression is immediately indicated. Pulmonary hypoplasia and pulmonary hypertension with right-to-left shunting are common with resultant hypoxemia.

The old management strategy of immediate surgery is now replaced by physiologic stabilization and delayed surgery.

The introduction of less invasive therapeutic techniques such as high frequency oscillation ventilation, inhaled nitric oxide, surfactant, and perfluorocarbon liquid ventilation may replace the need for ECMO.

A long-term follow-up is essential.

Key Words: Congenital diaphragmatic hernia (CDH), ECMO, Endotracheal intubation, High frequency oscillation, Inhaled nitric oxide, Orogastric decompression, Perfluorocarbon liquid ventilation, Physiological stabilization, Surfactant.

INTRODUCTION

Congenital diaphragmatic hernia (CDH) is a lethal birth defect with a reported incidence of 1 in 3000 live births. Despite the advances in antenatal diagnosis almost 20–30% cases are diagnosed after birth or later presenting with respiratory distress. Diagnosis is confirmed on plain chest radiograph. Definitive treatment is surgery which is done electively after an initial period of stabilization and management of pulmonary hypertension. The mortality and morbidity in these infants is high due to lung hypoplasia, pulmonary hypertension and severe co-existent anomalies.

CASE SCENARIO

A 23-year-old primigravida mother delivered a male baby at 39 weeks gestation by spontaneous vaginal delivery. There were no significant antenatal problems. Prenatal ultrasonography had not been done.

Contd...

Contd...

Immediately following delivery, the baby appeared "normal" and cried immediately. However, at 1 minute of age, he remained cyanotic. At 5 minutes of age, the baby still remained very cyanotic, tachypneic and dyspneic, despite 100% oxygen via mask.

The neonatal resuscitation team started bag-mask positive pressure ventilation with 100% oxygen, but the baby became bradycardic. Therefore, he was immediately intubated and ventilated.

Auscultation of the lung revealed good breath sounds in the right chest, but no breath sounds in the left. The heart sounds seemed loudest in the right chest, and the abdomen appeared scaphoid. Ventilation was continued through the endotracheal tube. An orogastric tube was inserted and suction applied.

The baby is transferred to the NICU and chest X-ray is done immediately which reveals air-filled bowel loops in the left chest cavity and absent bowel gas shadow in the abdominal cavity (Fig. 29.1), confirming the diagnosis of congenital diaphragmatic.

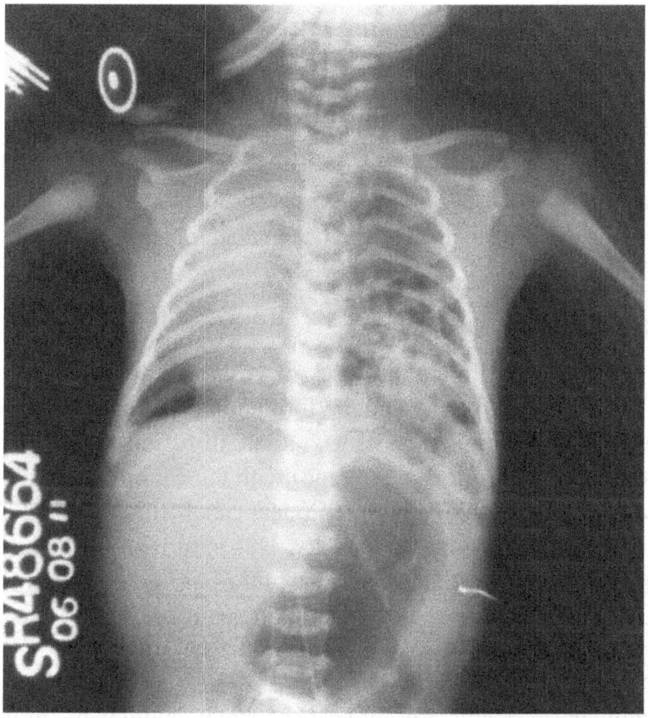

Fig. 29.1: X-ray chest showing left-sided congenital diaphragmatic hernia

CRITICAL CASE ANALYSIS

This neonate presenting with respiratory distress at birth or soon after birth, which continued to worsen despite resuscitation by bag mask ventilation, and was accompanied by mediastinal shift to right, absent breath sounds or presence of bowel sounds in the chest, was rightly suspected to have congenital diaphragmatic hernia.

Diagnosis was confirmed immediately by a plain chest X-ray which reveals air-filled bowel loops in the chest. Immediate neonatal management by endotracheal intubation and elective ventilation and gastric decompression were instituted as per standard protocol.

INTERACTIVE TOPIC DISCUSSION

How is CDH diagnosed antenatally?

CDH can predictably be diagnosed antenatally by ultrasonography at approximately 20 weeks' gestation.

At the time of prenatal diagnosis, it is important to exclude the presence of other anomalies and also the degree of pulmonary hypoplasia should be assessed.The presence of liver in the chest in left-sided CDH indicates severe pulmonary hypoplasia. The lung-to-head ratio (LHR – the area of the right lung at the level of the four-chamber view divided by the head circumference) has been shown to be a predictable estimation of the degree of pulmonary hypoplasia.

Currently, intrauterine lung measurement by MRI is being investigated as a means of estimating lung size.

What are the commonly associated anomalies with CDH?

Associated anomalies occur in 15–25% cases of CDH. Most common are cardiovascular anomalies (PDA, VSD, vascular rings, coarctation of aorta). Chromosomal anomalies (trisomy 13), CNS malformations (neural tube defects, anencephaly, encephalocele) and pulmonary sequestration are other anomalies seen with CDH.

What is the embryogenesis of CDH?

The diaphragm develops between 4th and 8th week of gestation and by the end of the 12th week the fetal bowel returns to the abdominal cavity and the formation of the diaphragm is complete, separating the intrathoracic from the intra-abdominal contents. Failure of fusion of the peripheral muscular part of diaphragm (arising from pleuroperitoneal membrane) with the central tendinous part (arising from the transverse septum) results in a persistent pleuroperitoneal canal (foramen of Bochdalek), which allows the intra-abdominal viscera to occupy the chest cavity. This in turn prevents the lungs from developing, resulting in lung hypoplasia which is worse on the side of the hernia. As the left side of diaphragm closes after the right side, hence, most CDH (85–90%) occur on the left side.

What is the clinical presentation of CDH?

If undiagnosed prenatally, these infants present as a "neonatal emergency" in the delivery room. They do not respond to the typical steps of neonatal resuscitation, and usually get worse with bag-mask ventilation (BMV). With left-sided CDH, breath sounds are diminished or absent in the left chest and because the mediastinum is displaced to the opposite side, the heart sounds are heard louder in the right chest. As the stomach and bowel fill with gas, (made worse by BMV), respiration and cardiac action are further compromised, and hypoxia and respiratory acidosis worsens. The neonate exhibits progressive respiratory distress, cyanosis and ultimately bradycardia. Because the abdominal contents are displaced into the chest, the abdomen often is scaphoid. Occasionally, the infants with CDH may remain relatively asymptomatic in the early hours and days of life and present later with respiratory distress.

What is the differential diagnosis of CDH?

CDH can be misdiagnosed as left tension pneumothorax, with acute respiratory distress. Occasionally, cystic adenomatoid malformation (CCAM) or intra-lobar sequestration of the lower lobe may be confused with CDH. Absence of the stomach bubble in the left upper quadrant of the abdomen on X-ray abdomen is an important radiologic clue to make the diagnosis of CDH.

What is the preoperative management in CDH?

Preoperative management includes orogastric decompression of the stomach and intestine, along with mechanical ventilation to reduce hypercarbia, hypoxemia and acidosis; and hyperventilation ("gentle" positive pressure ventilation) to induce respiratory alkalosis; and vasodilators to improve pulmonary artery hypertension. Appropriate fluid management and use of inotropes, sedation and analgesia is important. Inotropic agents (dopamine and dobutamine) help increase systemic arterial pressure and thereby reduce right-to-left shunting. Pulse oximetry helps in evaluating oxygenation and using two probes (one on right hand and other on lower leg) shunting can be detected. Monitoring of arterial blood gas levels (pre-ductal and post-ductal) is essential for evaluating response to management and assessing the degree of shunting. The main goal of preoperative management is to stabilize pulmonary circulation and manage pulmonary hypertension. If standard mechanical ventilation fails then other measures such as high frequency ventilation, inhaled nitric oxide and ECMO are used.

How has the ventilatory management strategy changed in CDH?

Conventionally mechanical ventilation with high pressures and hyperventilation were used to reverse ductal shunting and cause alkalinisation. This has now been replaced with newer ventilatory techniques utilizing the concepts of permissive hypercapnia and high frequency oscillation (HFO) ventilation. The complications of mechanical ventilation including air leaks, barotrauma and consequent broncho-pulmonary dysplasia are reduced because of these newer techniques. The goal is to reverse the persistent pulmonary hypertension causing right to left shunting through the ductus arteriosus and foramen ovale.

What is the role of inhaled nitric oxide in management of CDH?

The use of inhaled nitric oxide (iNO) is a recent development in treatment of CDH. Endogenous nitric oxide is an important modulator of vascular tone in the pulmonary circulation. It results in a reduction in pulmonary hypertension, with improvement in oxygenation but no change in the systemic vascular resistance. It is usually used as an adjunct to conventional mechanical ventilation and HFOV while preparing for extracorporeal membrane oxygenation (ECMO) cannulation.

What is the role of ECMO in management of CDH? What are the other adjunctive treatment modalities?

Extracorporeal membrane oxygenation (ECMO) has been shown to salvage some of the most severely affected neonates who do not improve despite aggressive therapy. Venovenous or venoarterial bypass is used, depending on the infant's hemodynamic stability. Bypass is continued until the pulmonary hypertension is reversed and lung function is improved, usually between 7 and 10 days of age. Approximately 60% of infants with CDH who are supported by ECMO survive.

The use of surfactant and perfluorocarbon liquid ventilation, are other newer adjunctive treatment modalities.

Sildenafil, a phosphodiesterase inhibitor, appears promising as a pulmonary vasodilator with success reported in some cases of CDH.

What is the right time for surgical repair?

The surgical repair should be undertaken as a semi-elective procedure when following criteria are met:

- Mean arterial blood pressure is normal for gestational age.
- Preductal saturation level is between 85–95% with a $FiO_2 < 50\%$.
- Serum lactate <3 mmol/l.
- Urine production >2 ml/kg/h.

What is the surgical management of CDH?

The CDH is usually repaired transabdominally through left subcostal incision. The hernia is reduced gently by withdrawing the viscera from the chest (Fig. 29.2).

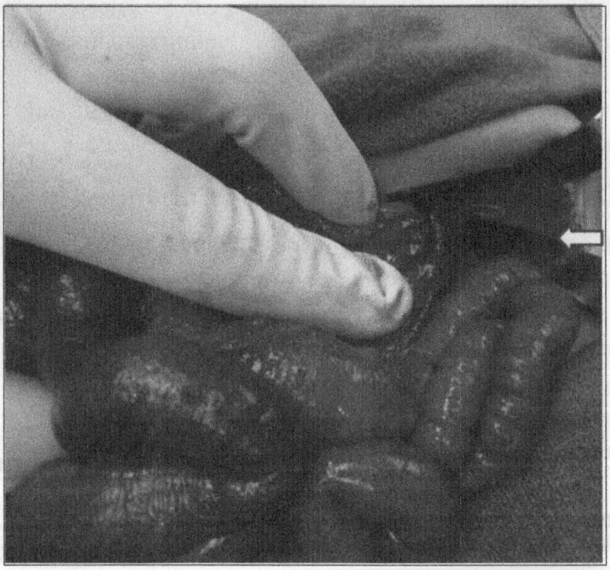

Fig. 29.2: Intraoperative picture of left diaphragmatic defect shown by arrow

Usually there is enough diaphragmatic tissue to complete a direct suture repair, but, if a large portion of the diaphragm is missing, prosthetic material must be used to repair the defect. A chest tube is usually placed in the left hemithorax and brought out through an intercostal space. As the abdominal contents have been in the thorax for most of fetal period, the abdomen often does not have enough room for the "missing" contents. Forcing the contents into the abdomen will compress the vena cava and compromise respirations by pushing up on the diaphragm. The surgeon may be forced to omit total anatomic closure of the abdominal wall, and instead perform a skin only repair creating a ventral hernia. The final repair is then completed after the infant has been weaned off the ventilator and is clinically stable. Transthoracic approach has disadvantage of inability to correct associated intestinal malrotation and to create a ventral hernia if necessary to relieve intra-abdominal pressure. Minimally invasive thoracoscopic repair of CDH in neonates has also been done successfully.

What is the status of fetal surgery in CDH?

Open fetal surgery has proven too invasive to be justified for the treatment of CDH. Progress in postnatal therapy (including ECMO and newer adjunctive modalities) has dramatically improved the neonatal outcome in all but the most severely affected infants. Fetal tracheal occlusion as a means of improving survival in CDH is currently being investigated.

What are the prognostic factors in CDH?

The variables that predict perinatal mortality and help in deciding eligibility to prenatal intervention are presence of other lethal malformations and chromosomal aberrations which should be excluded. In isolated left-sided CDH, herniation of the liver into the chest has been shown to be a predictor of high mortality. The lung-head ratio (LHR) has been shown to adequately predict outcome in left-sided, 'liver-up' CDH. An LHR <1.0 is associated with 100% mortality, whereas all patients with an LHR >1.4 survived. Currently, fetal MRI as a means of measuring lung volume and thereby predicting pulmonary hypoplasia is being investigated. Postnatal prediction of pulmonary hypoplasia and survival in infants with CDH is more difficult to ascertain. $PaCO_2<40$ mm Hg, preductal $PaO_2>60–80$ mm Hg and a ventilatory index <1000 (VI = mean airway pressure × respiratory rate) has been shown to have the best survival rate.

What is the outcome of CDH?

The outcome of CDH differs depending on the stage of the fetus or infant's life (i.e., antenatal, immediate postnatal, and postoperative). The median overall mortality is 58% for babies diagnosed in utero, 48% if born alive, and 33% postoperatively.The lower mortality in the postoperative group is because of the fact that they were stable enough to reach surgery. An earlier intrauterine diagnosis, before 25 weeks of gestation, is not found to be uniformly a bad prognostic indicator (median mortality 60%). The outcome is worse for fetus with associated congenital anomalies (median mortality 93%). ECMO appears to improve survival and the median mortality for all ECMO-treated infants is 44%.

What is the long-term outcome in survivors of CDH?

Survivors of CDH usually have persistent pulmonary and non-pulmonary problems to deal with. Many of these patients require bronchodilators, oxygen, diuretics, and corticosteroids for obstructive airway disease and bronchopulmonary dysplasia. They are at high risk from respiratory syncytial virus (RSV) and should receive RSV immuno-prophylaxis. Developmental delay and hearing loss, both probably due to prolonged hypoxia, have been reported in patients with CDH. A significant number of survivors report gastrointestinal symptoms, including gastroesophageal reflux, which may be symptomatic and incapacitating well beyond the neonatal period. Recurrence of the hernia may lead to rapid deterioration in respiratory function, as well as gastrointestinal symptoms.

CONCLUSIONS

CDH presents as a neonatal emergency in the delivery room with a normal appearing infant not responding to resuscitation, if it has not been diagnosed by antenatal sonography. Endotracheal intubation with gentle ventilation, followed by orogastric decompression is immediately indicated. Pulmonary hypoplasia and pulmonary hypertension with right-to-left shunting are common with resultant hypoxemia. The old management strategy of immediate surgery is now replaced by physiologic stabilization and delayed surgery. The introduction of less invasive therapeutic techniques such as high frequency oscillation ventilation, inhaled nitric oxide, surfactant, and perfluorocarbon liquid ventilation may replace the need for ECMO.

TAKE HOME MESSAGES

- Avoid bag mask ventilation in infants with CDH.
- Elective gentle ventilation with permissive hypercapnia should be practised to avoid barotrauma.
- Delayed surgery after stabilization of labile physiology is preferred.
- Patients should have a long-term follow-up.

FURTHER READING

1. Badillo A, Gingalewski C. Congenital diaphragmatic hernia: Treatment and outcomes. *Semin Perinatol* 2014; 38:92–96.
2. Losty PD. Congenital diaphragmatic hernia: Where and what is the evidence? *Semin Pediatr Surg* 2014; 23:278–282.
3. Menon SC, Tani LY, Weng HY, Lally PA, Lally KP, Yoder BA, Congenital Diaphragmatic Hernia Study Group. Clinical characteristics and outcomes of patients with cardiac defects and congenital diaphragmatic hernia. *J Pediatr* 2013;162:114–119.

Chapter

30 Abdominal Wall Defects

Alpana Prasad

ABSTRACT

Gastroschisis and omphalocele are the most frequently encountered congenital abdominal wall defects. Prenatal diagnosis of omphalocele and gastroschisis may impact timing, mode and location of delivery.

Major focus of neonatal resuscitation is temperature stability, fluid resuscitation, placement of an orogastric tube for intestinal decompression, care of eviscerated bowel and examination for presence of associated anomalies.

Major focus of surgical management is closure of the abdominal wall without injury to the viscera either directly or due to increased intra-abdominal pressure. The choice between primary and staged closure should be based on this balance.

Principal cause of morbidity and mortality in infants with omphalocele is presence and severity of associated anomalies. In infants with gastroschisis, morbidity and mortality is related to the degree of bowel injury as a result of exposure to amniotic fluid or atresia.

INTRODUCTION

The most frequently encountered congenital abdominal wall defects are gastroschisis and omphalocele. There is a reported increase in the incidence of these anomalies particularly gastroschisis in the recent years probably due to widespread use of antenatal ultrasound. The early detection of these defects and the related associated anomalies allows better parental counselling and planning of delivery at a specialized centre. Presently, the repair of these defects is always possible in single or multiple stages along with the management of the associated cardiac, urinary and gastrointestinal anomalies. Long-term outcome of these neonates is generally favorable.

CASE SCENARIO

A baby girl is born to a 21-year-old primigravida mother at 36 weeks gestation by Cesarean section.

Prenatal ultrasonography done at 32 weeks gestation revealed intestinal loops free floating in the amniotic fluid, coming from the anterior abdominal wall suggestive of abdominal wall defect. The

Contd...

Contd...

mother underwent a cesarean section delivery at 36 weeks gestation after fetal lung maturation was assured.

At birth, the baby weighs 2430 gm and is otherwise normal except for intestinal loops coming through an anterior abdominal wall defect just to the right of the umbilical cord (Fig. 30.1) The bowel loops are edematous and distended. Diagnosis of gastroschisis is confirmed.

Treatment in the delivery room includes evaluation of the ABCs. The intestines are wrapped with saline soaked sterile gauze, followed by dry sterile dressings to minimize heat loss. An orogastric tube is placed to decompress the stomach and intestines and the baby is transferred to NICU.

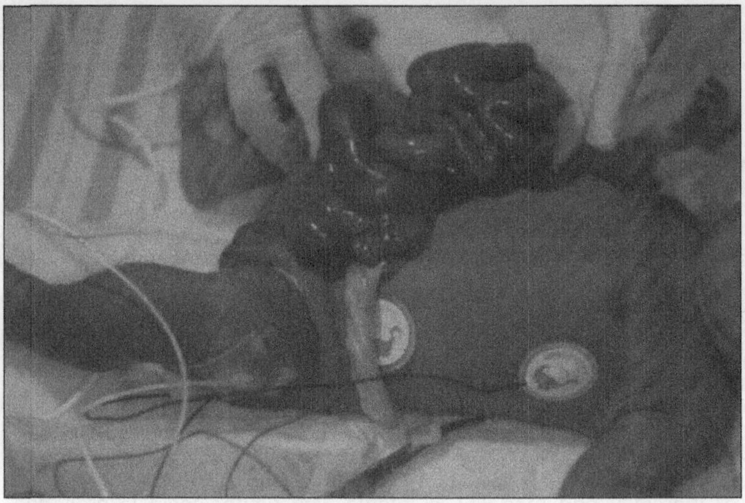

Fig. 30.1: Gastroschisis

CRITICAL CASE ANALYSIS

A neonate presenting with a defect in the abdominal wall with intestinal loops lying outside is quite obviously diagnosed as gastroschisis. Possibility of an omphalocele with ruptured sac has to be excluded as incidence of associated malformations is higher in infants with omphalocele.

The delivery room management to prevent hypothermia and fluid loss in these neonates is important.

Antenatal diagnosis helps in counselling and planning the delivery and better postnatal care.

INTERACTIVE TOPIC DISCUSSION

What is an abdominal wall defect? What is its incidence?

It is a defect in the development of abdominal wall which allows the intestine and other abdominal viscera to herniate outside the abdominal cavity. The two most common congenital abdominal wall defects are gastroschisis (herniated bowel loops are lying around free) and omphalocele (herniated viscera covered by a sac) (Fig. 30.2).

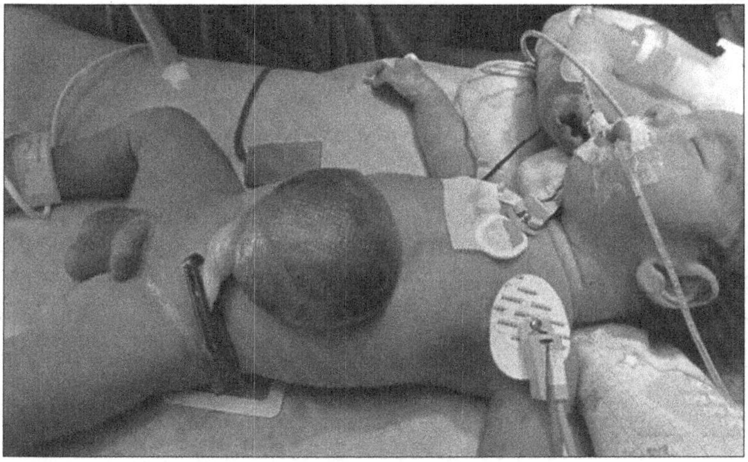

Fig. 30.2: Omphalocele

Both these conditions are obvious at birth and are usually associated with abnormal rotation and fixation of intestine.

Omphalocele occurs in one out of 5000 live births and affects boys more commonly than girls. Gastroschisis occurs in one out of 3000–3500 livebirths and equally affects both sexes. Gastroschisis is more common than omphalocele with a ratio of 1.5:1 to 2:1. There is a 10 to 20-fold increase in the overall incidence of gastroschisis in all age groups over the past 2 decades. Gastroschisis appears to occur more commonly in young mothers, especially those younger than 20 years of age.

What is the embryology of the abdominal wall defects?

Omphalocele is a central defect at the umbilical ring resulting from failure of the bowel to return to the abdomen secondary to delayed closure of the lateral folds. The eviscerated bowel loops and liver are covered by a sac consisting of peritoneum, Wharton's jelly, and amnion. Although the midgut is usually non-rotated, complications secondary to this including volvulus are infrequent, and duodenal obstruction from Ladd's bands is rare.

Failure of the cephalic fold to close leads to lower sternal abnormalities and an epigastric omphalocele, which is commonly associated with cardiac defects, pericardial absence, and a diaphragmatic defect together known as pentalogy of Cantrell. Failure of the caudal fold to close leads to a hypogastric omphalocele, often associated with bladder or cloacal exstrophy.

Gastroschisis is thought to result from a vascular accident involving the right omphalomesenteric artery leading to a defect lateral to the base of the umbilicus (usually on the right side), through which intestinal loops escape and lie free without a covering sac.

What is the etiology of these defects?

The exact etiology of these defects is not known. Omphalocele may have a genetic component, as suggested by the high incidence of associated anomalies and chromosomal abnormalities. A number of vasoactive drugs have been implicated in the causation of gastroschisis.

What are the associated anomalies in abdominal wall defects?

Associated anomalies are seen in up to two-thirds of patients with omphalocele. Of these, 18–24% are cardiac, with tetralogy of Fallot and atrial septal defects being the most common. Chromosomal abnormalities, most commonly trisomies 13, 18 and 21, occur in up to 49% of fetuses diagnosed with omphalocele. Beckwith-Wiedemann syndrome (gigantism, macroglossia and umbilical defect) occurs in 12% of cases. Pulmonary hypoplasia is also commonly associated with giant omphalocele.

Associated anomalies are less common in gastroschisis with majority involving the gastrointestinal tract. Intestinal atresia occurs in 10–15% of cases. Meckel's diverticulum and intestinal duplications have also been noted. Rarely, gastroschisis may be associated with Limb-body wall defect syndrome which includes limb abnormalities, meningocele, abnormal genitalia, intestinal atresias, and umbilical cord abnormalities.

How is abdominal wall defect diagnosed antenatally?

An abdominal wall defect is often suspected on routine screening because of elevation of the maternal serum alpha-fetoprotein (MSAFP), which is elevated in 90% of mothers carrying babies with omphalocele, and 100% of those with gastroschisis. Using a combination of maternal serum screening and ultrasound, the sensitivity and specificity for prenatal diagnosis of abdominal wall defect is 100%. In omphalocele, antenatal scan shows bowel loops and liver lying within a sac outside the fetal abdomen at the umbilicus. In such cases additional anomalies should be looked for on ultrasound, fetal echocardiography and karyotype analysis is done by amniocentesis or chorionic villous sampling. In gastroschisis, antenatal scan shows dilated bowel loops lying free in amniotic fluid adjacent to umbilical insertion.

What is the antenatal management of abdominal wall defects?

Presently, antenatal repair for either gastroschisis or omphalocele is not recommended. Prenatal diagnosis may impact the timing, location, and mode of delivery. Most infants with omphalocele should be delivered at term, whereas, infants with gastroschisis may benefit from early delivery to minimize the damage from exposure of the bowel to amniotic fluid. Mostly delivery is done at 37 weeks' gestation after documenting lung maturity. Use of routine cesarean delivery for both omphalocele and gastroschisis remains controversial. Giant omphalocele which are likely to rupture during vaginal delivery may benefit from cesarean delivery. All infants with an abdominal wall defect should undergo institutional delivery, where immediate neonatal and surgical expertise is available.

What is the management of a neonate with abdominal wall defect?

The initial treatment of a newborn with omphalocele or gastroschisis is similar and consists of fluid resuscitation, orogastric decompression of intestine, avoidance of hypothermia, and local care of the exteriorized viscera. If the size of the abdominal wall defect in gastroschisis is causing vascular compromise, the defect should be enlarged immediately. The bowel should be wrapped in warm saline-soaked gauze, supported on the anterior abdominal wall, and covered with a waterproof dry sterile dressing to minimize heat loss. Fluid requirement in neonates with gastroschisis is two and half to three times of a normal newborn on day one of life and averages approximately 175 ml/kg/day. Monitoring of acid-base and electrolytes is important as metabolic acidosis is common due to poor perfusion related to hypovolemia. Parenteral antibiotics are started and parenteral nutrition, preferably through a central venous catheter, should be initiated. No attempt should be made to reduce the eviscerated intestinal loops back into abdominal cavity. It is essential that optimal resuscitation is done and adequate urine output is established prior to surgery.

What is the surgical management of omphalocele and gastroschisis?

The goal of surgical management for both omphalocele and gastroschisis is to place the herniated viscera back into the abdomen and to provide primary closure without hemodynamic or respiratory compromise. The bowel should be inspected to look for associated atresia in gastroschisis and for evidence of a rotation abnormality. If the viscera do not fit into the abdomen without a significant increase in intra-abdominal pressure, a silastic 'silo' can be placed and the herniated contents gradually reduced back into the abdomen over the next few days. Bedside placement of a spring-loaded silo without the need for a general anesthetic is also an option. In giant omphalocele, non-operative escharotic management is usually done which involves covering the sac with silver sulfadiazine leading to formation of granulation tissue and ultimately in epithelialization. The resulting ventral hernia can be repaired at any time, when the child is medically stable. Patients with primary closure have better survival rates, reduced risk of sepsis and overall, a shorter hospital stay.

What is the outcome of infants with gastroschisis and omphalocele?

The outcome of infants born with gastroschisis depends on the condition of the intestine and is excellent in over 90% of cases. Mortality is mostly related to sepsis or late complications in babies with atresia or short bowel syndrome. They have high incidence of gastroesophageal reflux (GER) (40–50%) for which they should be closely monitored. A significant number of these patients require additional surgery, usually for adhesive intestinal obstruction, and a small group of children suffer from short bowel syndrome or long-term motility disorders which ultimately require small bowel transplantation. The outcome for infants with omphalocele is dependent on the size of defect, prematurity, intactness of sac and presence and severity of associated malformations. Overall mortality ranges between 30% and 60%. In the absence of severe pulmonary or cardiac anomalies, the majority of these children survive.

Any role of parenteral nutrition.

Considerable! Parenteral nutrition and intensive care have markedly improved survival in infants with abdominal wall defects.

CONCLUSIONS

Omphalocele or gastroschisis are congenital defects of the anterior abdominal wall. An omphalocele arises within the umbilical ring as a central defect, while a gastroschisis involves the base of the umbilical stalk, with the defect in the abdominal wall always occurring lateral to the umbilicus. The diagnosis of both types is frequently made on antenatal ultrasound. If missed, they are readily apparent at birth, where striking differences between the two are obvious. The survival rate of patients with abdominal wall defects has gradually improved and the outcome is largely dependent on coexisting anomalies. Although surviving children have a good quality of life, late surgical problems are seen, and close long-term follow-up is essential.

TAKE HOME MESSAGES

- Prenatal diagnosis of omphalocele and gastroschisis may influence timing, mode and location of delivery.
- Neonatal resuscitation should focus on temperature stability, fluid resuscitation, placement of an orogastric tube for intestinal decompression, care of eviscerated bowel and examination for presence of associated anomalies.
- The goal of surgical management is to close the abdominal wall without injury to the viscera either directly or due to increased intra-abdominal pressure. The choice between primary and staged closure should be based on this balance.
- The main cause of morbidity and mortality in infants with omphalocele is presence and severity of associated anomalies, whereas, in infants with gastroschisis, it is the degree of bowel injury as a result of exposure to amniotic fluid or atresia.

FURTHER READING

1. Gamba P, Midrio P. Abdominal wall defects: Prenatal diagnosis, newborn management, and long-term outcomes. *Semin Pediatr Surg* 2014;23:283–290.
2. Gomella TL, Cunningham MG, Eyal FG. *Neonatology,* 7th edn. New Delhi: McGraw Hill 2013.
3. Wilson EW. *Pediatric Surgery.* London: Smithson 2014.

Chapter

31 Intestinal Obstruction

Alpana Prasad

ABSTRACT

Neonatal intestinal obstruction invariably presents with bilious vomiting, often in association with abdominal distention and aberration in passage of meconium. Common causes include intestinal atresia – duodenal, jejunoileal, or rarely colonic – malrotation with or without volvulus, meconium ileus, meconium plug syndrome, Hirschsprung's disease or its variant total colonic aganglionosis or adynamic ileus related to sepsis.

Diagnosis is usually confirmed on plain abdominal X-ray. Contrast studies are required for incomplete obstruction or for excluding other causes of large bowel obstruction.

Definitive treatment is surgical. Nevertheless, preceding surgery, fluid and electrolyte correction is mandatory.

In the absence of other major associated anomalies, the outcome in infants with intestinal obstruction is good. In the absence of prematurity, low birthweight and major associated anomalies the overall outcome of these neonates is excellent.

Key Words: Abdominal distention, Adynamic ileus, Bilious vomiting, Hirschsprung's disease, Intestinal atresia, Malrotation, Meconium plug syndrome, Meconium ileus, Neonatal intestinal obstruction.

INTRODUCTION

Intestinal obstruction in neonates presents with vomiting which is usually bilious, abdominal distention and delayed, scanty or no passage of meconium. Plain X-ray abdomen is diagnostic in most of the cases showing "Double bubble" in duodenal obstruction, few air-fluid levels beyond duodenum indicates jejunal atresia, many gas filled loops indicates some form of distal ileal or colonic obstruction. Contrast enema differentiates the various types of distal bowel obstruction. Common causes of neonatal intestinal obstruction are intestinal atresia – duodenal, jejunoileal, or rarely colonic, malrotation with or without volvulus, meconium ileus, meconium plug syndrome, Hirschsprung's disease or its variant total colonic aganglionosis or adynamic ileus related to sepsis. Maternal polyhydramnios and Down's syndrome may be associated in some cases. Family history of Hirschsprung's disease, intestinal atresia or maternal diabetes may be present. Definitive treatment is surgical but prior to that fluid and electrolyte correction is mandatory. In the absence of other major associated anomalies, the outcome in infants with intestinal obstruction is good.

CASE SCENARIO

A 23-year-old primigravida mother delivers a male baby at 39 weeks gestation via normal spontaneous vaginal delivery. There were no significant antenatal or perinatal problems. Immediately following delivery, the baby appears "normal". He cries immediately and is shifted to mother's side. Oral feeds are started which baby tolerates initially. On day 2, baby presents with bilious vomiting following every feeding attempt. Hence, he is shifted to NICU. He has not passed meconium at 36 hours. On examination, the abdomen is distended and the anus is patent. A nasogastric tube is passed which drains bilious fluid. A plain X-ray abdomen is done and surgical consultation taken. X-ray abdomen shows multiple air-fluid levels suggestive of small intestinal obstruction, likely jejunoileal atresia. On detailed clinical examination no other apparent associated congenital anomaly is detected.

CRITICAL CASE ANALYSIS

This newborn presenting with bilious vomiting, abdominal distention and non-passage of meconium classically fits into the diagnosis of intestinal obstruction. Usually a plain X-ray abdomen confirms the diagnosis as was in this case. Contrast studies are not usually required. These are done only when there is a doubt in the diagnosis or when we need to differentiate between various causes of distal intestinal obstruction. The dictum is: "bilious vomiting in a neonate indicates intestinal obstruction until proven otherwise".

INTERACTIVE TOPIC DISCUSSION

INTESTINAL ATRESIA

What is the incidence of intestinal atresia?

Intestinal atresias are congenital defect in the continuity of the intestine. Jejunoileal atresias are common and account for approximately one third of all cases of neonatal intestinal obstruction. Colonic atresia is rare. The incidence of jejunoileal atresia varies from 1 in 400 live births to 1 in 3500 live births and affects both sexes equally. Isolated jejunal atresia has a higher prevalence in twins and infants with low birthweight. One third of jejunal atresia, one-fourth of ileal atresia and 50% of multiple atresia babies are of low birthweight. Small intestinal atresia is equally distributed between jejunum (51%) and ileum (49%). Involvement of proximal jejunum (31%) is more frequent than distal jejunum (20%), whereas in ileum distal (36%) involvement is more frequent than proximal (13%). Majority (>90%) of atresias are single; however, in 10% cases multiple atresia are seen.

What is the etiology of intestinal atresia?

Jejunoileal atresias are thought to occur because of an intrauterine mesenteric vascular ischemic event of the intestine such as intussusception, volvulus, malrotation, arterial occlusion, internal hernia or strangulation due to an abdominal wall defect such as an omphalocele or in gastroschisis. This may result in a focal infarction resulting in an atretic portion of bowel. These atresias are also associated with meconium ileus which occurs in newborns with cystic fibrosis.

Is an antenatal diagnosis of intestinal atresia possible?

Yes, jejunoileal atresia can be diagnosed by prenatal ultrasound in less than one-third of the cases. The presence of multiple distended loops of bowel with vigorous peristalsis seen on an ultrasound is suggestive of intestinal atresia. Also, echogenic bowel may be seen which is non-specific and is associated with any gastrointestinal malformation. About one-fourth of all infants with jejunoileal atresia have a history of maternal polyhydramnios which is more common (38%) in proximal jejunal atresia.

What are the different types of jejunoileal atresia?

There are four different types of intestinal atresias. Type I is mucosal obstruction that is caused by an epithelial intraluminal membrane, but the proximal and distal ends of the bowel are intact. In type I, which accounts for 20% of jejunoileal atresias, the bowel wall and the mesentery of the intraluminal membrane are both intact. Type II is characterized by the connection of the blind ends of the bowel by a fibrous cord with an intact mesentery and constitutes 35% of intestinal atresias. Type III is subdivided into Type IIIa and IIIb. In type IIIa, the blind ends of the bowel are completely separated by a mesenteric defect that is V-shaped. It accounts for 35% of all atresias. Type IIIb, also known as "apple peel" or "Christmas tree" deformity, describes a loss of the normal blood supply to the distal bowel and is associated with a significant mesenteric defect. It appears that there is a genetic predisposition to Type IIIb atresia. Type IV comprises 5% of all bowel atresias and is characterized by multiple bowel atresias which resemble a string of sausages (Fig. 31.1).

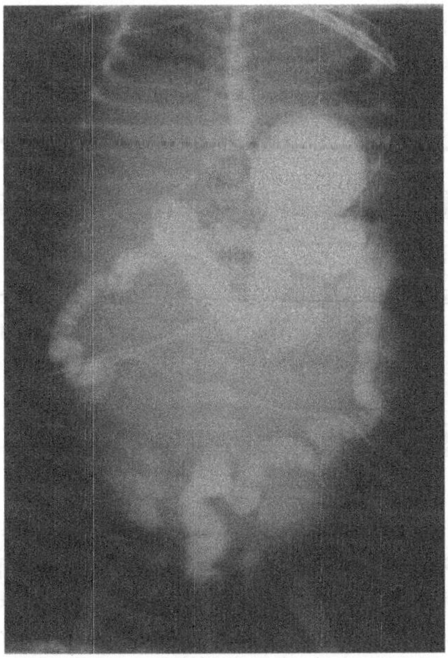

Fig. 31.1: Type IV jejunal atresia

What are the associated congenital anomalies?

As occurrence of jejunoileal atresia is related to late intrauterine vascular insult, hence, overall there is a low incidence (7%) of associated extraintestinal anomalies in these infants. Instead they may have coexisting intestinal anomalies such as malrotation, meconium peritonitis, meconium ileus, total colonic aganglionosis and neuronal intestinal dysplasia. Other congenital abnormalities are more common with duodenal and jejunal atresias as compared to ileal atresia.

What is the clinical presentation?

The majority of newborns with jejunoileal atresia present clinically with bilious vomiting or bilious gastric aspirate, abdominal distention, jaundice and failure to pass normal amount of meconium within the first 24 hours of life. However, passage of small amount of meconium does not rule out intestinal atresia because a third of infants with jejunoileal atresia may pass some meconium prior to development of obstructive symptoms. In proximal jejunal obstruction bilious vomiting is more common and presents earlier than in ileal atresia. Abdominal distension is usually more obvious in the upper abdomen in proximal jejunal atresia whereas it is more generalized in distal ileal and colonic atresia. Abdominal distension noted immediately at birth suggests the presence of giant cystic meconium peritonitis. Jaundice is also more common in jejunal (30%) than in ileal (20%) atresia and is associated with indirect hyperbilirubinemia.

How is the diagnosis of intestinal atresia confirmed?

The diagnosis is usually confirmed by a plain X-ray of abdomen in erect and supine position which may show air-fluid levels or peritoneal calcifications. The greater is the number of air-fluid levels, the more distal is the obstruction. Peritoneal calcification is seen in 12% cases and signifies meconium peritonitis secondary to intrauterine bowel perforation. Contrast enema study is useful to distinguish between ileal and colonic obstruction, shows the presence of unused colon "microcolon" in jejunoileal atresia and determines the position of caecum which may be abnormal if there is an associated malrotation. Intestinal malrotation is seen in 10% of cases. Upper GI contrast study is rarely done and is indicated only in partial or incomplete obstruction (stenosis).

What is the differential diagnosis of intestinal atresia?

The differential diagnosis of intestinal atresia will include all the conditions presenting as intestinal obstruction in neonates. These are: malrotation with or without volvulus, meconium ileus, internal hernia, colonic atresia, meconium plug, total colonic aganglionosis, Hirschsprung's disease and adynamic ileus related to sepsis. Contrast enema studies help in diagnosis of distal aganglionosis and colonic atresia.

What is the treatment of jejunoileal atresia?

Immediate management involves starting intravenous fluids for correcting fluid and electrolyte imbalance, nasogastric decompression, temperature maintenance and starting intravenous antibiotics. Monitoring of oxygen saturation by pulse oximetry and ensuring adequate urine output prior to surgery is essential. Definitive treatment requires resection of the dilated atretic portion of the bowel with an end-to-oblique anastomosis. Besides this, tapering enteroplasty is done in some cases of proximal jejunal atresia. Postoperatively, nutritional support is provided by parenteral hyperalimentation until bowel function is restored. Prognosis is determined by the length and function of the remaining bowel.

What is the outcome in infants with intestinal atresia?

In infants with intestinal atresia early mortality is related to pneumonia, peritonitis or sepsis. Postoperative complications are functional intestinal obstruction at anastomosis site or anastomosis leak. Overall survival is >90%. Mortality is higher in multiple and apple peel atresia (50–70%) and when there is associated meconium ileus, meconium peritonitis and gastroschisis. Factors affecting mortality and morbidity are prematurity, associated anomalies, respiratory distress, postoperative bowel obstruction and short bowel syndrome.

Long-term complications include malabsorption, feeding intolerance and bacterial overgrowth. Multiple atretic segments may result in a short gut syndrome with insufficient or marginal total bowel nutrition absorptive capacity.

DUODENAL ATRESIA

What is the etiology of duodenal atresia?

Duodenal atresia results from a failure of vacuolization and recanalization that occurs after the solid phase of intestinal development during week 4 and 5 of gestation. It may also be caused by local ischemia and may have a genetic component.

What is the epidemiology and different types of duodenal atresia?

Duodenal atresia occurs in 1/10,000 live births. Approximately 50% of infants with duodenal atresia are born prematurely and are of low birthweight. Duodenal atresia occurs most frequently (80%) in the second part of duodenum distal to the ampulla of Vater.

There are three types of duodenal atresia: Type I is a mucosal web with normal muscular wall. Type II describes a short, fibrous cord that connects two ends of the atretic duodenum. Type III represents complete separation of the atretic ends. Type I is the most common (65%) and type III is the least common.

What are the associated anomalies in duodenal atresia?

Down's syndrome (trisomy 21) is seen in 30% of infants with duodenal atresia. Other associated anomalies are annular pancreas, congenital heart disease, malrotation, esophageal atresia, urinary tract anomalies and anorectal malformations. Vertebral and musculoskeletal anomalies are uncommon.

What are the characteristic clinical features of duodenal atresia?

Duodenal atresia classically presents with bilious vomiting without abdominal distention on the first day of life. Other manifestations include maternal polyhydramnios which is present in 50% of cases, jaundice and intolerance to feeding. Uncommonly the vomiting may be non-bilious if the obstruction is pre-ampullary (20%).

How is the diagnosis of duodenal atresia confirmed?

Diagnosis is confirmed on plain X-ray of abdomen by the presence of the "double-bubble sign" which results from accumulation of gas in the stomach and proximal duodenum (Fig. 31.2). Because of the atresia, bowel gas does not enter the remainder of the bowel until after the first day of life. Duodenal atresia can be diagnosed prenatally by fetal ultrasonography. Early prenatal diagnosis of duodenal atresia should lead to karyotype analysis for trisomy 21 and detailed screening to exclude other associated anomalies.

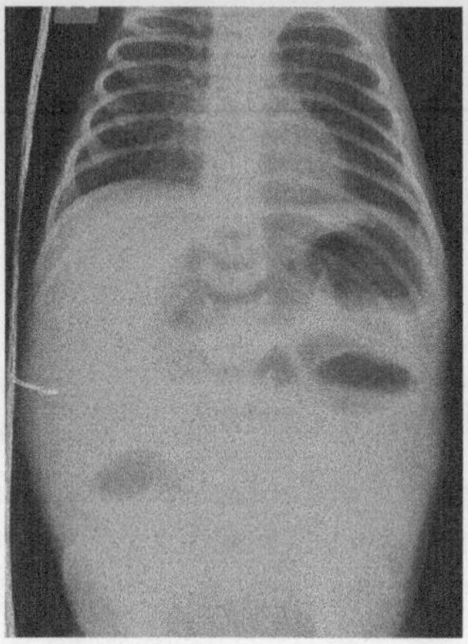

Fig. 31.2: Dodenal atresa: Double bubble sign

What is the management of a neonate with duodenal atresia?

Initial treatment consists of nasogastric decompression of stomach along with IV fluid replacement to correct fluid and electrolyte derangements. Hypothermia and hypoglycemia should be avoided. Prior to surgical correction of duodenal atresia, an evaluation for associated life-threatening congenital abnormalities should be done. Duodenal atresia is usually surgically repaired by duodeno-duodenostomy which bypasses the obstruction.

What is the outcome in duodenal atresia?

Early complications are related to anastomosis, prolonged adynamic ileus, wound infection, pneumonia or congestive heart failure. Late complications are duodenal dysmotility (megaduodenum), gastroesophageal reflux and adhesive bowel obstruction. Mortality, morbidity and long-term prognosis is determined by the presence of associated congenital abnormalities, prematurity and low birthweight. In the absence of major associated anomalies overall survival in infants with duodenal atresia is 95%.

MALROTATION

What are the characteristic clinical features of malrotation in neonates?

Malrotation in neonates presents with recurrent episodes of subacute obstruction with intermittent bilious vomiting or with sudden onset of bilious vomiting in a previously healthy neonate. Vomitus may contain altered blood and this may be accompanied with abdominal distension, abdominal tenderness, melena and shock. As bowel gangrene progresses, it may lead to perforation, peritonitis, edema and erythema of anterior abdominal wall. About 50% of infants with malrotation present within first week of life, 80% present within the first month and 90% within the first year. It may coexist with other major congenital anomalies like omphalocele and congenital diaphragmatic hernia. It may result in duodenal obstruction, volvulus, internal hernia and failure to thrive. Suspect acute volvulus secondary to malrotation if the baby has signs of shock, metabolic acidosis or peritonitis.

What are the characteristic radiological features of malrotation?

In malrotation plain X-ray of abdomen is often non-diagnostic. A "gasless" appearance with air in stomach and duodenum and little or no gas in rest of the intestine may be seen on a plain X-ray in midgut volvulus (Fig. 31.3). Diagnosis is confirmed by upper GI contrast study which shows abnormal configuration of duodenum with duodenojejunal flexure to the right side of midline and small bowel loops on right side of abdomen. In presence of volvulus, duodenum and upper jejunum show a "corkscrew" appearance. Contrast enema shows caecum and appendix in abnormal position usually in right hypochondrium or mid-abdomen.

A color doppler ultrasound is useful to determine the relationship of superior mesenteric vessels which is reversed in malrotation (SMV is to the left of SMA in malrotation).

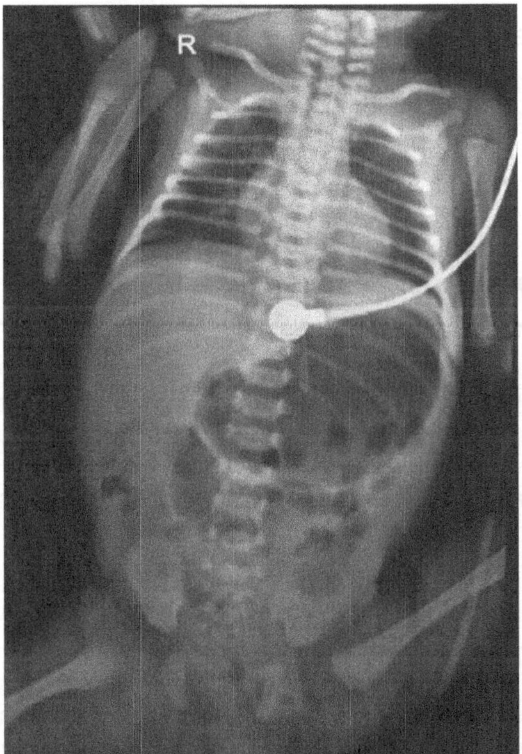

Fig. 31.3: Midgut volvulus

What are the associated anomalies in malrotation?

Associated anomalies seen with malrotation are congenital diaphragmatic hernia, Gastroschisis, Omphalocele, duodenal atresia, prune-belly syndrome and heterotaxia syndrome.

What is the management of neonates with malrotation?

Operative correction of malrotation in neonates is a surgical emergency and hence it should be undertaken after a brief period of intensive resuscitation with intravenous fluid and plasma infusion, nasogastric decompression of bowel and broad-spectrum antibiotics. Surgery involves immediate laparotomy, untwisting of bowel in counter-clockwise rotation (midgut volvulus evident by clockwise twist) and Ladd's procedure (division of bands across second part of duodenum) with appendectomy. Postoperatively, parenteral nutrition may be required if massive small bowel resection has been done.

What is the outcome in neonates with malrotation?

Recurrence of midgut volvulus after surgical correction is rare. Adhesive intestinal obstruction is not uncommon and occurs with a relative risk of 8–10%. Mortality is associated primarily with peritonitis from extensive intestinal necrosis in midgut volvulus, late nutritional complications or sepsis.

MECONIUM ILEUS

What is meconium ileus?

Intestinal obstruction in a newborn occurring due to the presence of thick and tenacious meconium throughout the distal small and large intestine is known as meconium ileus. Majority (80%) of infants with meconium ileus have cystic fibrosis and the remaining non-cystic fibrosis infants may be either full-term, healthy neonate or very low birthweight and small for gestational age. Out of all babies born with cystic fibrosis about 10–20% present with meconium ileus.

What is the genetic basis of meconium ileus?

Cystic fibrosis is an autosomal recessive disease with a reported incidence of 1 in 2000 live births in Caucasian population. The defective gene is localized to long-arm of chromosome 7. The most common mutation is the ΔF508 mutation in the CFTR (cystic fibrosis transmembrane regulator) protein. A cystic fibrosis modifier locus for meconium ileus has been found on chromosome 19.

What is the characteristic presentation of meconium ileus before and after birth?

About half of these infants present with features of intestinal obstruction: generalized abdominal distension, bilious vomiting, and failure to pass meconium in the first 24–48 hours after birth, as a result of simple luminal obstruction by meconium, known as "simple meconium ileus". The other half present with "complicated meconium ileus" secondary to volvulus, atresia, gangrene or perforation. Giant cystic meconium peritonitis occurs following an antenatal intestinal perforation which has become loculated. Antenatal ultrasound showing distended bowel loops with an echogenic bowel wall in the second or third trimester is suggestive of meconium ileus. Presence of fetal ascites, calcification and bowel dilatation are signs suggestive of meconium peritonitis. Most of the infants present at birth with grossly distended abdomen, bilious gastric aspirates and patent anus. On examination visible or palpable loops of distended intestine is present with infrequent bowel sounds and meconium may be palpable as a doughy substance in the dilated loops of distended bowel. Rectal examination shows anus and rectum are typically narrow with little mucoid stools. Family history of cystic fibrosis is not uncommon. Maternal history of polyhydramnios is present in 20% cases.

What are the radiological features of meconium ileus?

On a plain X-ray abdomen distended air-filled loops of intestine are seen; bowel contents have a "soap-bubble appearance" in right lower quadrant due to air mixed with meconium in the distal ileum. This is known as "Neuhauser's sign" and is strongly suggestive of meconium ileus. Calcification on abdominal X-ray is seen in about 13% cases and usually indicates meconium peritonitis (Fig. 31.4). Contrast enema shows narrow, unused "microcolon" with inspissated meconium proximally. Abdominal ultrasound may show intraperitoneal cyst or fluid.

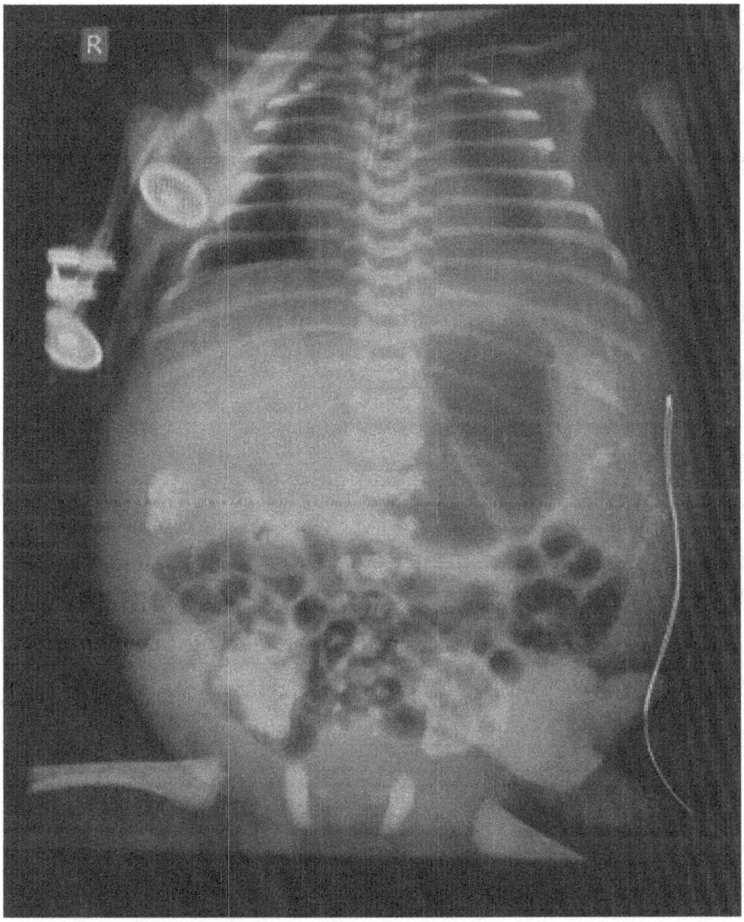

Fig. 31.4: Meconium peritonitis

What is the management of an infant with meconium ileus?

Primary management comprises nasogastric decompression with administration of intravenous fluid and broad spectrum antibiotics. Thereafter, gastrografin enemas are given. These have a success rate of 35–65%. Multiple enemas may be required. There is a 10% reported risk of perforation with enema. Surgery is indicated if gastrografin enemas do not relieve the obstruction or infant appears too ill to delay operation or diagnosis of meconium ileus is uncertain. In complicated meconium ileus with persistent or worsening abdominal distension, persistent bowel obstruction, enlarging abdominal mass, suspected intestinal atresia, volvulus or perforation, or meconium pseudocyst formation with peritonitis or suspected bowel necrosis immediate surgery is indicated.

What is the outcome in meconium ileus?

Infants with meconium ileus have excellent (100%) survival with present day advanced neonatal intensive, surgical and anesthetic care. Postoperative complications like adhesive obstruction and prolonged ileus are reported. Gastrointestinal complications of meconium ileus include an increased incidence of intussusception, rectal prolapse, acute or chronic appendicitis, calculous cholecystitis, malabsorption and colonic strictures. The early morbidity and mortality in meconium ileus is of pulmonary origin including bacterial sepsis and bronchopneumonia. Mortality may also be related to intraperitoneal sepsis from unrecognized leakage or short bowel syndrome with complicating liver failure.

CONCLUSIONS

Neonatal intestinal obstruction usually presents with bilious vomiting. Abdominal distension and non-passage of meconium is not always present. Diagnosis is usually confirmed on plain abdominal X-ray and contrast studies are required for incomplete obstruction or for excluding other causes of large bowel obstruction. In the absence of prematurity, low birthweight and major associated anomalies the overall outcome of these neonates is excellent.

TAKE HOME MESSAGE

- Bilious vomiting in a neonate is usually due to a surgical cause until proven otherwise.
- Fluid and electrolyte imbalance should be corrected before proceeding to surgery.
- Associated congenital malformations should always be looked for before definitive surgery.
- In the absence of major associated anomalies the overall outcome of neonates with intestinal obstruction is excellent.

FURTHER READING

1. Adams SD, Stanton MP. Malrotation and intestinal atresias. *Early Hum Dev* 2014;90:921–925.

2. Applebaum H, Sydorak R. Duodenal atresia and stenosis—Annular pancreas. In: Coran AG (ed): *Pediatric Surgery*, 7th edn. Philadelphia: Elsevier/Saunders 2012;1051–1057.

3. Conforti A, Morini F, Bagolan P. Difficult esophageal atresia: Trick and treat. *Semin Pediatr Surg* 2014; 23:261–269.

4. Frischer JS, Azizkhan RG. Jejunoileal atresia and stenosis. In: Coran AG (ed): *Pediatric Surgery*, 7th ed. Phildelphia: Elsevier/Saunders 2012;1059–1071.

5. Ziegler MM. Meconium Ileus. In: Coran AG (ed): *Pediatric Surgery*, 7th edn. Philadelphia; Elsevier/Saunders 2012;1073–1083.

Chapter

32 Hirschsprung's Disease

Alpana Prasad

ABSTRACT

Hirschsprung's disease, one of the common causes of neonatal intestinal obstruction, should be suspected in any neonate presenting with abdominal distention, feeding intolerance and delayed passage of meconium beyond 48 hours. Rectal examination may reveal a patent but tight anus. The diagnosis is confirmed by radiographic studies, anorectal manometry and a rectal biopsy. Contrast enema is usually diagnostic and shows both the transition zone and the length of the distal aganglionic segment of bowel. Rectal biopsy is the gold standard for diagnosing Hirschsprung's disease and shows absence of ganglion cells in myenteric and submucosal plexuses and presence of hypertrophied nerve trunks. Treatment involves bowel decompression and resection of distal aganglionic bowel with pull-through of ganglionated proximal bowel to the anal verge. A wide spectrum of complications has been reported following definitive repair of Hirschsprung's disease. Enterocolitis remains the most serious late complication following definitive repair, others being chronic constipation, incontinence and encopresis. The majority (94%) of infants with Hirschsprung's disease do quite well following definitive operation regardless of the technique employed.

Key Words: Chronic constipation, Congenital intestinal agangliosis, Congenital megacolon, Down syndrome, Encopresis, Enterocolitis, Hirschsprung's disease, Incontinence, Rectal biopsy, Total intestinal gangliosis.

INTRODUCTION

Hirschsprung's disease (also known as congenital megacolon or congenital intestinal aganglionosis) is one of the important causes of neonatal intestinal obstruction exceeded only by intestinal atresia, malrotation and meconium ileus. It has a reported incidence of 1 in 5000 live births with a 4:1 predominance in boys. It is characterized by the absence of ganglion cells in the distal bowel beginning at the internal sphincter and extending proximally for varying distances. The most frequently involved areas of aganglionosis are the rectum and sigmoid, with decreasing incidence progressing cephalad. Aganglionosis is confined to rectosigmoid in 75% of cases; proximal sigmoid or splenic flexure in 17%; total colonic with short segment of ileum in 8%. Total intestinal aganglionosis is the most rare form. Long segment involvement is common in girls with M:F ratio of 1.5–2:1.

CASE SCENARIO

A 3-day-old term male infant had an uneventful perinatal course and was discharged to home at 24 hours of age after a normal vaginal delivery. His mother noted that he initially fed well but developed bilious vomiting on day 3 of life and passed very small amount of meconium for the first time on day 3 after rectal stimulation. On examination he is alert and active; vital signs are normal, weight 3.4 kg; capillary refill is <2 seconds, lungs are clear; no cardiac murmur; abdomen is diffusely distended and non-tender; bowel sounds are very active but not obstructive in nature. No abdominal masses or organomegaly is appreciated. Anus is patent and normally located. Digital rectal examination is followed by prompt evacuation of a large amount of meconium. An abdominal X-ray reveals large dilated loops of bowel but no air in the rectum. A hand injected contrast enema done after 48 hours shows no distinct transition zone. A further 24-hour delayed film shows significant retention of contrast. A rectal biopsy reveals absence of ganglion cells and presence of hypertrophied nerve fibers consistent with the diagnosis of Hirschsprung's disease. Rectal irrigations are not successful in decompressing the colon leading to surgery and the establishment of a descending colonic stoma placed under biopsy guidance.

CRITICAL CASE ANALYSIS

A term neonate presenting with history of feeding intolerance, generalized abdominal distention and delayed passage of meconium on rectal stimulation after a couple of days after birth should be suspected to have distal intestinal obstruction. On digital rectal examination, presence of empty rectum and prompt evacuation of meconium following it, suggests Hirschsprung's disease (HD). Plain abdominal X-ray usually shows dilated bowel loops and if rectal gas shadow is absent then there is high probability of HD. Contrast enema with a 24 hours plain film showing significant retention of contrast or a transition zone is suggestive of HD. The diagnosis is confirmed on rectal biopsy (suction mucosal or full-thickness) which reveals absence of ganglion cells and presence of hypertrophied nerve fibres.

INTERACTIVE TOPIC DISCUSSION

What is the etiology of Hirschsprung's disease?

The various factors attributed to the causation of Hirschsprung's disease are: failure of migration of neural crest cells (earlier is the arrest of migration, the longer is the aganglionic segment), altered distribution of extracellular matrix, abnormal expression of neurotrophic factors (NGF-nerve growth factor, NT-3 neurotrophic factor 3), neural cell adhesion molecule (NCAM), major histocompatibility complex (MHC) class-II antigens and genetic factors. There is a familial inheritance factor greatest among siblings but less common among children of parents with the disease. Hirschsprung's disease mutations have been mapped to RET proto-oncogenes at 10Q11.2, the recessive EDNRB gene at 13Q22, its ligand endothelin 3 (EDN3) and glial cell line-derived neurotrophic factor (GDNF). Although the majority of cases are multigenic or multifactorial, there are some conditions associated with Hirschsprung's disease.

Can you specify condition associated with Hirschsprung's disease?

Down's syndrome, Waardenburg syndrome, neurofibromatosis, neuroblastoma, pheochromocytoma, the MEN2B syndrome, etc. are the best known.

What is the pathophysiology of Hirschsprung's disease?

The pathophysiology of Hirschsprung's disease is not fully understood. Abnormal adrenergic, cholinergic, peptidergic and nitergic innervation leads to spasticity of aganglionic intestine. Abnormalities of nerve-supporting cells and altered distribution of interstitial cells in Cajal (ICC) in aganglionic bowel has been reported. The aganglionic bowel lacks normal peristalsis resulting in functional obstruction.

How does the Hirschsprung's disease present clinically?

Delayed passage of meconium beyond 48 hours is the cardinal symptom seen in up to 90% of neonates. Other common presenting symptoms are abdominal distension, poor feeding, bilious vomiting and constipation during early neonatal period. More than 90% of infants are symptomatic and diagnosed in neonatal period. Failure to thrive is usually seen beyond the neonatal period.

A temperature probe may be gently inserted to prove anal patency. One-third of infants present with diarrhea which is almost always suggestive of enterocolitis. Sudden onset of marked abdominal distension, bilious vomiting, fever, signs of dehydration and shock along with explosive expulsion of gas and foul smelling stools on rectal examination suggests "toxic megacolon" and is the commonest cause of death. The diagnosis of Hirschsprung's disease is based on clinical history, radiological studies, anorectal manometry and histopathological examination of rectal biopsy.

Any role of per rectum examination.

Syndrome may be seen in 4-5% of cases.

A digital rectal examination in a neonate is usually not helpful. In fact, it may prevent an accurate contrast enema study.

What are the radiological features of Hirschsprung's disease?

In Hirschsprung's disease plain abdominal X-ray usually shows dilated loops of intestine with air-fluid levels and a gasless rectum (Fig. 32.1). Pneuomoperitoneum may be present occasionally suggesting the presence of intestinal perforation. A hand injected contrast enema should be obtained to outline the rectum and sigmoid colon. Intestines should not be overfilled which may lead to obscuring of the transition zone. Contrast enema demonstrates narrow spastic rectum and distal intestinal segment with dilated proximal bowel (Figs. 32.2 and 32.3). Significant retention of contrast on a 24 hours delayed film strongly suggests the diagnosis despite the absence of a definite transition area. Hirschsprung's disease is diagnosed on barium enema with 75–80% accuracy. Contrast enemas in infants less than 2 months old may be non-diagnostic in over 20% of cases.

What is the pathology in Hirschsprung's disease?

The characteristic gross pathological feature is dilatation and hypertrophy of proximal colon with abrupt or gradual transition to narrow distal bowel. When clinical and radiographic findings are unable to make a definitive diagnosis, a rectal biopsy (suction mucosal biopsy or full thickness rectal biopsy) becomes necessary. **A full thickness rectal biopsy is the gold standard for the diagnosis of Hirschsprung's disease.** It shows absence of ganglion cells in myenteric and submucosal plexuses and presence of hypertrophied non-myelinated nerve trunks. There is marked increase in acetylcholinesterase activity in lamina propria and muscularis which is evident as coarse, discreet cholinergic nerve fibres stained

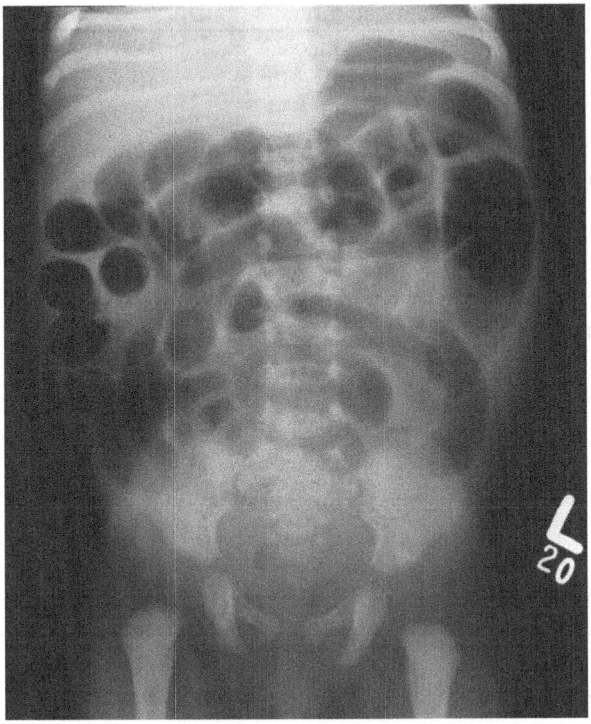

Fig. 32.1: Plain X-ray abdomen with dilated bowel loops and absent rectal gas shadow suggestive of Hirschsprung's disease

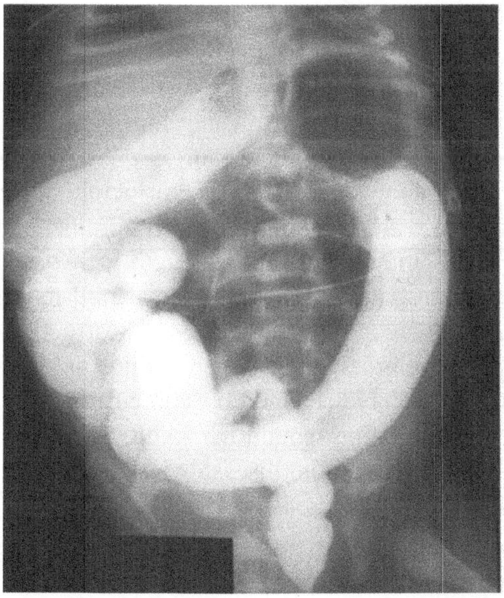

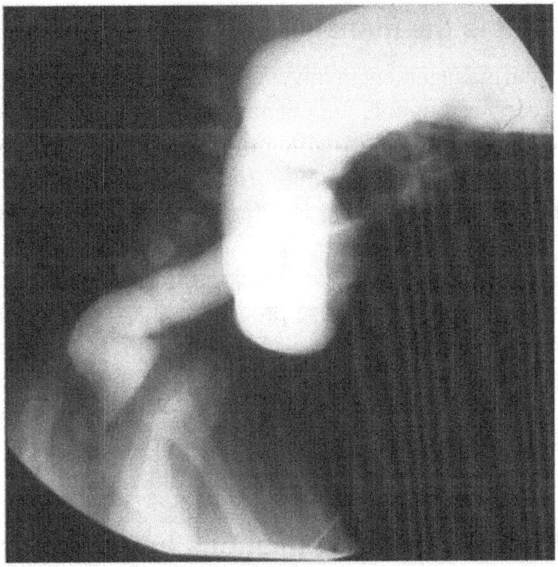

Figs. 32.2 and 32.3: Barium enema showing rectosigmoid transition zone suggestive of Hirschsprung's disease

brown to black. Proximally there is hypoganglionic segment of varying length with reduced number of ganglion cells and nerve fibres. A rectal mucosal suction biopsy of Meissner's plexus located in the muscularis propria (i.e., performed more superficially and less invasively) is the preferred biopsy technique in neonates. Ganglion cells are absent in the most distal 2 centimeters of the normal rectum which is of importance when performing the biopsy and in the determination of an ultra-short segment Hirschsprung's disease (i.e., the rectal biopsy should ideally be obtained proximal to this region).

What is the role of anorectal manometry in the diagnosis of Hirschsprung's disease?

Anorectal manometry measures the resting anal sphincter pressure which is elevated in infants with Hirschsprung's disease. The normal physiologic pressure in the anal canal during defecation involves a decrease in internal sphincter pressure (relaxation) with rectal distention, thus allowing passage of the fecal bolus. In an infant with Hirschsprung's disease this relaxation of the involuntary internal sphincter does not occur, which can be assessed by anorectal manometry. Although anorectal manometry is an excellent screening method for exclusion of Hirschsprung's disease, it is difficult and less reliable in neonates.

What is the differential diagnosis of Hirschsprung's disease?

The most common differential diagnoses of Hirschsprung's disease are:

- Mechanical obstruction – in meconium ileus, distal ileal or colonic atresia or stenosis, low imperforate anus.
- Functional obstruction – in prematurity, sepsis and electrolyte imbalance, hypothyroidism, small left colon syndrome, meconium plug syndrome, or neuronal intestinal dysplasia.

What is the management of Hirschsprung's disease?

Initial management involves correction of fluid and electrolyte imbalance along with bowel decompression as early as possible. Parenteral nutrition and effective antibiotics are started. Bowel decompression may be done by rectal irrigation or a levelling colostomy just above the transition zone in the ganglionic intestine. A definitive pull-through procedure is done at 6–12 months age. The basic principle of pull-through surgery involves resection of aganglionated intestine with restoration of fecal continence by means of anastomosis of ganglionated bowel to the anal verge. Commonly used procedures are Swenson's rectosigmoidectomy, Duhamel's retrorectal transanal procedure and Soave's endorectal pull-through procedure. Each of these procedures has been successful in overcoming the functional obstruction in the great majority of cases. Recently with the introduction of minimally invasive procedures involving laparoscopic dissection and various stapling devices, techniques have changed but the basic concepts for overcoming the non-relaxing, functionally obstructive distal colon remain the same. Single stage transanal pull-through surgery is being done in neonates with rectosigmoid disease who are stable and diagnosed early. In the very small, critically ill infant multistage procedure is preferred.

What are the complications in Hirschsprung's disease?

Complications can be grouped as early and late. **Early complications** are wound infection, bleeding, anastomotic complications (leak, pelvic abscess, cuff abscess), wound dehiscence, retraction of pull-through segment and stoma related complications. **Late complications** are enterocolitis, constipation, adhesive intestinal obstruction, anastomotic strictures, fecal incontinence, perianal excoriation, sphincter achalasia and voiding and sexual dysfunction.

Enterocolitis, characterized by abdominal distension and pain, fever, explosive watery diarrhea with foul smelling stools and vomiting is the most common complication. It may occur prior to colostomy or after a pull-through procedure. It occurs in a quarter to a third of cases and its spectrum varies from mild infection to fulminant gram-negative septicaemia. It should be treated early and aggressively with rectal irrigations to decompress the colon along with antibiotics, anal dilatations, intravenous support and bowel rest as death may occur if it is neglected. Although fever and signs of infection may be present, stool cultures are often not helpful. Each of the pull-through procedure has its own complications. About 5% of infants who have undergone Swenson procedure experience anastomotic leaks. Incomplete emptying of the aganglionic portion of the pouch occurs in some infants following Duhamel procedure and presents with persistent constipation. Patients who have undergone Soave endorectal pull-through may suffer from cuff abscesses and may require continued dilatations. A limited number of Hirschsprung's patients may have coexisting neuronal intestinal dysplasia that may explain continued postoperative morbidity and persistent constipation in some cases. In HD mortality is low (<2%). Apart from children who die of associated cardiac anomalies or other major anomalies, toxic enterocolitis remains the most common cause of disease-related postoperative death. Other causes of death include sepsis, abscess, hemorrhage, pneumonia and embolism.

What is the outcome in Hirschsprung's disease?

Most patients continue to improve bowel control for several years postoperatively and majority achieves satisfactory continence and function with time. Long-term outcome depends on the intensity of bowel training, social background and respective intelligence of patients. Continued advances in our understanding of the disturbances in bowel motility and the immunological and neurohormonal forces involved in this disorder will result in an improvement in its prognosis.

CONCLUSIONS

Hirschsprung's disease is one of the common causes of neonatal intestinal obstruction. It should be suspected in any neonate presenting with abdominal distension, feeding intolerance and delayed passage of meconium beyond 48 hours. Rectal examination may reveal a patent but tight anus. The diagnosis is confirmed by radiographic studies, anorectal manometry and a rectal biopsy. Contrast enema is usually diagnostic and shows both the transition zone and the length of the distal aganglionic segment of bowel. Rectal biopsy is the gold standard for diagnosing Hirschsprung's disease and shows absence of ganglion cells in myenteric and submucosal plexuses and presence of hypertrophied nerve trunks. Treatment involves bowel decompression and resection of distal aganglionic bowel with pull-through of ganglionated proximal bowel to the anal verge. A wide spectrum of complications has been reported following definitive repair of Hirschsprung's disease. Enterocolitis remains the most serious late complication following definitive repair, others being chronic constipation, incontinence and encopresis. The majority (94%) of infants with Hirschsprung's disease do quite well following definitive operation regardless of the technique employed.

TAKE HOME MESSAGES

- Any neonate presenting with abdominal distension, feeding intolerance and delayed passage of meconium beyond 48 hours should be suspected to have Hirschsprung's disease.
- Contrast enema demonstrating distal narrow rectum and abrupt transition of dilated colon proximally, is diagnostic in up to 80% cases. Significant retention of contrast in delayed 24 hours film is suggestive of Hirschsprung's disease in neonates.
- Rectal biopsy is the gold standard for diagnosis of Hirschsprung's disease showing absence of ganglion cells in distal spastic segment.
- Treatment involves early bowel decompression by rectal irrigation or levelling colostomy just above the transition zone followed by definitive pull-through surgery which may be done as single staged or multi-staged procedure.

FURTHER READING

1. Gomella TL, Cunningham MD, Eyal FG. *Neonatology*. New Delhi: McGraw Hill/Lange 2013.
2. Langer JC. Hirschsprung's disease. In: Coran AG (ed): *Pediatric Surgery*, 7th edn. Philadelphia; Elsevier/Saunders, 2012;1265–1278.
3. Wilson EW. *Pediatric Surgery*. London: Smithson 2014.

Chapter

33 Esophageal Atresia and Tracheoesophageal Fistula

Alpana Prasad

ABSTRACT

Amongst the congenital anomalies of the esophagus, esophageal atresia with a distal TEF tops the list in frequency. A newborn presenting with excessive salivation and respiratory distress at birth should be suspected of this diagnosis. Failure to pass a 10 Fr stomach tube beyond 10 cm. from the lips confirms the diagnosis.

Such factors as prematurity, low birth weight associated life-threatening cardiac and other anomalies, superimposed pneumonia and presence of long-gap atresia are important prognostic factors.

A good perioperative care, meticulous surgical technique and aggressive management of associated anomalies improve the survival in these infants. Long-term follow-up of these infants is imperative for improved quality of life in such infants.

Key Words: Distal tracheoesophageal fistula, Long gap esophageal atresia, Low birthweight, Prematurity, Superimposed pneumonia, Quality of life, Tracheoesophageal fistula.

INTRODUCTION

Esophageal atresia (EA), with or without tracheoesophageal fistula (TEF), is the most common congenital anomaly of the esophagus. In the current era, due to advances in neonatal intensive care, neonatal anesthesia, better surgical technique and prenatal diagnosis, the mortality in these infants is minimal. Prematurity, low birthweight, associated life-threatening cardiac and other anomalies, pneumonia and presence of long-gap atresia are important prognostic factors. Though the outcome is generally good, this is a technically challenging anomaly for the surgeon.

CASE SCENARIO

A baby girl was born to a 25-year-old primigravida mother at 36 weeks gestation by an uneventful vaginal delivery. Mother had polyhydramnios on antenatal ultrasound scan done just prior to delivery.

The baby looked normal at birth. However, excessive salivation is noticed when the baby is being shifted to nursery. An attempt to pass orogastric tube in to the stomach, fails. A plain abdominal

Contd...

Contd...

radiograph is done with a size 10 red rubber catheter passed per orally in to the upper esophagus. X-ray reveals the blind ending upper esophagus with the catheter in-situ and presence of bowel gas shadows in abdomen (Fig. 33.1).

The baby's symptoms along with the radiographic findings are suggestive of esophageal atresia with distal tracheoesophageal fistula.

Immediately frequent suctioning of blind upper esophageal pouch is initiated along with supplemental oxygen by nasal cannula. Pulse oximeter is placed for monitoring oxygen saturation which remains between 92 and 98% as long as frequent suctioning is done. No other obvious congenital abnormality is noticed and the baby is transferred to NICU for further evaluation and management.

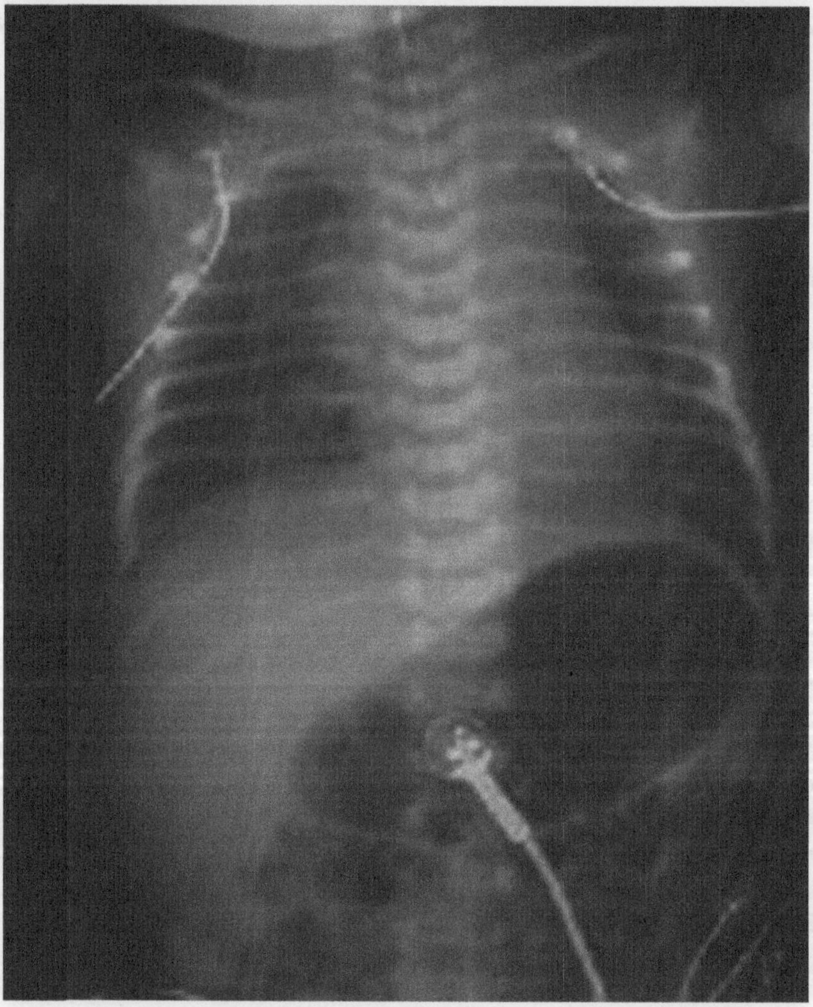

Fig. 33.1: Esophageal atresia with tracheoesophageal fistula

CRITICAL CASE ANALYSIS

A newborn presenting with respiratory distress at birth along with excessive oral secretions despite frequent oral suctioning should be suspected to have esophageal atresia. History of maternal polyhydramnios further supports the diagnosis but may not be present in all cases. Clinical confirmation of diagnosis is possible at bedside by gently passing a 10 Fr stiff orogastric catheter which gets arrested at about 10 cm distance, confirming the blind ending upper esophagus. A plain X-ray chest and abdomen with catheter in place confirms the diagnosis of esophageal atresia which may be with or without a tracheoesophageal fistula (TEF). The presence of TEF is confirmed by seeing air-filled bowel loops in abdomen on an X-ray. Other associated congenital malformations are absent in the infant.

INTERACTIVE TOPIC REVIEW

What is the incidence of esophageal atresia? What are the different types of EA and their relative frequency?

The incidence of esophageal atresia (EA) varies from 1 in 3000–4500 live births, with a slight male preponderance. Approximately one-third of infants with esophageal atresia are born prematurely. The most common type is EA with distal TEF seen in 87%, followed by isolated EA in 8% and H-type TEF in 4%. Uncommon types of EA with both proximal and distal fistulas and EA with proximal fistula are seen in <1% each (Fig. 33.2).

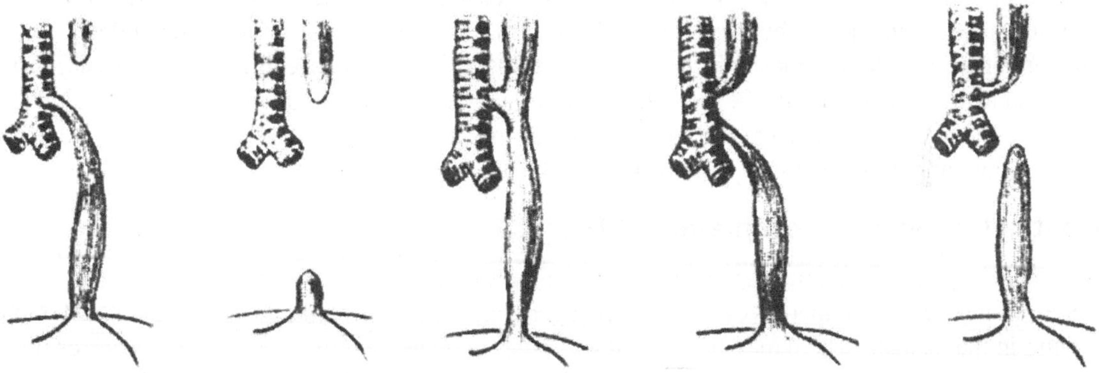

87% 8% 4% <1% <1%

Fig. 33.2: Types of esophageal atresia with tracheoesophageal fistula

What is the etiology of EA? What is its risk of recurrence?

The etiology of EA is multifactorial and involves multiple genes and complex gene-environment interactions. Exposure to teratogenic drugs during pregnancy has been implicated, including thalidomide, progesterone and estrogen. The estimated risk of recurrence for parents of a single affected child is 0.5–2.0%, rising to 20% if another sibling is born with EA. The vertical transmission risk is 3–4%.

What is the embryology of EA?

It is believed that EA occurs as a result of the failure of the primitive foregut to recanalize. When EA is accompanied by a fistula, these tracheoesophageal fistulas (TEF) occur due to the failure of the lung bud to separate from the foregut in the 4th week of gestation. Another theory suggests that the pathogenesis of EA may be related to defective pharyngeal arch development.

How can EA be diagnosed antenatally and what is the advantage of antenatal diagnosis?

The absence of stomach bubble and associated polyhydramnios (from inability of the fetus to swallow and absorb amniotic fluid) are classical antenatal ultrasound features of EA. Rate of antenatal diagnosis is only 20–40%, and there is a high false-positive rate. The ultrasound finding of an anechoic area in the middle of the fetal neck along with maternal polyhydramnios and a small stomach increases the accuracy of antenatal diagnosis. A careful search for associated chromosomal or cardiac anomalies is important as presence of a chromosomal abnormality may have implications for termination of pregnancy.

Fetal diagnosis is advantageous, as delivery can be planned at a specialist center with full neonatal surgical facility. Also, it reduces the likelihood of inadvertent feeding and aspiration pneumonitis.

What are the associated anomalies in EA?

Between 50 and 70% of infants with EA have at least one associated congenital malformation. Cardiovascular anomalies (PDA, VSD, ASD, TOF) occur most frequently in 29–35%, followed by genitourinary (absent kidney, hypospadias) in 24%, gastrointestinal (imperforate anus, duodenal atresia, annular pancreas, pyloric stenosis) in 15–24%, musculoskeletal (hemivertebrae, limb dysplasia) in 13–22%, and neurological in 12%. The incidence of VACTERL association (vertebral, anal atresia, cardiac, tracheo-esophageal, renal defects and limb dysplasia) in EA is approximately 25–30%. The anomalies are most common in isolated EA (without TEF) and least in H-type TEF.

What is the clinical presentation of EA?

Esophageal atresias should be suspected if there is history of maternal polyhydramnios or excessive oral secretions in a neonate or there is cyanosis, choking, regurgitation or coughing occurring with attempted feeding in the neonate. There may be respiratory distress due to aspiration of oral secretions or due to reflux of gastric secretions through the distal tracheoesophageal fistula. Abdomen may be distended in EA with TEF due to air trapping in stomach and intestine especially if bag mask ventilation had been done. In isolated EA without TEF, the abdomen is usually scaphoid.

How is the diagnosis of EA confirmed?

The diagnosis of an EA can be confirmed by passing a firm catheter per orally into the esophagus until it meets resistance. Then a plain X-ray of chest and abdomen is taken which shows the arrest of the tube in the proximal esophageal pouch. A gasless abdomen is suggestive of isolated EA without a TEF (Fig. 33.3). Presence of gas in the stomach and bowel confirms a distal TEF. Figure 33.4 shows air fluid levels suggestive of jejunal atresia. Contrast studies are not required and should not be done. Bronchoscopy is usually done for suspected H-type TEF.

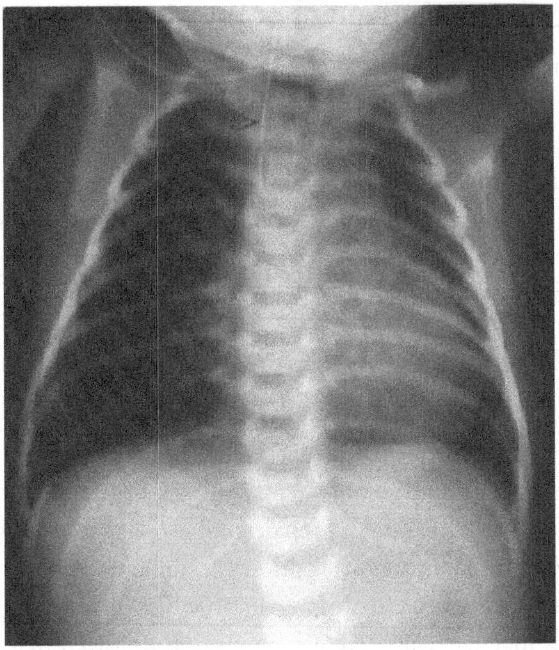

Fig. 33.3: Isolated esophageal atresia with gasless abdomen

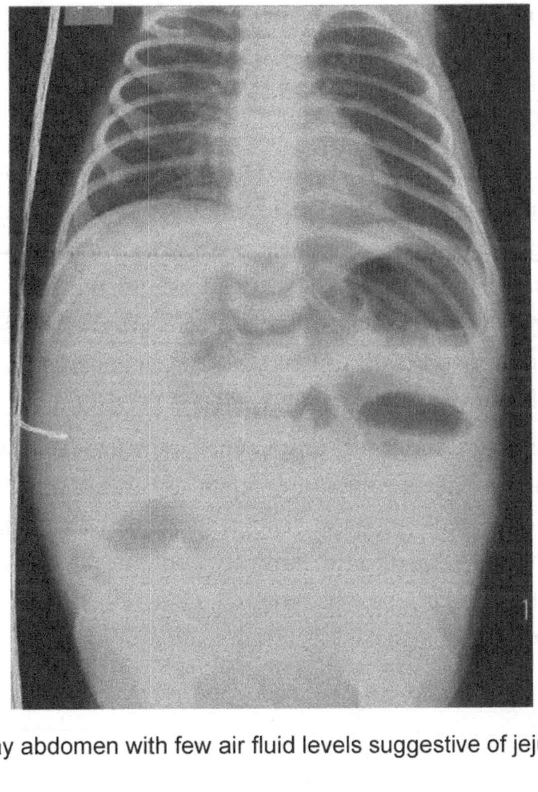

Fig. 33.4: X-ray abdomen with few air fluid levels suggestive of jejunoileal atresia

What is the preoperative management of EA with TEF?

Newborns with EA require gentle, frequent suctioning of the blind upper esophageal pouch. A double-lumen Replogle type of catheter is best for this purpose. Neonate should be placed in the head-up (30^0 elevated) and prone position to minimize both the risk of aspiration of oral secretions and the flow of gastric contents into the lungs. Oral intake should be discontinued and intravenous fluids and broad-spectrum antibiotics should be started. Bag mask ventilation or nasal CPAP should be avoided. Oxygen by nasal cannula may be given to maintain oxygen saturation >90%. A work-up to rule out associated anomalies (echocardiography, renal ultrasound, X-ray spine, chromosomal analysis) should be done.

What is the surgical management of EA?

The goal of surgical treatment is to achieve complete primary repair. The operative approach depends on the specific type of EA and the presence of associated anomalies. In EA with distal TEF, right thoracotomy and ligation of TEF and primary repair of esophagus is usually done. In long gap EA with TEF or isolated EA without TEF, delayed repair until esophageal ends come closer, or esophageal replacement surgery are the available surgical options. In preterm infants with significant respiratory distress, staged approach is preferred. Staged repair involves initial gastrostomy and upper pouch suctioning for 1–2 months together with parenteral nutrition followed by delayed complete definitive repair. Routine cervical esophagostomy is avoided if possible.

Postoperatively, an esophagogram should be performed before feeding is resumed to determine the integrity of the esophageal anastomosis.

What are the complications of EA?

The complications in infants with EA can be divided in to early and late. Early complications are anastomotic leak, anastomotic stricture and recurrent tracheoesophageal fistula. Anastomotic leak occurs in 15–20% of cases and up to 95% of these leaks close spontaneously with adequate drainage and nutritional support. Anastomotic stricture requiring dilatation may occur in up to 80% cases. Those which do not respond to repeated esophageal dilatation are usually associated with severe GER and require surgical resection of stricture with esophageal reanastomosis. Recurrent TEF occurs in up to 10% of cases and almost always requires surgical repair if it persists beyond 4 weeks.

Late complications are gastroesophageal reflux (GER), tracheomalacia and disordered esophageal peristalsis. Reflux occurs in 30–70% of babies after repair of EA. Initially, it can be managed medically but those that fail to respond will require fundoplication surgery. Symptomatic tracheomalacia is seen in 10–25% of infants after repair of EA with TEF. It mostly improves with time but if the patient has acute life threatening apneic spells then aortopexy is required. Other complications of the disease are failure to thrive, slow feeding, esophageal stenosis, recurrent aspiration pneumonia, reactive airway disease, coughing and choking.

What is the outcome of infants with EA?

The overall survival rates for infants with EA with or without TEF, is 85–95%. Survival in good-risk category (term neonate with birthweight >1500 gm, no significant pneumonia and no major cardiac disease) is almost 100%. The risk of mortality and long-term morbidity is higher in preterm or low birthweight infants (<1500 gm), in infants with major congenital heart disease, severe associated anomalies or ventilator dependency or if there is a long gap between the two esophageal ends. Prognosis is also determined by the extent of pulmonary aspiration and severity of pneumonia. Patients with EA commonly have structural malformations of the trachea, such as, degeneration of elastic, cartilage and connective tissue of the trachea (tracheomalacia). However, tracheal development is normal if it is an isolated EA without a TEF.

What is an H-type TEF?

Uncommonly, infants have a tracheoesophageal fistula (TEF) without an EA. This is known as H-type TEF (also known as N-type as the connection between the trachea and esophagus is more oblique like an N). It usually presents with choking on feeds and cyanotic episodes in a neonate. Older children may present with recurrent coughing, repeated chest infections along with aspiration pneumonia. H-type TEF is commonly diagnosed in childhood or sometimes even later, by esophageal instillation of methylene blue followed by bronchoscopy to look for dye entering the trachea. Once identified, H-type TEF requires surgical correction.

What is the long-term outcome in infants with EA?

Symptoms of asthma and bronchitis are frequent, especially in the young child, and may persist into adolescence. Tracheobronchial inflammation and airway narrowing have been demonstrated by bronchoscopy in one-third of patients. Long-term follow-up studies have shown that only 10% of adults have severely deranged lung functions. Esophageal dysmotility is a significant factor in long-term morbidity. Less severe symptoms of dysphagia have been reported in 20% of adolescents and in 48% of adults in long-term follow-up studies. GER may persist into adult life. Incidence of symptoms of heartburn and acid brash ranges between 18 and 50%. Medical treatment for GER in all EA infants might reduce the incidence of long-term respiratory complications. Chest wall deformities and scoliosis is reported in about 20% cases. Scoliosis is more common in those with vertebral anomalies. The long-term outcomes have also generally been favorable.

CONCLUSIONS

Esophageal atresia with a distal TEF is the most common congenital anomaly of the esophagus. It should be suspected in any newborn presenting with excessive salivation and respiratory distress at birth. Diagnosis is confirmed by inability to pass a 10 Fr stomach tube beyond 10 cm from the lips. Improvements in perioperative care, meticulous surgical technique and aggressive management of associated anomalies, has led to increased survival in these infants. Long-term follow-up of these infants tends to improve their quality of life.

TAKE HOME MESSAGES

- Antenatal diagnosis in EA is uncommon and should be suspected in presence of maternal polyhydramnios and small or absent fetal stomach on antenatal scan.
- Institutional delivery is a must if antenatal diagnosis is suspected.
- Bag mask ventilation and nasal CPAP should be avoided.
- Frequent, gentle suctioning of upper pouch is essential to maintain the airway and prevent aspiration pneumonia.
- Single stage or staged delayed repair of esophagus should be done as far as possible.
- Long-term follow-up in multidisciplinary clinics is important to improve the outcome in these infants.

FURTHER READING

1. Conforti A, Morini F, Bagolan P. Difficult esophageal atresia: Trick and treat. *Semin Pediatr Surg* 2014; 23:261–269.
2. De Long E, Felix JF, De Klein A, *et al.* Etiology of esophageal atresia and tracheoesophageal fistula: "Mind the gap". *Curr Gastroenterol Rep* 2010;12:215–222.
3. Harmon CM, Coran AG. Congenital anomalies of the esophagus. In: Coran AG (ed): *Pediatric Surgery*, 7th edn., Philadelphia: Elsevier/Saunders 2012; 893–918.
4. Kunisaki SM, Foker JE. Surgical advances in the fetus and neonate: Esophageal atresia. *Clin Perinatol* 2012;39:349–361.

Index